# Geriatric Emergencies

*Editors*

KALPANA N. SHANKAR
BRENDAN G. MAGAURAN Jr
JOSEPH H. KAHN


# EMERGENCY MEDICINE CLINICS OF NORTH AMERICA

www.emed.theclinics.com

*Consulting Editor*
AMAL MATTU


August 2016 • Volume 34 • Number 3

**ELSEVIER**

1600 John F. Kennedy Boulevard • Suite 1800 • Philadelphia, Pennsylvania, 19103-2899
http://www.theclinics.com

**EMERGENCY MEDICINE CLINICS OF NORTH AMERICA Volume 34, Number 3**
**August 2016 ISSN 0733-8627, ISBN-13: 978-0-323-45961-7**

Editor: Patrick Manley
Developmental Editor: Casey Jackson

*Emergency Medicine Clinics of North America* (ISSN 0733-8627) is published quarterly by Elsevier Inc., 360 Park Avenue South, New York, NY, 10010-1710. Months of issue are February, May, August, and November. Business and Editorial Offices: 1600 John F. Kennedy Boulevard, Suite 1800, Philadelphia, PA 19103-2899. Customer Service Office: 6277 Sea Harbor Drive, Orlando, FL 32887-4800. Periodicals postage paid at New York, NY, and additional mailing offices. Subscription prices are $100.00 per year (US students), $320.00 per year (US individuals), $579.00 per year (US institutions), $220.00 per year (international students), $450.00 per year (international individuals), $711.00 per year (international institutions), $220.00 per year (Canadian students), $385.00 per year (Canadian individuals), and $711.00 per year (Canadian institutions). International air speed delivery is included in all *Clinics'* subscription prices. All prices are subject to change without notice. **POSTMASTER:** Send address changes to *Emergency Medicine Clinics of North America*, Elsevier Periodicals Customer Service, 11830 Westline Industrial Drive, St. Louis, MO 63146. Customer Service (orders, claims, online, change of address): Elsevier Periodicals **Customer Service, 11830 Westline Industrial Drive, St. Louis, MO 63146. Tel: 1-800-654-2452 (U.S. and Canada); 314-453-7041 (outside U.S. and Canada). Fax: 314-453-5170. E-mail: journalscustomerservice-usa@elsevier.com (for print support);** journalsonlinesupport-usa@elsevier.com (for online support).

*Reprints.* For copies of 100 or more of articles in this publication, please contact the Commercial Reprints Department, Elsevier Inc., 360 Park Avenue South, New York, NY 10010-1710. Tel.: 212-633-3874; Fax: 212-633-3820; E-mail: reprints@elsevier.com.

*Emergency Medicine Clinics of North America* is covered in *MEDLINE/PubMed (Index Medicus), Current Contents/Clinical Medicine, EMBASE/Excerpta Medica, BIOSIS, SciSearch, CINAHL, ISI/BIOMED,* and *Research Alert.*

# Contributors

## CONSULTING EDITOR

**AMAL MATTU, MD, FAAEM, FACEP**
Professor and Vice Chair, Department of Emergency Medicine, University of Maryland School of Medicine, Baltimore, Maryland

## EDITORS

**KALPANA N. SHANKAR, MD, MSc, MSHP**
Assistant Professor of Emergency Medicine, Boston Medical Center, Boston University School of Medicine, Boston, Massachusetts

**BRENDAN G. MAGAURAN Jr, MD, MBA**
Assistant Chief Medical Officer, Boston Medical Center, Assistant Clinical Professor of Emergency Medicine, Boston University School of Medicine, Boston, Massachusetts

**JOSEPH H. KAHN, MD, FACEP**
Associate Professor of Emergency Medicine, Boston Medical Center, Boston University School of Medicine, Boston, Massachusetts

## AUTHORS

**ANDREW R. BARBERA, MD**
Chief Resident, Department of Emergency Medicine, Jacobi/Montefiore Medical Centers, Albert Einstein College of Medicine, Bronx, New York

**STEPHEN TYLER CONSTANTINE, MD**
University of Chicago Medicine, Chicago, Illinois

**ALEXIS CORTIJO-BROWN, MD**
Emergency Medicine, Montefiore/Jacobi Medical Centers, Bronx, New York

**AOKO DORIS CRAIN, MD**
University of Chicago Medicine, Chicago, Illinois

**BENJAMIN GRIMMNITZ, MD**
Department of Emergency Medicine, Boston Medical Center, Boston, Massachusetts

**ROHIT GUPTA, MD**
Attending Physician, Department of Emergency Medicine, Advocate Christ Medical Center, Oak Lawn, Illinois

**TERESITA M. HOGAN, MD, FACEP**
Director, Geriatric Emergency Medicine, University of Chicago Medicine; Associate Professor, Department of Medicine, Divisions of Emergency Medicine, and Geriatrics and Palliative Care, Chicago, Illinois

**MICHAEL P. JONES, MD**
Associate Residency Director, Assistant Professor, Department of Emergency Medicine, Jacobi/Montefiore Medical Centers, Albert Einstein College of Medicine, Bronx, New York

**JOSEPH H. KAHN, MD, FACEP**
Associate Professor of Emergency Medicine, Boston Medical Center, Boston University School of Medicine, Boston, Massachusetts

**STEPHEN Y. LIANG, MD, MPHS**
Assistant Professor of Medicine, Divisions of Emergency Medicine and Infectious Diseases, Washington University School of Medicine, St Louis, Missouri

**BRENDAN G. MAGAURAN Jr, MD, MBA**
Assistant Chief Medical Officer, Boston Medical Center, Assistant Clinical Professor of Emergency Medicine, Boston University School of Medicine, Boston, Massachusetts

**PHILLIP D. MAGIDSON, MD, MPH**
Departments of Emergency Medicine and Medicine, University of Maryland Medical Center, Baltimore, Maryland

**JOSEPH P. MARTINEZ, MD, FAAEM, FACEP**
Associate Professor, Departments of Emergency Medicine and Medicine, Assistant Dean for Student Affairs, University of Maryland School of Medicine, Baltimore, Maryland

**ALYSSIA McEWAN, DO**
Department of Emergency Medicine, Albert Einstein College of Medicine, Bronx, New York

**RON MEDZON, MD**
Associate Professor, Emergency Medicine; Director, Solomont Center for Clinical Simulation and Nursing Education, Boston Medical Center, Boston University School of Medicine, Boston, Massachusetts

**ROBERT MUNOZ, MD**
Resident, Department of Emergency Medicine, Advocate Christ Medical Center, Oak Lawn, Illinois

**MARK B. MYCYK, MD**
Department of Emergency Medicine, Cook County Health and Hospitals System, Chicago, Illinois

**LAUREN M. NENTWICH, MD**
Director of Quality and Patient Safety, Department of Emergency Medicine, Boston Medical Center; Assistant Professor of Emergency Medicine, Boston University, Boston, Massachusetts

**JONATHAN S. OLSHAKER, MD, FACEP, FAAEM**
Professor and Chairman, Department of Emergency Medicine; Chief, Boston Medical Center, Boston University School of Medicine, Boston, Massachusetts

**JASON E. ONDREJKA, DO**
Director of Ultrasound, Department of Emergency Medicine, Clinical Instructor of Emergency Medicine, Summa Health System-Akron City Hospital, Northeastern Ohio Medical University, Akron, Ohio

**THOMAS PERERA, MD**
Emergency Medicine, Montefiore/Jacobi Medical Centers, Bronx, New York

**CASPER RESKE-NIELSEN, MD**
Chief Resident, Emergency Medicine, Boston Medical Center, Boston University School of Medicine, Boston, Massachusetts

**LYNNE ROSENBERG, PhD**
President, CEO, Practical Aspects LLC, Denville, New Jersey; Department of Emergency Medicine, St. Joseph's Healthcare System, Paterson, New Jersey

**MARK ROSENBERG, DO, MBA**
Chairman, Department of Emergency Medicine and Chief Population Health, St. Joseph's Healthcare System, Paterson New Jersey; Associate Professor Clinical Emergency Medicine, New York Medical College, Valhalla, New York

**KALPANA N. SHANKAR, MD, MSc, MSHP**
Assistant Professor of Emergency Medicine, Boston Medical Center, Boston University School of Medicine, Boston, Massachusetts

**JOSHUA Z. SILVERBERG, MD**
Assistant Professor, Department of Emergency Medicine, Albert Einstein College of Medicine, Bronx, New York

**KATHERINE LOUISE WELKER, MD, MPH**
Department of Emergency Medicine, Cook County Health and Hospitals System, Chicago, Illinois

**SCOTT T. WILBER, MD, MPH**
Chair, Department of Emergency Medicine, Professor of Emergency Medicine, Summa Health System-Akron City Hospital, Northeastern Ohio Medical University, Akron, Ohio

# Contents

The number of geriatric visits to United States emergency departments
continues to rise. This article reviews demographics, statistics, and future
projections in geriatric emergency medicine. Included are discussions of
US health care spending, geriatric emergency departments, prehospital
care, frailty of geriatric patients, delirium, geriatric trauma, geriatric
screening and prediction tools, medication safety, long-term care, and
palliative care.

The geriatric population makes up a large portion of the emergency patient
population. Geriatric patients have less reserve and more comorbid diseases. They are frequently on multiple medications and are more likely
to require aggressive treatment during acute illness. Although it may not
be obvious, it is important to recognize the signs of shock as early as
possible. Special care and monitoring should be used when resuscitating
the elderly. The use of bedside ultrasound and monitoring for coagulopathies are discussed. Clinicians should be constantly vigilant and reassess
throughout diagnosis and treatment. Ethical considerations in this population need to be considered on an individual basis.

The aging population of the United States creates pharmaceutical challenges for the practicing emergency physician. Polypharmacy, drug-drug
and drug-disease interactions, and other pharmaceutical complications
from the pathophysiologic changes associated with aging need to be
recognized in order to optimize outcomes in the elderly. Effective strategies
that improve patients outcomes include a better understanding of the physiologic and pharmacologic changes that occur with aging, integrated use of
clinical emergency department pharmacists, and choosing nonpharmacologic treatment options when possible.

Older patients who present to the emergency department frequently have acute or chronic alterations of their mental status, including their level of consciousness and cognition. Recognizing both acute and chronic changes in cognition are important for emergency physicians. Delirium is an acute change in attention, awareness, and cognition. Numerous life-threatening conditions can cause delirium; therefore, prompt recognition and treatment are critical. The authors discuss an organized approach that can lead to a prompt diagnosis within the time constraints of the emergency department.

As the geriatric population increases in the United States, there is an increase in number of visits to emergency departments for end-of-life and palliative care. This provides the emergency physician with a unique opportunity to alleviate and prevent further suffering in this vulnerable population. Competency in communication strategies that support shared decision making and familiarity with medicolegal terminology increase physician confidence about addressing complaints at the end of life. Familiarity with evidence-based recommendations for symptom management of pain at the end of life aids the emergency physician in creating a positive experience for the patient and their loved ones.

# EMERGENCY MEDICINE
# CLINICS OF NORTH AMERICA

**FORTHCOMING ISSUES**

*November 2016*
Neurologic Emergencies
Jonathan Edlow and Michael Abraham,
*Editors*

*February 2017*
Severe Sepsis Care in the Emergency
Department
Jack Perkins and Michael E. Winters,
*Editors*

*May 2017*
Wilderness and Environmental Medicine
Eric Weiss and Doug Sward, *Editors*

**RECENT ISSUES**

*May 2016*
Abdominal and Gastrointestinal Emergencies
Joseph P. Martinez and
Autumn C. Graham, *Editors*

*February 2016*
Respiratory Emergencies
Robert J. Vissers and Michael A. Gibbs,
*Editors*

*November 2015*
Psychiatric and Behavioral Emergencies
Veronica Tucci and Dick Kuo, *Editors*

**RELATED INTEREST**

*Clinics in Geriatric Medicine,* May 2016 (Vol. 32, Issue 2)
Managing Chronic Conditions in Older Adults with Cardiovascular Disease
Michael W. Rich, Cynthia Boyd, and James T. Pacala, *Editors*

## PROGRAM OBJECTIVE
The goal of *Emergency Medicine Clinics of North America* is to keep practicing emergency medicine physicians and emergency medicine residents up to date with current clinical practice in emergency medicine by providing timely articles reviewing the state of the art in patient care.

## LEARNING OBJECTIVES
Upon completion of this activity, participants will be able to:
1. Review the evaluation and management of geriatric emergencies such as chest pain and syncope.
2. Recognize protocols in treating trauma and infections in geriatric patients in the emergency department.
3. Discuss current trends in geriatric emergency care, as well as palliative care in the emergency department.

## ACCREDITATION
The Elsevier Office of Continuing Medical Education (EOCME) is accredited by the Accreditation Council for Continuing Medical Education (ACCME) to provide continuing medical education for physicians.

The EOCME designates this enduring material for a maximum of 15 *AMA PRA Category 1 Credit*(s)™. Physicians should claim only the credit commensurate with the extent of their participation in the activity.

All other health care professionals requesting continuing education credit for this enduring material will be issued a certificate of participation.

## DISCLOSURE OF CONFLICTS OF INTEREST
The EOCME assesses conflict of interest with its instructors, faculty, planners, and other individuals who are in a position to control the content of CME activities. All relevant conflicts of interest that are identified are thoroughly vetted by EOCME for fair balance, scientific objectivity, and patient care recommendations. EOCME is committed to providing its learners with CME activities that promote improvements or quality in healthcare and not a specific proprietary business or a commercial interest.

**The planning committee, staff, authors and editors listed below have identified no financial relationships or relationships to products or devices they or their spouse/life partner have with commercial interest related to the content of this CME activity:**
Andrew R. Barbera, MD; Stephen Tyler Constantine, MD; Alexis Cortijo-Brown, MD; Aoko Doris Crain, MD; Anjali Fortna; Benjamin Grimmnitz, MD; Rohit Gupta, MD; Teresita M. Hogan, MD, FACEP; Michael P. Jones, MD; Joseph H. Kahn, MD, FACEP; Indu Kumari; Stephen Y. Liang, MS, MPHS; Brendan G. Magauran, MD, MBA; Phillip D. Magidson, MD, MPH; Patrick Manley; Joseph P. Martinez, MD, FAAEM, FACEP; Amal Mattu, MD, FAAEM, FACEP; Alyssia McEwan, DO; Ron Medzon, MD; Robert Munoz, MD; Mark B. Mycyk, MD; Lauren M. Nentwich, MD; Jonathan S. Olshaker, MD, FACEP, FAAEM; Jason E. Ondrejka, DO; Thomas Perera, MD; Casper Reske-Nielsen, MD; Mark Rosenberg, DO, MBA; Lynne Rosenberg, PhD; Erin Scheckenbach; Kalpana Narayan Shankar, MD, MSc, MSHP; Katherine Louise Welker, MD, MPH; Scott T. Wilbur, MD, MPH.

**The planning committee, staff, authors and editors listed below have identified financial relationships or relationships to products or devices they or their spouse/life partner have with commercial interest related to the content of this CME activity:**
**Joshua Z. Silverberg, MD** has stock ownership in Johnson & Johnson Services, Inc. and Pfizer Inc.

## UNAPPROVED/OFF-LABEL USE DISCLOSURE
The EOCME requires CME faculty to disclose to the participants:
1. When products or procedures being discussed are off-label, unlabelled, experimental, and/or investigational (not US Food and Drug Administration [FDA] approved); and
2. Any limitations on the information presented, such as data that are preliminary or that represent ongoing research, interim analyses, and/or unsupported opinions. Faculty may discuss information about pharmaceutical agents that is outside of FDA-approved labelling. This information is intended solely for CME and is not intended to promote off-label use of these medications. If you have any questions, contact the medical affairs department of the manufacturer for the most recent prescribing information.

## TO ENROLL
To enroll in the *Emergency Medicine Clinics* Continuing Medical Education program, call customer service at 1-800-654-2452 or sign up online at http://www.theclinics.com/home/cme. The CME program is available to subscribers for an additional annual fee of $235 USD.

**METHOD OF PARTICIPATION**

In order to claim credit, participants must complete the following:

1. Complete enrolment as indicated above.
2. Read the activity.
3. Complete the CME Test and Evaluation. Participants must achieve a score of 70% on the test. All CME Tests and Evaluations must be completed online.

**CME INQUIRIES/SPECIAL NEEDS**

For all CME inquiries or special needs, please contact elsevierCME@elsevier.com.

# Foreword

# Geriatric Emergency Medicine

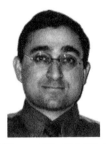

Amal Mattu, MD, FAAEM, FACEP
*Consulting Editor*

Patients over the age of 65 years represent the fastest growing segment of the US population. They account for 10% to 15% of emergency department (ED) visits. They have a longer length of ED stay and undergo more laboratory and radiologic testing than younger patients. Despite these more extensive workups, the elderly account for a disproportionate number of hospital and intensive care unit admissions; they have a higher misdiagnosis rate, and they suffer a higher rate of morbidity and mortality from similar diseases than younger patients.[1,2]

There are many reasons elderly patients fare worse than younger patients. History-taking often poses a challenge in these patients, especially when communication problems are present. Presentations are often atypical in this group, and classic physical examination findings are frequently absent. Vital signs may be altered by chronic medications, which may lead to misdiagnoses. Laboratory testing can also be unreliable in the elderly, and radiologic tests and electrocardiograms are typically more difficult to interpret because of chronic baseline abnormalities. In addition, there are a handful of deadly diseases that occur almost exclusively in the elderly and can easily be missed if the practitioner is unaware of this set of diseases. Just as pediatricians often preach that children are not simply little adults, experts in geriatric emergency medicine state that the elderly are not simply old adults. There are so many special considerations in this group of patients that they deserve their own curriculum, just as children do.

In this issue of *Emergency Medicine Clinics of North America*, guest editors Drs Kalpana Shankar, Brendan Magauran, and Joseph Kahn have stepped forward to provide us with this much-needed geriatric emergency medicine curriculum. They have assembled an outstanding group of authors who have addressed emergency medical issues in the elderly from top to bottom. Basic demographic information is provided so that the reader can understand the scope of the problems we face in caring for elderly patients in the ED. They discuss reasons for misdiagnosis, including the challenges of relying on typical historical, examination, and laboratory features of many common diseases. They discuss many of the most

Emerg Med Clin N Am 34 (2016) xv–xvi
http://dx.doi.org/10.1016/j.emc.2016.06.002
0733-8627/16/$ – see front matter © 2016 Published by Elsevier Inc.

emed.theclinics.com

typical presentations, including altered mental status, chest pain, and abdominal pain. Along the way, they discuss the diagnosis and treatment of deadly conditions that occur more commonly in the elderly than younger patients and the actual need to have a *different* differential in older patients for any given chief complaint.

Care of the elderly patient in the ED has recently become an area of great focus within many emergency medicine organizations. Dedicated geriatric EDs have sprung up around the country; major conferences are routinely including lectures and symposia focused on geriatric emergency medicine, and national guidelines pertaining to elder care have been created. Residency programs in emergency medicine, including our own, have created dedicated geriatric emergency medicine curricula to enlighten ED care providers about how to optimally diagnose and treat elderly patients. This issue of *Emergency Medicine Clinics of North America* is an invaluable addition to this "movement" regarding geriatric emergency medicine education and care. This issue should be considered must-reading for any acute care provider who routinely cares for the elderly. Our sincere thanks go to the guest editors and the authors for their time and commitment to this important issue.

Amal Mattu, MD, FAAEM, FACEP
Department of Emergency Medicine
University of Maryland School of Medicine
Baltimore, MD 21201, USA

E-mail address:
amalmattu@comcast.net

## REFERENCES

1. Spangler R, Pham TV, Khoujah D, et al. Abdominal emergencies in the geriatric patient. Int J Emerg Med 2014;7:43. Available at: http://www.intjem.com/content/7/1/43.
2. Caterino JM. Evaluation and management of geriatric infections in the emergency department. Emerg Med Clin North Am 2008;26:319–43.

# Preface

# Geriatric Emergencies

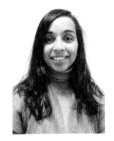
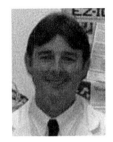
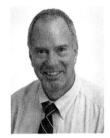

| Kalpana N. Shankar, MD, MSc, MSHP | Brendan G. Magauran Jr, MD, MBA | Joseph H. Kahn, MD, FACEP |

*Editors*

The elderly patient is becoming an increasingly larger demographic who seeks care in the emergency department (ED). According to the Census Bureau, in 2010, there were 40.3 million people aged 65 and above in the United States, comprising 13% of the overall population. By 2050, projections indicate the population over 65 will comprise 20.9% of the population. The elderly ED patient represents 43% of all admissions and just under 50% of intensive care unit admissions. This patient population is often quite complex, requires longer ED visits compared with their younger counterparts, undergoes far more testing, and often challenges us with ethical questions when they present with life-threatening disease. In short, the older adult is an expensive demographic to treat in the ED and requires the physician to understand their unusual presentations and unique treatment needs given their comorbidities and social circumstances.

In this issue, we attempt to provide a framework on the state of geriatric emergency care and topics unique to geriatric care, including the geriatric ED, acute resuscitation and medication management as well as trauma and falls, altered mental status, delirium, and palliative care. Furthermore, it is well-established that our pathophysiology for disease manifestation changes as we age. Because the older adult often presents atypically with significant illness, we are providing readers with a nuanced approach in the evaluation of common ED complaints, including sepsis, chest pain, dyspnea, abdominal pain, neurologic emergencies, and syncope. We hope that the content provides guidance in the delivery of care in the most effective and efficient means possible but in a manner that is in line with the patient's safety and goals of care.

We wish to thank all of the authors who wrote, researched, and edited the various articles included in this issue of *Emergency Medicine Clinics of North America*. We would also like to express our gratitude to Amal Mattu, Patrick Manley, Casey Jackson, and the staff at Elsevier for their guidance and support. Last, we wish to

Emerg Med Clin N Am 34 (2016) xvii–xviii
http://dx.doi.org/10.1016/j.emc.2016.06.001
0733-8627/16/$ – see front matter © 2016 Published by Elsevier Inc.

emed.theclinics.com

thank our families for their support in the hours needed to create, write, revise, and compile this issue.

Kalpana N. Shankar, MD, MSc, MSHP
Department of Emergency Medicine
Boston University School of Medicine
Boston, MA, USA

Brendan G. Magauran Jr, MD, MBA
Department of Emergency Medicine
Boston Medical Center
Boston University School of Medicine
Boston, MA, USA

Joseph H. Kahn, MD, FACEP
Department of Emergency Medicine
Boston Medical Center
Boston University School of Medicine
1 Boston Medical Center Place
Boston, MA 02118, USA

E-mail addresses:
kns1@bu.edu (K.N. Shankar)
brendan.maguaran@bmc.org (B.G. Magauran)
jkahn@bu.edu (J.H. Kahn)

# Current Trends in Geriatric Emergency Medicine

Joseph H. Kahn, MD*, Brendan G. Magauran Jr, MD, MBA, Jonathan S. Olshaker, MD, Kalpana N. Shankar, MD, MSc, MSHP*

## KEYWORDS

- Geriatric emergency medicine • US health spending • Geriatric screening
- Geriatric trauma • Palliative care

## KEY POINTS

- As the number (and percentage) of Americans 65 years and older continues to grow, the number (and percentage) of geriatric emergency department (ED) visits will continue to rise significantly.
- The aging of the United States population is a force that is driving up the cost of health care.
- There is a growing movement in the United States to incorporate features into EDs to make them friendlier for elderly patients.
- Geriatric patients are often sicker than their younger counterparts and may be lacking many classic features of disease states.
- Recognizing delirium in the elderly ED patient is an essential component of geriatric emergency medicine.

## BACKGROUND

According to the Administration on Aging (AoA), US Department of Health and Human Services, 14.1% of the population in the United States, totaling 44.7 million Americans, was 65 years of age or older in 2013. AoA projects that older Americans will make up 21.7% of the population by 2040 and that there will be 98 million older persons living in America by 2060[1] (**Fig. 1**).

The National Center for Health Statistics of the Centers for Disease Control reports 136.3 million emergency department (ED) visits in 2011,[2] of which 20.4 million (15%) were senior citizens (age ≥65 years) (**Table 1**).[3] More recent statistics estimate the current percentage of ED visits of patients older than 65 years at 18%[4], with patients 75 and older having the highest visit rate compared with all other demographics.[5]

Disclosures: None.
Department of Emergency Medicine, Boston University School of Medicine, Boston Medical Center, 1 Boston Medical Center Place, Boston, MA 02118, USA
* Corresponding author.
E-mail addresses: Joseph.kahn@bmc.org; Kalpana.Narayan@bmc.org

Emerg Med Clin N Am 34 (2016) 435–452
http://dx.doi.org/10.1016/j.emc.2016.04.014           emed.theclinics.com
0733-8627/16/$ – see front matter © 2016 Elsevier Inc. All rights reserved.

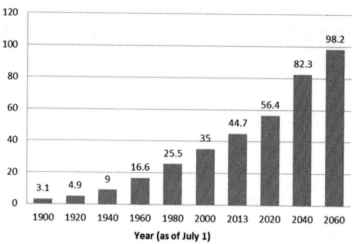

**Fig. 1.** This chart shows the large increases in the older population from 3.1 million people in 1900 to 44.7 million in 2013 and projected to be 98.2 million in 2060. Source: U.S. Census Bureau, Population Estimates and Projections.

Senior citizens presenting to the ED are more likely to be triaged to higher levels of urgency (levels 1, 2, and 3) (**Table 2**), spend more time in the ED for diagnostic testing, and use more resources compared with their younger counterparts.[6]

A review of hospital administrative data for the 10-year period from 2002 to 2012 in Switzerland revealed a 27.6% overall increase in ED visits, with 42.3% increase in the subset of patients older than 65 years.[7]

## UNITED STATES HEALTH SPENDING

The Center for Medicare and Medicaid Services reported in *Health Affairs* in 2015 that US health spending is expected to increase by 5.8% per year over the next 10 years due to faster economic growth, aging of the population, and expanded insurance coverage through the Affordable Care Act (ACA).[8,9] *Health Affairs* further reports that health care spending will consume 19.6% of US gross domestic product in 2024, up from 17.4% in 2013.[8]

## GERIATRIC EMERGENCY DEPARTMENTS

EDs are often not designed with the care of the elder patient in mind. The bright lights, bright floors, high noise level, uncomfortable stretchers, and lack of easily accessible bathrooms may unsettle an elderly patient who has fewer coping skills than younger people. Emergency care itself is not generally geared toward the elderly. The rapid pace of triage, evaluation, and treatment may overwhelm the elderly patient, who may have been sent to the ED and may not even know why she or he is there.[10] In response to this need, many US hospitals have developed geriatric-friendly EDs. Many hospitals do not have the resources to build a geriatric ED but can still make the existing ED geriatric-friendly.

The American College of Emergency Physicians, The American Geriatrics Society (AGS), Emergency Nurses Association, and Society for Academic Emergency Medicine have developed "Geriatric Emergency Department Guidelines" to serve as a framework for creating senior-friendly EDs.[11] These guidelines outline not only the physical plans that are conducive to emergency care but also review the recommended staffing needed to make the geriatric ED work. Additional resources needed for

**Table 1**
**Emergency department visits by patient age, sex, and residence: United States, 2011**

| Selected Patient Characteristics | Number of Visits in Thousands (Standard Error in Thousands) | | Percent Distribution (Standard Error of Percent) | | Number of Visits per 100 Persons per Year[a] (Standard Error of Rate) | |
|---|---|---|---|---|---|---|
| All visits | 136,296 | (6413) | 100.0 | — | 44.5 | (2.1) |
| Age[a] | | | | | | |
| Younger than 15 y | 24,823 | (1724) | 18.2 | (0.9) | 40.6 | (2.8) |
| Younger than 1 y | 3485 | (303) | 2.6 | (0.2) | 87.3 | (7.6) |
| 1–4 y | 9773 | (737) | 7.2 | (0.4) | 60.5 | (4.6) |
| 5–14 y | 11,565 | (823) | 8.5 | (0.4) | 28.2 | (2.0) |
| 15–24 y | 22,150 | (1140) | 16.3 | (0.3) | 51.7 | (2.7) |
| 25–44 y | 39,124 | (1997) | 28.7 | (0.6) | 48.7 | (2.5) |
| 45–64 y | 29,828 | (1537) | 21.9 | (0.5) | 36.4 | (1.9) |
| 65 y and older | 20,372 | (1172) | 14.9 | (0.5) | 50.8 | (2.9) |
| 65–74 y | 8208 | (518) | 6.0 | (0.2) | 36.9 | (2.3) |
| 75 y and older | 12,163 | (729) | 8.9 | (0.3) | 68.2 | (4.1) |
| Sex and age[a] | | | | | | |
| Female | 74,621 | (3622) | 54.7 | (0.4) | 47.6 | (2.3) |
| Younger than 15 y | 11,385 | (820) | 8.4 | (0.5) | 38.1 | (2.7) |
| 15–24 y | 13,289 | (746) | 9.8 | (0.2) | 62.6 | (3.5) |
| 25–44 y | 22,534 | (1192) | 16.5 | (0.4) | 55.1 | (2.9) |
| 45–64 y | 15,381 | (862) | 11.3 | (0.3) | 36.4 | (2.0) |
| 65–74 y | 4353 | (296) | 3.2 | (0.2) | 36.6 | (2.5) |
| 75 y and over | 7678 | (498) | 5.6 | (0.2) | 72.1 | (4.7) |
| Male | 61,676 | (2890) | 45.3 | (0.4) | 41.2 | (1.9) |
| Younger than 15 y | 13,439 | (945) | 9.9 | (0.5) | 43.0 | (3.0) |
| 15–24 y | 8861 | (463) | 6.5 | (0.2) | 41.0 | (2.1) |
| 25–44 y | 16,590 | (906) | 12.2 | (0.3) | 42.1 | (2.3) |
| 45–64 y | 14,446 | (768) | 10.6 | (0.3) | 36.4 | (1.9) |
| 65–74 y | 3855 | (283) | 2.8 | (0.1) | 37.2 | (2.7) |
| 75 y and older | 4485 | (293) | 3.3 | (0.2) | 62.4 | (4.1) |
| Patient residence | | | | | | |
| Private residence[a] | 126,297 | (5984) | 92.7 | (0.4) | 41.2 | (2.0) |
| Nursing home[b] | 2557 | (184) | 1.9 | (0.1) | 74.2 | (5.3) |
| Homeless[c] | 1092 | (160) | 0.8 | (0.1) | 171.7 | (25.1) |
| Other | 1401 | (135) | 1.0 | (0.1) | 0.5 | (0.0) |
| Unknown or blank | 4949 | (475) | 3.6 | (0.3) | 1.6 | (0.2) |

—, Category not applicable. 0.0. Quantity more than zero but less than 0.05. Note: numbers may not add to totals because of rounding.

[a] Visit rates for age, sex, and private residence are based on the July 1, 2011, set of estimates of the civilian noninstitutionalized population of the United States as developed by the Population Division, US Census Bureau.

[b] Visit rates for nursing home residents are based on the 2011 population denominators from the Center for Clinical Standards and Certification Group, Centers for Medicare and Medicaid Services.

[c] Visit rates for the homeless people are based on The 2011 Annual Homeless Assessment Report to Congress by the US Department of Housing and Urban Development.

*Data from* CDC/NCHS. National Hospital Ambulatory Medical Care Survey. Available at: http://www.cdc.gov/nchs/fastats/emergency-department.htm. Accessed October 14, 2015.

**Table 2**
Triage status of emergency department visits, by selected patient characteristics: United States, 2011

| Patient and Visit Characteristics | Number of Visits in Thousands | Total | Level 1 (Immediate) | | Level 2 (Emergent) | | Level 3 (Urgent) | | Level 4 (Semiurgent) | | Level 5 (Nonurgent) | | No triage[1] | |
|---|---|---|---|---|---|---|---|---|---|---|---|---|---|---|
| | | | Percent distribution (standard error of percent) | | | | | | | | | | | |
| All visits | 136,296 | 100.0 | 1.2 | (0.2) | 10.7 | (0.6) | 42.3 | (1.1) | 35.5 | (1.0) | 8.0 | (0.7) | *2.2 | (0.8) |
| Age | | | | | | | | | | | | | | |
| Younger than 15 y | 24,823 | 100.0 | 0.7 | (0.2) | 6.2 | (0.9) | 31.1 | (1.5) | 47.0 | (1.6) | 13.1 | (1.5) | *1.9 | (0.7) |
| Younger than 1 y | 3485 | 100.0 | * | | 6.5 | (1.9) | 31.7 | (2.3) | 46.5 | (2.6) | 13.1 | (2.0) | * | — |
| 1–4 y | 9773 | 100.0 | * | | 5.1 | (0.8) | 31.8 | (1.9) | 47.4 | (2.0) | 13.3 | (1.5) | *1.5 | (0.6) |
| 5–14 y | 11,565 | 100.0 | * | | 6.9 | (0.9) | 30.3 | (2.0) | 46.8 | (1.9) | 13.0 | (1.6) | *2.3 | (0.8) |
| 15–24 y | 22,150 | 100.0 | 1.1 | (0.3) | 7.6 | (0.7) | 40.1 | (1.5) | 39.8 | (1.3) | 9.0 | (1.0) | *2.4 | (1.0) |
| 25–44 y | 39,124 | 100.0 | 1.1 | (0.2) | 8.9 | (0.7) | 42.8 | (1.3) | 37.0 | (1.0) | 8.0 | (0.9) | *2.1 | (0.8) |
| 45–64 y | 29,828 | 100.0 | 1.3 | (0.3) | 14.8 | (1.0) | 45.3 | (1.3) | 30.3 | (1.2) | 6.1 | (0.7) | *2.2 | (0.8) |
| 65 y and older | 20,372 | 100.0 | *1.9 | (0.6) | 17.1 | (1.0) | 53.0 | (1.6) | 21.8 | (1.4) | 3.7 | (0.6) | *2.4 | (0.9) |
| 65–74 y | 8208 | 100.0 | *2.2 | (0.9) | 17.9 | (1.3) | 50.3 | (1.8) | 23.2 | (1.5) | 4.0 | (0.7) | *2.4 | (1.0) |
| 75 y and older | 12,163 | 100.0 | *1.7 | (0.5) | 16.6 | (1.2) | 54.9 | (1.9) | 20.9 | (1.6) | 3.6 | (0.6) | *2.4 | (0.9) |
| Sex | | | | | | | | | | | | | | |
| Female | 74,621 | 100.0 | 0.9 | (0.2) | 10.1 | (0.7) | 44.2 | (1.3) | 35.0 | (1.2) | 7.6 | (0.7) | *2.2 | (0.8) |
| Male | 61,676 | 100.0 | 1.6 | (0.3) | 11.4 | (0.7) | 40.0 | (1.0) | 36.2 | (0.9) | 8.6 | (0.8) | *2.1 | (0.8) |

| | | | | | | | | | | | | | |
|---|---|---|---|---|---|---|---|---|---|---|---|---|---|
| **Race[2,3]** | | | | | | | | | | | | | |
| White | 98,147 | 100.0 | 1.3 | (0.3) | 11.2 | (0.7) | 42.5 | (1.3) | 34.6 | (1.1) | 8.0 | (0.8) | *2.4 (0.9) |
| Black or African American | 32,627 | 100.0 | 1.0 | (0.2) | 9.4 | (0.8) | 41.6 | (1.4) | 38.3 | (1.5) | 8.5 | (0.9) | *1.3 (1.1) |
| Other | 5523 | 100.0 | * | — | 9.2 | (1.3) | 43.4 | (2.6) | 35.9 | (2.2) | 6.7 | (1.3) | *3.8 (2.6) |
| **Ethnicity and race[2,3]** | | | | | | | | | | | | | |
| Hispanic or Latino | 19,206 | 100.0 | 0.8 | (0.2) | 9.3 | (1.0) | 41.4 | (2.0) | 37.2 | (1.7) | 10.0 | (1.4) | *1.3 (1.0) |
| Not Hispanic or Latino | 117,091 | 100.0 | 1.3 | (0.3) | 10.9 | (0.7) | 42.5 | (1.2) | 35.3 | (1.0) | 7.7 | (0.7) | *2.3 (0.8) |
| White | 81,185 | 100.0 | 1.4 | (0.3) | 11.6 | (0.8) | 42.8 | (1.4) | 34.2 | (1.2) | 7.6 | (0.8) | *2.5 (0.9) |
| Black or African American | 31,514 | 100.0 | 1.0 | (0.2) | 9.6 | (0.8) | 41.4 | (1.5) | 38.3 | (1.6) | 8.4 | (0.9) | *1.4 (1.2) |
| Other | 4392 | 100.0 | * | — | 9.3 | (1.3) | 44.8 | (2.9) | 34.5 | (2.2) | 5.9 | (1.2) | *4.5 (3.2) |
| **Expected sources of payment[4]** | | | | | | | | | | | | | |
| Private insurance | 47,600 | 100.0 | 1.3 | (0.4) | 11.9 | (0.7) | 45.3 | (1.4) | 32.6 | (1.1) | 6.8 | (0.8) | *2.2 (0.8) |
| Medicaid or CHIP[5] | 43,327 | 100.0 | 0.8 | (0.2) | 9.6 | (0.9) | 38.7 | (1.3) | 38.4 | (1.4) | 9.8 | (1.0) | *2.6 (1.1) |
| Medicare | 25,060 | 100.0 | 1.7 | (0.5) | 16.4 | (1.0) | 50.2 | (1.4) | 24.8 | (1.4) | 4.4 | (0.5) | *2.6 (1.1) |
| Medicare and Medicaid[6] | 5771 | 100.0 | * | — | 16.3 | (1.7) | 46.8 | (2.2) | 27.0 | (2.2) | 5.3 | (0.8) | *3.4 (1.8) |
| No insurance[7] | 21,744 | 100.0 | 1.4 | (0.3) | 9.2 | (0.8) | 39.7 | (1.3) | 39.2 | (1.2) | 8.7 | (1.0) | *1.9 (0.8) |
| Workers' compensation | 1503 | 100.0 | * | — | * | — | 22.1 | (3.0) | 57.7 | (3.5) | * | — | * — |
| Other | 5592 | 100.0 | * | — | 10.3 | (1.1) | 44.5 | (2.6) | 37.1 | (1.6) | 6.4 | (1.3) | * — |
| Unknown or blank | 7867 | 100.0 | * | — | 7.5 | (1.3) | 42.2 | (2.5) | 37.3 | (2.1) | 10.1 | (1.3) | * — |

—, Category not applicable.

* Figure does not meet standards of reliability or precision (see author's note on page 447).

Data from National Hospital Ambulatory Medical Care Survey: 2011 Emergency Department Summary Tables. Available at: http://www.cdc.gov/nchs/fastats/emergency-department.htm. Accessed October 14, 2015.

geriatric assessments are discussed, including access to pharmacists, social workers, and case managers, who are all needed in the facilitation of clinical care and care transitions, which are the pillars of quality geriatric care. Finally, these guidelines review the importance of screening tools for geriatric patients, the appropriate use of urinary catheters, medication management, fall assessment, delirium and dementia assessments, and the introduction of palliative care. Modern Healthcare reports that "more than 50 US hospitals have opened EDs for elderly patients since 2011 and at least 150 more have senior-specific EDs in development," according to Emergency Care Research Institute.[12] The financial implications of developing a geriatric ED are potentially promising but are unclear at this time.

## FRAIL SENIORS

Frailty encompasses a decline in resilience and physiologic reserves and ultimately places an elder at increased risk of poor outcomes.[13] One component of frailty is mobility, a question commonly asked by ED staff, particularly at the time of discharge. Based on a recent study by Dr Timothy Platts-Mills in Annals of Emergency Medicine, self-reporting may not be an accurate method of assessing seniors' mobility.[14] In this study, 12% of independently-living senior citizens who reported that they could get out of bed, walk 10 feet, turn around, and return to bed without assistance, actually needed help to complete this task. Of seniors who stated that they could complete the task independently with the aid of a cane or walker, 48% actually needed assistance or could not complete the task.[15] Dr Platts-Mills recommends direct observation of mobility of seniors being discharged to live independently.[14,15]

Toosizadeh and Mohler[16] (2015) report an objective measure of frailty that does not depend on gait. Slowness of elbow flexion, weakness, exhaustion, and flexibility were measured using wireless sensors. This technology may be applicable to older nonambulatory individuals in the ED. Soong and colleagues[17] (2015) found that frailty syndromes based on hospital data alone can be a good predictor of mortality, institutionalization, and ED recidivism; however, further prospective studies are needed to assess its use.

## PREHOSPITAL CARE

Another issue facing the future of health care with the aging of the population is how it will affect emergency medical service (EMS) usage. Elders use EMS more often than their younger counterparts. This was confirmed in a recent Canadian study by Goldstein and colleagues,[18] who found that close to 50% of the EMS call volume over a 1-year period was for people age older than 65 years.

Kodadek and colleagues[19] undertook a study to determine whether older trauma victims are appropriately triaged by reviewing the 2011 Nationwide Emergency Department Sample. After comparing new injury severity score with triage to levels 1 and 2 trauma centers or elsewhere, his analysis demonstrates a significant undertriage of trauma patients of age older than 55 years.

Nelson-Williams and colleagues[20] recently reviewed the Nationwide Emergency Department Sample from 2006 to 2010 of isolated hip fracture patients older than 65 years. He concludes that patients with isolated hip fractures triaged to higher level trauma centers (levels 1 and 2) do not have a significant difference in mortality or discharge disposition when compared with those triaged to a level 3 trauma center or nondesignated trauma center.

Currently, there is an ongoing program evaluation underway in Ontario, Canada, to reduce EMS calls and improve health care in seniors' apartment buildings. Through he Community Health Assessment Programme with EMS, paramedics have weekly sessions in which they assess risk for cardiovascular disease, diabetes, and falls, and communicate with the person's primary care provider.[21] This is an ongoing study with no published results yet.

## SCREENING AND PREDICTION TOOLS

There are multiple screening and prediction tools that have been developed to help determine the outcome of elderly patients after discharge from the ED.

Functional assessment tools include Activities of Daily Living and Instrumental Activities of Daily Living, both of which are incorporated into Older American Resources and Services. Other screening tools for functional assessment are the "get up and go" test and the short performance physical battery, among others.[22]

There are numerous tools used to predict functional decline after discharge from the ED, including identification of seniors at risk (ISAR), brief risk identification for geriatric health tool, and triage risk screening tool, among others.[22] The ISAR tool was recently reviewed by Yao and colleagues[23] to determine its predictive validity. In this systematic review, the ISAR tool was found to have poor validity related to ED return visits and hospital readmission.

Most recently, a large systematic review and meta-analysis performed by Carpenter and colleagues[24] determined that, although absence of dependency reduces the risk of 1-year mortality, no individual risk factor, frailty construct, or risk assessment instrument accurately predicts risk of adverse outcomes in older ED patients.

The Mayo Ambulatory Geriatric Evaluation questionnaire can be completed by elders during primary care provider visits to determine the relationship between geriatric symptoms and ED visits and/or hospitalization within 1 year.[25] Several symptoms were found to be associated with ED visits and/or hospitalization within 1 year: advanced age, self-report of worsening health, 2 or more falls, weight loss, and depressed mood.[25]

Launay and colleagues[26] recently used artificial neural networks to analyze a 10-item brief geriatric assessment in older ED patients admitted to an acute care hospital. The purpose was to determine which admitted seniors would have prolonged hospital stays. The investigators concludes that the 10-item assessment accurately predicts which patients will have prolonged length of stay, with the presence of chronic conditions being the most important contributor to predictive accuracy of the screening tool.

Inzitari and colleagues[27] recently reviewed 3 screening tools to help determine which elders can be transferred directly from the ED to intermediate care facilities instead of admission to acute care hospitals. The investigators reviewed ISAR, Silver Code, and the Walter indicator, and concluded that ISAR was independently associated with transfer to intermediate care from the ED but that predictive validity was poor and that further research is needed on this determination. Regardless of the tool selected, it is important for older adults discharged from the ED, either to home or to inpatient status, to receive a geriatric assessment. These assessments not only identify risk factors for poor outcomes but also increase the likelihood of a patient being alive and in their own home at up to 12 months.[28,29] An important question is who should perform geriatric screenings? Can screenings be performed by social workers or case mangers as opposed to emergency medicine clinicians? Although there is limited evidence in this area, future research is needed to understand these limitations and what ED instruments can be developed that use alternative variables such as a variety of social determinants of health, health literacy, and dementia, which are often clinically occult.

Finally, it is important to incorporate a caregiver's input into the decision-making process of admission or discharge because they often understand the patient's ability to successfully thrive in the outpatient setting far better than the transient snapshot ED providers obtain during their visit. Ae and colleagues[30] report that a caregiver daily impression rating instrument may detect illness severity beyond physical findings and propose that, once validated, it could be used by caregivers as part of their daily assessments.

## MEDICATION SAFETY

The AGS reports that 35% of older adults living in the community experience an adverse drug event (ADE) every year, and that 2 out of 3 people living in skilled nursing facilities experience an ADE over 4 years. AGS further reports that nearly 1 of 3 hospital admissions in senior citizens is caused by an ADE. Risk factors for an ADE include multiple chronic diseases, multiple prescription medications, multiple medication doses per day, advanced age, and reduced creatinine clearance, among others.[31]

There are multiple age-related alterations in pharmacokinetics, which may predispose elderly people to an ADE. The frequency of bleeding events associated with anticoagulants, for example, increases with age. Medication review and reconciliation is essential in preventing ADEs in the elderly.[32] ED pharmacists can make a significant contribution to patient safety in elderly ED patients.

## DETECTING DELIRIUM

Delirium is a common syndrome in hospitalized older adults and is associated with increased mortality, hospital costs, and long-term cognitive and functional impairment.[33,34] Recognition of delirium in older patients during ED visits, and differentiating it from dementia, is challenging yet of paramount importance.[35] The International Statistical Classification of Diseases 10th Revision, 2015, defines delirium as "an etiologically nonspecific organic cerebral syndrome characterized by concurrent disturbances of consciousness and attention, perception, thinking, memory, psychomotor behavior, emotion, and the sleep-wake schedule, the duration is variable and the degree of severity ranges from mild to very severe."[36] Delirium is generally acute in onset and can be caused by medical conditions that are reversible, with improvement in mental status when the underlying medical problem is treated.[37] The longer a patient is delirious, the worse the outcome, including an increase in the risk of death at 3 months.[37]

Extensive work on detecting delirium early in the ED can potentially reduce inpatient morbidity. Informal assessments of delirium are known to be inadequate[38] with several formal delirium tools being too cumbersome. Modified versions of the Confusion Assessment Method show good promise as a short, effective, and feasible tool that can be easily implemented in EDs[38–40] However, their sensitivity for older adults, particularly the intensive care unit version remains modest at best.[39]

Dementia, on the other hand, develops more gradually, presents with progressive cognitive deficits, and is generally not reversible.[41] It is particularly challenging to recognize delirium in the setting of pre-existing dementia.

The Richmond Agitation Sedation Scale (RASS), a rapid assessment tool for level of consciousness, was recently evaluated by Han and colleagues[42] for its use in detecting delirium in the ED. RASS is scored from minus 5 (unarousable) to plus 4 (combative), with 0 being alert and calm (**Table 3**). The investigators conclude that a RASS score greater than plus 1 or less than minus 1 is highly sensitive and specific for diagnosing delirium.[42]

**Table 3**
**Richmond agitation-sedation scale**

| | | Step 1 Level of Consciousness Assessment | |
|---|---|---|---|
| Scale | Label | Description | |
| +4 | Combative | Combative, violent, immediate danger to staff | |
| +3 | Very agitated | Pulls to remove tubes or catheters, aggressive | |
| +2 | Agitated | Frequent nonpurposeful movement, fights ventilator | |
| +1 | Restless | Anxious, apprehensive, movements not aggressive | |
| 0 | Alert & calm | Spontaneously pays attention to caregiver | |
| −1 | Drowsy | Not fully alert but has sustained awakening to voice (eye opening & contact >10 s) | Voice |
| −2 | Light sedation | Briefly awakens to voice (eyes open & contact <10 s) | |
| −3 | Moderate sedation | Movement or eye opening to voice (no eye contact) If RASS is ≥ −3 proceed to CAM-ICU (Is patient CAM-ICU positive or negative?) | |
| −4 | Deep sedation | No response to voice but movement or eye opening to physical stimulation | Touch |
| −5 | Unarousable | No response to voice or physical stimulation If RASS is −4 or −5 → Stop (patient unconscious), recheck later | |

*From Refs.*[72–74]

## TRAUMA AND FALLS

The American College of Surgeons (ACS) has developed Geriatric Trauma Management Guidelines, in which ACS reports that "traumatic injury in the geriatric population is increasing in prevalence and is associated with higher mortality and complication rates compared with younger patients" (**Fig. 2**). There are also data to suggest that victims of falls are subject to poor outcomes and ED recidivism.[43] The ACS guidelines suggest a lower threshold of trauma team activation for elderly trauma victims (**Fig. 3**, **Table 4**).

ACS reported in 2013 that traumatic injuries in elderly patients are often underestimated.[44] Because of this, elderly trauma victims are sometimes not taken to trauma

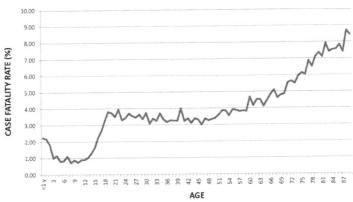

**Fig. 2.** Case fatality rate by age. (*Data from* NTDB 2013 Annual Report. Available at: www.facs. org/~/media/files/quality%20programs/trauma/ntdb/ntdb%20annual%20report%202013. ashx. Accessed October 14, 2015.)

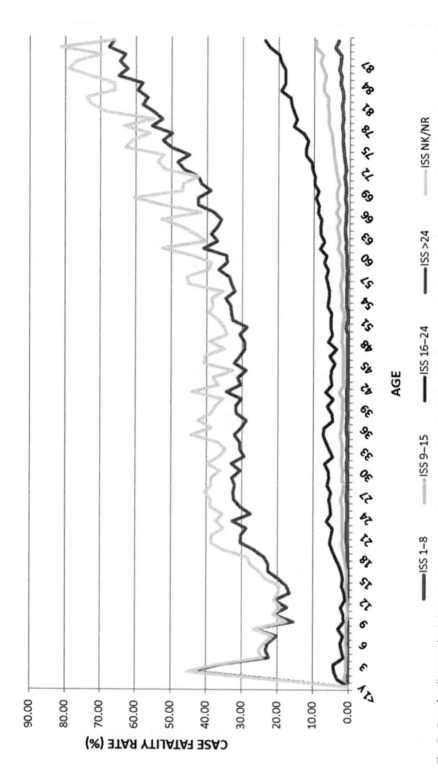

**Fig. 3.** Case fatality rate by injury severity score and age. Injury Severity Score definitions can be found in Appendix B. (*Data from* NTDB 2013 Annual Report. Available at: www.facs.org/~/media/files/quality%20programs/ntdb/ntdb%20annual%20report%202013.ashx, http://www.icudelirium. org/docs/RASS.pdf. Accessed October 14, 2015.)

**Table 4**
Case fatality rate by injury severity score and age

| Age | ISS 1–8 Case Fatality Rate | ISS 9–15 Case Fatality Rate | ISS 16–24 Case Fatality Rate | ISS >24 Case Fatality Rate | ISS NK/NR Case Fatality Rate |
|---|---|---|---|---|---|
| <1 y | 0.24 | 0.95 | 2.00 | 18.98 | 1.06 |
| 1–4 | 0.19 | 0.43 | 2.46 | 29.49 | 1.34 |
| 5–9 | 0.14 | 0.40 | 1.45 | 19.34 | 0.78 |
| 10–14 | 0.12 | 0.35 | 1.14 | 16.84 | 2.03 |
| 15–19 | 0.39 | 0.96 | 2.68 | 21.94 | 6.02 |
| 20–24 | 0.60 | 1.26 | 3.35 | 24.82 | 7.09 |
| 25–34 | 0.56 | 1.44 | 3.86 | 25.89 | 6.81 |
| 35–44 | 0.63 | 1.31 | 3.32 | 25.81 | 7.53 |
| 45–54 | 0.62 | 1.30 | 3.35 | 26.31 | 5.65 |
| 55–64 | 0.86 | 1.71 | 4.47 | 29.03 | 8.61 |
| 65–74 | 1.21 | 2.48 | 6.30 | 33.40 | 7.19 |
| 75–84 | 2.11 | 4.09 | 9.84 | 40.51 | 8.90 |
| >84 | 3.43 | 6.50 | 13.11 | 44.98 | 8.38 |
| NK/NR | 33.33 | 58.33 | 12.50 | 88.89 | 100.00 |

Abbreviations: ISS, injury severity score; NK/NR, not known/not reported.
From National Trauma Databank 2013 Annual Report. Available at: www.facs.org/~/media/files/quality%20programs/trauma/ntdb/ntdb%20annual%20report%202013.ashx. Accessed October 14, 2015.

centers, even though their injuries are severe enough for trauma center evaluation and management. That said, the overall mortality of all geriatric trauma patients over the last 20 years is declining, in part due to streamlined trauma care whether at a trauma center or a nontrauma center.[45]

ACS further reports that the leading cause of traumatic injuries for the elderly is falls (**Fig. 4**, **Table 5**). This statistical has remained unchanged over the years, with data to suggest that victims of falls are subject to poor outcomes and ED recidivism.[43] There are many evidence-based falls prevention and fear of falling prevention programs in the community such as Tai Chi, Otago, Stepping On, and Matter of Balance.[46–52] Many referrals for these programs come from clinics but further studies are needed to assess the feasibility of referring patients from the ED and measuring the associated outcomes.

## LONG-TERM CARE AND HOME HEALTH CARE

Long-term care encompasses home health care, skilled nursing facilities, hospices, residential care communities, and adult daycare centers.[53] A 2010 cross-sectional study demonstrated that nearly one-quarter of long-term care residents visit an ED within 6 months, with 24.6% of these presenting with an ambulatory sensitive condition (many ED visits resulted in hospitalization) and 11% presenting with a low acuity complaint. Until better access for other venues of ambulatory care and/or higher acuity services within long-term care facilities become available, EDs will still remain the source of their care.[54]

It is anticipated that the number of Americans requiring some form of long-term care will reach 27 million by 2050 (up from 13 million in 2000).[53] With the increasing number of people coming to EDs from long-term care facilities and being transferred back to these

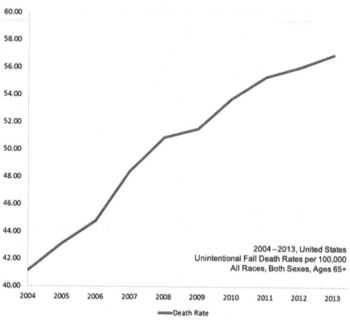

**Fig. 4.** Unintentional fall death rates, adults 65 years and older. (*Data from* www.cdc.gov/ injury/wisqars. Accessed October 14, 2015.)

**Table 5**
**Incidents by selected mechanism of injury and age**

| Age | Fall | Motor Vehicle Traffic | Struck by, Against | Transport, Other | Firearm | Cut or Pierce |
|---|---|---|---|---|---|---|
| <1 y | 5249 | 460 | 423 | 38 | 43 | 45 |
| 1–4 | 13,803 | 3435 | 2194 | 628 | 173 | 487 |
| 5–9 | 14,422 | 4784 | 2204 | 1604 | 180 | 507 |
| 10–14 | 9403 | 6007 | 4497 | 3681 | 634 | 719 |
| 15–19 | 7863 | 23,423 | 6940 | 5132 | 5727 | 3502 |
| 20–24 | 8041 | 32,213 | 7471 | 4468 | 8563 | 6280 |
| 25–34 | 15,785 | 41,958 | 11,597 | 6287 | 10,182 | 10,005 |
| 35–44 | 18,113 | 31,775 | 8704 | 5514 | 4860 | 6757 |
| 45–54 | 31,624 | 34,825 | 8901 | 5927 | 3122 | 5363 |
| 55–64 | 42,195 | 26,739 | 4663 | 4153 | 1561 | 2506 |
| 65–74 | 44,660 | 14,996 | 1731 | 2166 | 646 | 901 |
| 75–84 | 63,458 | 9589 | 1007 | 1124 | 297 | 390 |
| >84 | 64,182 | 3933 | 585 | 473 | 167 | 133 |
| NK/NR | 8 | 27 | 3 | — | 7 | 4 |
| Total | 338,806 | 234,164 | 60,920 | 41,195 | 36,162 | 37,599 |

*From* National Trauma Databank 2013 Annual Report. Available at: www.facs.org/~/media/files/ quality%20programs/trauma/ntdb/ntdb%20annual%20report%202013.ashx. Accessed October 14, 2015.

facilities, communication between the sending facility and the ED is very important.[55] There are multiple studies demonstrating that poor communication during care transitions can lead to higher costs, increased health care use, and unnecessary duplication of services.[56–59] Therefore, developing a cohesive and organized method of information transfer is well established as an effective method to accomplishing this goal.[60]

Jones and colleagues[61] report, in a letter to the *Journal of the American Geriatrics Society*, that the number of home health care referrals for geriatric patients being released from acute care hospitals increased substantially from 2001 to 2012. This trend is partly fueled by Medicare imposing penalties for readmission of patients with heart failure, pneumonia, chronic obstructive pulmonary disease, and myocardial infarction within 30 days. Patients with heart failure had the highest percentage of home health care referrals in 2012.[61] For patients who are otherwise thriving in their home environment, these referrals are often beneficial and can frequently be initiated in the ED.

## PALLIATIVE CARE

Public and professional awareness of palliative care has increased significantly over the past 10 years.[62] Palliative care is defined as "interdisciplinary care (medicine, nursing, social work, chaplaincy, and other specialties when appropriate) that focused on improving quality of life for persons of any age who are living with any serious illness and their families."[62] Hospice care, on the other hand, provides palliative care to dying individuals in their final months of life. Recent research in palliative care interventions in the ED show benefits in reduced hospital stays, hospice referrals, patient satisfaction, less intensive care utilization, and cost savings.[63–66] Although palliative care interventions are infrequently initiated in the ED, a systematic review described the feasibility of a screening and referral for palliative care consultation in the ED setting.[67]

Palliative care may be delivered at home, in long-term care settings, and in hospitals. Community-based palliative care is growing since the implementation of the ACA.[62]

Palliative care and hospice care are not synonymous with advance directives. Advance directives allow people to record their wishes about end-of-life care.[68] A living will allows people to state in advance what treatments they wish to receive when they are dying or irreversibly comatose. The durable power of attorney allows an individual to name a health care proxy, who will be empowered to make health care decisions for the individual if she or he becomes incapacitated.[68] Although physician orders for life-sustaining treatment forms are widely recognized, the implementation and acceptance has been slow and wrought with its own challenges.[69] That said, grassroots-level education and dissemination does show an improvement in uptake, especially in areas in which there is an active coalition to promote its use but work is still needed to expand this in lower income areas and in areas in and around for-profit hospitals.[70,71]

## SUMMARY

In summary, the aging of the population, both in the United States and the rest of the world, presents many challenges and opportunities for improvement in the delivery of health care in the ED and across all medical disciplines.

## AUTHOR'S NOTE

1 A visit which occurred in an emergency service area that does not conduct nursing triage. 2 The race groups, white, black or African American, and other include persons of Hispanic and not Hispanic origin. Persons of Hispanic origin may be of any race. For 2011, race data were missing for 14.8 percent of visits, and

ethnicity data were missing for 18.5 percent of visits. The National Center for Health Statistics uses model-based single imputation for NHAMCS race and ethnicity data. The race imputation is restricted to three categories (white, black, and other) based on research by an internal work group and on quality concerns with imputed estimates for race categories other than white and black. The imputation technique is described in more detail in the 2011 NHAMCS Public Use Data File documentation, available at: ftp://ftp.cdc.gov/pub/Health_Statistics/NCHS/Dataset_Documentation/NHAMCS/doc11.pdf. 3 Other race includes the categories of Asian, Native Hawaiian or other Pacific Islander, American Indian or Alaska Native, and persons with more than one race. 4 Total exceeds "all visits" because more than one source of payment may be reported per visit. 5 CHIP is the Children's Health Insurance Program. 6 The visits in this category are also included in both the Medicare and the Medicaid or CHIP categories. 7 "No insurance" is defined as having only self-pay, no charge, or charity as payment sources. The individual self-pay and no-charge or charity categories are not mutually exclusive. NOTES: The 2011 Patient Record Form (PRF) requested responses using a 1–5 scale. PRF responses were evaluated with reference to responses on the Ambulatory Unit Record, completed during induction, to the question, "How many levels are in this emergency service area's (ESA) triage system?" ESAs using 3 or 4 level triage systems had their responses rescaled to fit the 5 level system, such that, for 3-level ESAs, responses of 1, 2, and 3 were recoded to 2, 3, and 4. For ESAs using a 4–level system, responses were recoded from 1–4 to 2–5. The rescaling method was determined in consultation with subject matter experts and based on record analysis. Rescaling was required for about 12.0 percent of records. Also, missing responses (17.9%) were imputed to levels 1–5 using a hot deck (ie, current year's data) to identify donor records. Matching was based on the number of levels in the ESA's triage system, 3-digit ICD-9-CM code for primary diagnosis, the hospital's ED volume, and geographic region. This is unlike years 2005–2008 when "no triage" and "unknown," checkboxes used on the PRF in those years, were also valid imputation categories. Numbers may not add to totals because of rounding. SOURCE: CDC/NCHS, National Hospital Ambulatory Medical Care Survey.

## REFERENCES

1. Administration for Community Living (ACL). Administration on Aging (AoA), aging statistics. Washington, DC: U.S. Department of Health and Human Services; 2014. Available at: http://www.aoa.acl.gov/Aging_Statistics/index.aspx. Accessed September 23, 2015.

2. Centers for Disease Control and Prevention. National Center for Health Statistics (NCHS). Atlanta (GA): U.S. Department of Health and Human Services; 2015. Available at: http://www.cdc.gov/nchs/fastats/emergency-department.htm. Accessed September 23, 2015.

3. National Hospital Ambulatory Medical Care Survey. Emergency Department Summary Tables. 2011. Available at: http://www.cdc.gov/nchs/data/ahcd/nhamcs_emergency/2011_ed_web_tables.pdf. Accessed September 23, 2015.

4. Flomenbaum N. Unsung heroes: ED social workers. Emerg Med. Parsippany (NJ): Frontline Medical Communications Inc; 2015. p. 389. Available at: www.emed-journal.com.

5. Centers for Disease Control. National hospital ambulatory medical care survey: 2011 emergency department summary tables. National Center for Health Statistics; 2010. Available at: http://www.cdc.gov/nchs/data/ahcd/nhamcs_emergency/2011_ed_web_tables.pdf. Accessed September 23, 2015.

6. Aminzadeh F, Dalziel WB. Older adults in the emergency department: A systematic review of pattern of use, adverse outcomes, and effectiveness of interventions. Ann Emerg Med 2002;39:238–47.
7. Shaha M, Gmür S, Schoenenberger AW, et al. Trends and characteristics of attendance at the emergency department of a Swiss university hospital: 2002-2012. Swiss Med Wkly 2015;145:w14141.
8. Keehan SP, Cuckler GA, Sisko AM, et al. National health expenditure projections, 2014-24: spending growth faster than recent trends. Health Aff (Millwood) 2015; 34(8):1407–17.
9. McCarthy M. US healthcare spending will reach 20% of GDP by 2024. BMJ 2015; 351:h4204.
10. Hwang U, Morrison S. The Geriatric Emergency Department. J Am Geriatr Soc 2007;55(11):1873–6.
11. American College of Emergency Physicians. The American Geriatrics Society, Emergency Nurses Association, and the Society for Academic Emergency Medicine. Geriatric Emergency Department Guidelines. 2013. Available at: http://www.acep.org/geriEDguidelines/. Accessed September 23, 2015.
12. Lee J. Growth of senior-specific EDs holds quality promise but raises cost issues. Mod Healthc 2014;44(1):8.
13. Varadhan R, Seplaki CL, Xue QL, et al. Stimulus-response paradigm for characterizing the loss of resilience in homeostatic regulation associated with frailty. Mech Ageing Dev 2008;129(11):666–70.
14. Healthday. Seniors Often Underestimate their Frailty, Study Finds. 2015. Available at: http://consumer.healthday.com/general-health-information-16/emergencies-and-first-aid-news-227/seniors-often-overestimate-mobility-study-reports-702149. html. Accessed September 1, 2015.
15. Roedersheimer KM, Pereira GF, Jones CW, et al. Self-reported versus performance-based assessments of a simple mobility task among older adults in the emergency department. Ann Emerg Med 2015;67(2):151–6.
16. Toosizadeh N, Mohler J. Assessing upper extremity motion: an innovative method to identify frailty. J Am Geriatr Soc 2015;63:1181–6.
17. Soong J, Poots AJ, Scott S, et al. Developing and validating a risk prediction model for acute care based on frailty syndromes. BMJ Open 2015;5(10): e008457.
18. Goldstein J, Jensen JL, Carter AJ, et al. The epidemiology of prehospital emergency responses for older adults in a provincial EMS system. CJEM 2015;20:1–6.
19. Kodadek LM, Selvarajah S, Velopulos CG, et al. Undertriage of older trauma patients: is this a national phenomenon? J Surg Res 2015;199(1):220–9.
20. Nelson-Williams H, Kodadek L, Canner J, et al. Do trauma center levels matter in older isolated hip fracture patients? J Surg Res 2015;198(2):468–74.
21. Agarwal G, McDonough B, Angeles R, et al. Rationale and methods of a multicentre randomised controlled trial of the effectiveness of a Community Health Assessment Programme with Emergency Medical Services (CHAP-EMS) implemented on residents aged 55 years and older in subsidised seniors' housing buildings in Ontario, Canada. BMJ Open 2015;115(6):e008110.
22. Geriatric Emergency Management (GEM). An overview of delivery models, screening tools and practice guidelines. Ontario Hospital Association; 2003. Available at: http://rgp.toronto.on.ca/GEM/GEMOHA.pdf. Accessed October 1, 15.
23. Yao JL, Fang J, Lou QQ, et al. Systematic review of the identification of seniors at risk (ISAR) tool for the prediction of adverse outcome in elderly patients seen in the emergency department. Int J Clin Exp Med 2015;8(4):4778–86.

24. Carpenter CR, Shelton E, Fowler S, et al. Risk factors and screening instruments to predict adverse outcomes for undifferentiated older emergency department patients: a systematic review and meta-analysis. Acad Emerg Med 2015;22(1):1–21.

25. Chandra A, Crane SJ, Tung EE, et al. Patient-reported geriatric symptoms as risk factors for hospitalization and emergency department visits. Aging Dis 2015;6(3):188–95.

26. Launay CP, Rivière H, Kabeshova A, et al. Predicting prolonged length of hospital stay in older emergency department users: use of a novel analysis method, the Artificial Neural Network. Eur J Intern Med 2015;26(7):478–82.

27. Inzitari M, Gual N, Roig T, et al. Geriatric Screening Tools to Select Older Adults Susceptible for Direct Transfer From the Emergency Department to Subacute Intermediate-Care Hospitalization. J Am Med Dir Assoc 2015;16(10):837–41.

28. Deschodt M, Devriendt E, Sabbe M, et al. Characteristics of older adults admitted to the emergency department (ED) and their risk factors for ED readmission based on comprehensive geriatric assessment: a prospective cohort study. BMC Geriatr 2015;26(15):54.

29. Ellis G, Whitehead MA, O'Neill D, et al. Comprehensive geriatric assessment for older adults admitted to hospital. Cochrane Database Syst Rev 2011;(7):CD006211.

30. Ae R, Kojo T, Okayama M, et al. Caregiver daily impression could reflect illness latency and severity in frail elderly residents in long-term care facilities: a pilot study. Geriatr Gerontol Int 2015. http://dx.doi.org/10.1111/ggi.12524.

31. Caprio AJ, Biese K, Roberts E, et al. Medication use in the elderly patient: physiology, pharmacology, prescribing. The American Geriatrics Society. Available at: www.americangeriatrics.org; https://www.pogoe.org/sites/default/files/gsr/11_Medication_Use_in_the_Elderly_Patient.pdf. Accessed October 12, 2015.

32. Jansen PAF, Brouwers RBJ. Clinical Pharmacology in Old Persons. Scientifica (Cairo) 2012;2012:723678.

33. Siddiqi N, House AO, Holmes JD. Occurrence and outcome of delirium in medical in-patients: a systematic literature review. Age Ageing 2006;35(4):350–64.

34. Kennedy M, Enander RA, Tadiri SP, et al. Delirium risk prediction, healthcare use and mortality of elderly adults in the emergency department. J Am Geriatr Soc 2014;62(3):462–9.

35. Rosen T, Connors S, Clark S, et al. Assessment and Management of Delirium in Older Adults in the Emergency Department: Literature Review to Inform Development of a Novel Clinical Protocol. Adv Emerg Nurs J 2015;37(3):183–96.

36. ICD-10 Version. International Statistical Classification of Diseases and Related Health Problems 10th Revision (ICD-10)-2015-WHO Version. F05 Delirium, not induced by alcohol and other psychoactive substances. 2015. Available at: http://apps.who.int/classifications/icd10/browse/2015/en#/F05. Accessed October 11, 2015.

37. Han JH, Wilber ST. Altered mental status in older patients emergency department patients. Clin Geriatr Med 2013;29(1):101–36.

38. Grossmann FF, Hasemann W, Graber A, et al. Screening, detection and management of delirium in the emergency department – a pilot study on the feasibility of a new algorithm for use in older emergency department patients: the modified Confusion Assessment Method for the Emergency Department (mCAM-ED). Scand J Trauma Resusc Emerg Med 2014;22:19.

39. Han JH, Wilson A, Graves AJ, et al. Validation of the Confusion Assessment Method for the Intensive Care Unit in older emergency department patients. Acad Emerg Med 2014;21(2):180–7.

40. Han JH, Wilson A, Vasilevskis EE, et al. Diagnosing delirium in older emergency department patients: validity and reliability of the delirium triage screen and the brief confusion assessment method. Ann Emerg Med 2013;62(5):457–65.
41. Han JH, Zimmerman EE, Cutler N, et al. Delirium in Older Emergency Department Patients: Recognition, Risk Factors, and Psychomotor Subtypes. Acad Emerg Med 2009;16(3):193–200.
42. Han JH, Vasilevskis EE, Schnelle JF, et al. The diagnostic performance of the Richmond Agitation Sedation Scale for detecting delirium in older emergency department patients. Acad Emerg Med 2015;22(7):878–82.
43. Liu SW, Obermeyer Z, Chang Y, et al. Frequency of ED revisits and death among older adults after a fall. Am J Emerg Med 2015;33(8):1012–8.
44. ACS Traumatic Injuries in Elderly Patients are Often Underestimated. American College of Surgeons. Available at: https://www.facs.org/media/press-releases/jacs/elderly-trauma1013. Accessed October 12, 2015.
45. Maxwell CA, Miller RS, Dietrich MS, et al. The aging of America: a comprehensive look at over 25,000 geriatric trauma admissions to United States hospitals. Am Surg 2015;81(6):630–6.
46. Wolf SL, Barnhart HX, Kutner NG, et al. Reducing frailty and falls in older persons: an investigation of Tai Chi and computerized balance training. Atlanta FICSIT Group. Frailty and Injuries: Cooperative Studies of Intervention Techniques (see comments). J Am Geriatr Soc 1996;44:489–97.
47. Li F, Harmer P, Fisher KJ, et al. Tai Chi and fall reductions in older adults: A randomized controlled trial. J Gerontol A Biol Sci Med Sci 2005;60(2):187–94.
48. Campbell AJ, Robertson MC, Gardner MM, et al. Falls prevention over 2 years: a randomized controlled trial in women 80 years and older. Age Ageing 1999;28(6):513–8.
49. Clemson L, Cumming RG, Kendig H, et al. The effectiveness of a community-based program for reducing the incidence of falls in the elderly: a randomized trial. J Am Geriatr Soc 2004;52(9):1487–94.
50. Yardley L, Todd C, Beyer N, et al. Development and initial validation of the Falls Efficacy Scale International (FES-I). Age Ageing 2005;34:614–9.
51. Tennstedt S, Howland J, Lachman ME, et al. A randomized controlled trial of a group intervention to reduce fear of falling and associated activity restriction in older adults. J Gerontol B Psychol Sci Soc Sci 1998;53B:384–92.
52. Zijlstra GAR, van Haastregt JCM, Ambergen T, et al. Effects of a multicomponent cognitive behavioral group intervention on fear of falling and activity avoidance in community-dwelling older adults: Results of a randomized clinical trial. J Am Geriatr Soc 2009;57:2020–8.
53. National Center on Caregiving. Family caregiver alliance. Selected long-term care statistics. Available at: https://www.caregiver.org/selected-long-term-care-statistics. Accessed February 1, 2016.
54. Gruneir A, Bell CM, Bronskill SE, et al. Frequency and pattern of emergency department visits by long-term care residents - a population-based study. J Am Geriatr Soc 2010;58(3):510–7.
55. Callinan SM, Brandt NJ. Tackling communication barriers between long-term care facility and emergency department transfers to improve medication safety in older adults. J Gerontol Nurs 2015;41(7):8–13.
56. Boockvar K, Fishman E, Kyriacou CK, et al. Adverse events due to discontinuations in drug use and dose changes in patients transferred between acute and long-term care facilities. Arch Intern Med 2004;164(5):545–50.
57. Clancy CM. Care transitions: a threat and an opportunity for patient safety. Am J Med Qual 2006;21(6):415–7.

58. Coleman EA. Falling through the cracks: Challenges and opportunities for improving transitional care for persons with continuous complex care needs. J Am Geriatr Soc 2003;51(4):549–55.
59. Coleman EA, Min SJ, Chomiak A, et al. Posthospital care transitions: Patterns, complications, and risk identification. Health Serv Res 2004;39(5):1449–65.
60. The National Transitions of Care Coalition. Available at: http://www.ntocc.org/. Accessed February 1, 2016.
61. Jones CD, Ginde AA, Burke RE, et al. Increasing home healthcare referrals upon discharge from U.S. Hospitals: 2001-2012. J Am Geriatr Soc 2015;63(6):1265–6.
62. Kelley AS, Morrison RS. Palliative Care for the Seriously Ill. N Engl J Med 2015; 373(8):747–55.
63. Grudzen CR, Stone S, Morrison S. The palliative care model for emergency department patients with advanced illness. J Palliat Med 2011;14:945–50.
64. Meier D, Beresford L. Fast response is key to partnering with the emergency department. J Palliat Med 2007;10:641–5.
65. Beemath A, Zalenski R. Palliative emergency medicine: resuscitating comfort care. Ann Emerg Med 2009;54:103–4.
66. Penrod J, Deb P, Luhrs C, et al. Cost and utilization outcomes of patients receiving hospital-based palliative care consultation. J Palliat Med 2006;9:855–60.
67. George N, Phillips E, Zaurova M, et al. Palliative care screening and assessment in the emergency department: a systematic review. J Pain Symptom Manage 2015;51(1):108–19.e2.
68. National Institutes of Health. U.S. National Library of Medicine. MedlinePlus Advance Directives. Available at: https://www.nlm.nih.gov/medlineplus/advancedirectives. html. Accessed February 1, 2016.
69. Jesus JE, Geiderman JM, Venkat A, et al, ACEP Ethics Committee. Physician orders for life-sustaining treatment and emergency medicine: ethical considerations, legal issues, and emerging trends. Ann Emerg Med 2014;64(2):140–4.
70. Wenger NS, Citko J, O'Mally K, et al. Implementation of physician orders for life sustaining treatment in nursing homes in California: Evaluation of a novel statewide dissemination mechanism. J Gen Intern Med 2012;28:51–7.
71. Sugiyama T, Zingmond D, Lorenz KA, et al. Implementing physician orders for life-sustaining treatment in California hospitals: factors associated with adoption. J Am Geriatr Soc 2013;61(8):1337–44.
72. Choice of Analgesia and Sedation. Available at: http://www.icudelirium.org/ sedation.html. Accessed October 14, 2015.
73. Sessler CN, Gosnell MS, Grap MJ, et al. The Richmond Agitation-Sedation Scale: validity and reliability in adult intensive care unit patients. Am J Respir Crit Care Med 2002;166(10):1338–44.
74. Ely EW, Truman B, Shintani A, et al. Monitoring sedation status over time in ICU patients: reliability and validity of the Richmond Agitation-Sedation Scale (RASS). JAMA 2003;289(22):2983–91.

# Geriatric Resuscitation

Thomas Perera, MD*, Alexis Cortijo-Brown, MD

## KEYWORDS

- Geriatric • Ethics • Shock • Coagulopathies • Resuscitation

## KEY POINTS

- Do not use age as the sole criteria to perform or withhold any type of resuscitation.
- Early signs of shock may not be apparent in the elderly.
- Do not assume that the cause of shock is apparent. Always keep a high level of suspicion for hemorrhage and obstructive forms of shock.
- Use bedside ultrasound as an adjunct to diagnosis and care.
- Frequent reassessment is necessary to gauge the effectiveness of resuscitation.

## INTRODUCTION

The geriatric population is an ever growing demographic in the United States, and thus a significant representation of health care recipients. If 65 years of age is used as the demarcation, in 2010 a total of 13% of the US population was geriatric. Accordingly, by 2030 the percentage is projected to increase to more than 20%.[1] A significant portion of this population will become dependent on the health care system. By the time a person reaches 65 years of age they will have on average three chronic medical conditions and close to a 20% risk for hospitalization per year.[2] According to one source by the year 2050, a total of 39% of trauma admissions will be geriatric patients.[3] Currently, nearly two-thirds of intensive care unit beds are occupied by those greater than 65 years of age.[4] Emergency medical treatment of this expanding population is complicated by their relative fragility caused by nothing more than normal physiologic changes that occur with age. In general, these changes cause the individual to be at greater risk for illness and injury. In addition, many of these individuals have comorbidities that make resuscitation more complex. Trauma, sepsis, gastrointestinal (GI) bleeding, and cardiac arrest have all been shown to have an age-related increase in mortality. Most recent studies show that much of this increase is caused by comorbid disease states and not age alone. Comorbidities can decrease physiologic reserve and alter the body's ability to resist external insults.

Disclosures: None.
Emergency Medicine, Montefiore/Jacobi Medical Centers, 1400 Pelham Parkway South, Bronx, NY 10461, USA
* Corresponding author.
E-mail address: thomas.perera@nbhn.net

Emerg Med Clin N Am 34 (2016) 453–467
http://dx.doi.org/10.1016/j.emc.2016.04.002
0733-8627/16/$ – see front matter © 2016 Elsevier Inc. All rights reserved.

## ETHICAL CONSIDERATIONS

Before starting resuscitation a clinician should try to determine the patient's wishes, whether they have advance directives in place, and evaluate the patient's condition for medical futility. This is true in all populations but is more frequently an issue in the elderly. In a perfect world the patient or the patient's agent/proxy would be readily available to express the patient's wishes. More often the patient arrives by emergency medical service with limited information. The advance health care directives or advance directives were developed to provide a practical process for ensuring patient autonomy and self-determination at the end of life.[5] Even though there are distinctions, for this discussion advance directives are used interchangeably with living will, a do-not-resuscitate order, or a Physician Orders for Life-Sustaining Treatment. These directives allow physicians and family to make treatment decisions that reflect the decisions that the patient would have made for himself or herself. Advance directives are not simply about avoiding treatment that would prolong life in undesirable conditions. They have become increasingly detailed and specific, often containing patient preferences for a variety of medical treatments in hypothetical medical scenarios.[6] Most of the advance directives that affect the provider at this stage of resuscitation involve do-not-resuscitate or do-not-intubate orders.

When available and known, most physicians feel comfortable complying with these patient decisions. When physicians fail to comply with a patient's advance directive, the patient or their representative may bring a civil law suit for damages.[7] Unfortunately, the advance directives are often not known or not available at the initial stages of resuscitation. Often a call to the patient's home/facility or a call to the next of kin needs to be made to clarify the proper action. If there is no information available then resuscitation should proceed as the physician deems appropriate. If an action, such as intubation, is taken and later the patient's wishes to the contrary become known, it should be noted that there is little ethical distinction between not initiating care and withdrawing care. When patient's wishes become known the providers should make every effort to apply them. Physicians may override the advance directive, but this should only be done in rare instances where there is evidence that the patient's wishes have changed since the advance directives were written.[8]

Not every patient presenting to the emergency department should be resuscitated. If the medical providers believe that an intervention is futile or that it may only bring harm to the patient, they should choose not to perform that intervention. Arguments against providing care that is futile include potential harm to patients; family members or caregivers with little or no likely benefits; and to a lesser extent, the diversion of resources that might otherwise be used to provide care to those patients who could positively respond to such care. The physician's judgment should be unbiased, and should be based on available scientific evidence, and societal and professional standards. It should include an assessment of the likelihood that a patient could physically recover as a result of treatment, or the likelihood of such treatment to relieve a patient's suffering. The American College of Emergency Physicians has a policy statement that provides some guidance and protection to the physician.[9] The best course of action is to engage the patient and/or their proxies in the decision as to what is best for the patient and continue accordingly.

## RESUSCITATION

Once the decision to resuscitate has been made, the emergency physician should act rapidly. There is a tendency to treat older persons less aggressively. However, recognizing illness early and starting appropriate therapy is essential in the geriatric population. Aggressive, early treatment has been shown to improve survival in the elderly.[10] It is important to consider criteria other than just chronologic age, such as recent performance level, quality of life, comorbidities, and patient preference, when determining the aggressiveness of care. Efforts should be aimed at early recognition of shock states because the longer a patient is in extremis the lower the chance of full recovery. Elderly patients have less reserve and injuries and insults that seem minor in isolation may have catastrophic consequences in this population.

## Airway

The geriatric airway evaluation starts with making sure that the airway is clear and patent, evaluating the neck and tracheal area for injury, swelling, or crepitus. Make note of facial hair, dentures, or dental appliances. Geriatric patients are more difficult to bag-valve-mask ventilate, even in the absence of these obstructions.[11] There are several physiologic changes in the geriatric airway that should be noted. There is a loss of muscular pharyngeal support, making the elderly more susceptible to upper airway obstruction. There is also a decrease in respiratory effort in response to upper airway occlusion.[12] The protective mechanisms of coughing and swallowing also diminish with age, placing geriatric individuals at higher risk for aspiration.[13] Factors associated with a difficult airway that worsen with age include limited mouth opening caused by temporomandibular joint stiffening, limited mandibular protrusion, decreased thyromental distance, and decreased submandibular compliance. An individual's Mallampati score increases with age and neck mobility decreases.[14] These factors combine to make most geriatric airways by definition a difficult airway. If intubation becomes necessary the goals are to safely and quickly secure the airway, while minimizing the risk of aspiration without worsening shock. It is essential to prepare for a difficult airway with available fiberoptic and other airway adjuncts. Be prepared to use the LMA as a temporary or definitive airway when other options fail. Rapid sequence intubation or modified rapid sequence intubation is most commonly used to facilitate intubation and minimize the risk of active regurgitation.

## Breathing

The second step is to assess breathing and ventilation. Examine the patient visually and with a stethoscope. Palpate the chest wall, and look for old surgical scars, pacemakers, and ports that may give clues to the past medical history. When treating geriatric patients at this stage of the examination, there are several important physiologic changes to be noted. Weakened respiratory muscles and decreased elastic recoil of the lungs may lead to reduced vital capacity, functional residual capacity, and forced expiratory volume in 1 second. There is a significant increase in dead space, sometimes called "senile emphysema," which decreases the respiratory reserve. These changes indicate that this population is at increased risk for respiratory failure and acute lung injury, thus leading to intubation and support on mechanical ventilation.

The universal use of supplemental oxygen in patients with major illness has been the mainstay of the initial stabilization. However, recent studies have called this practice into question. Studies on diseases, such as myocardial infarction (MI) and congestive heart failure, have shown an increase in mortality with the use of supplemental oxygen. Furthermore, the geriatric population has more comorbid diseases, such as chronic obstructive pulmonary disease, which predispose to hypercarbia when patients are on supplemental oxygen. Depending on the case, when an oxygen saturation level becomes available, supplemental oxygen can be given to maintain oxygen saturation in the low 90% range or a $Pao_2$ greater than or equal to 60 mm Hg. However, oxygen may not be needed in patients with normal oxygenation.

When available, use continuous pulse oximetry and capnometry or capnography to assess oxygenation and ventilation. Elderly patients often have a diminished response to hypercarbia, hypoxia, and acidosis.[15] They may have a normal respiratory rate because it takes them longer to compensate. While examining the chest be aware of the increased fragility of the chest wall in geriatric patients. The elderly have a decreased ability to tolerate chest wall trauma. These patients are more likely to sustain injuries, such as rib fractures, sternal fractures, flail chest, hemopneumothorax, and pulmonary contusion and/or cardiac contusion.

### Intubation

Intubation may be considered for a variety of reasons, including respiratory failure, patient fatigue, and airway protection. Although the decision is usually determined by clinical criteria, intubation should be considered when patients have a respiratory rate of greater than 40 breaths per minute, or a $Pao_2$ less than 60 mm Hg or a $Paco_2$ greater than 50 mm Hg. The decision to intubate is always an important one, but this is especially true in the elderly. For this population there is a higher rate of aspiration, ventilator-associated pneumonia, and failure to wean from the ventilator.[16] Consider noninvasive ventilation when attempting to delay or avoid intubation. It has been proven beneficial despite difficulty securing the appropriately fitting mask because of poor dentition, dental appliances, and altered mental status. Noninvasive ventilation has proven beneficial for chronic obstructive pulmonary disease where it has been shown to drastically reduce symptoms and the need for intubation.[17] It has symptomatic benefit in congestive heart failure and may be advantageous in other respiratory processes.[18]

Once the decision to intubate is made, orotracheal intubation using neuromuscular blockade should be used in most cases. Doses for neuromuscular blocking agents do not have to be altered in the elderly, regardless of their renal function. Consider reducing the dosage when administering sedatives. The dose of benzodiazepines, etomidate, and barbiturates should be reduced by as much as half because renal and liver function affects their clearance. Reduced clearance may lead to complications, such as hypotension and prolonged sedation. Lower dosages of ketamine should also be considered because of increased duration of action and reduced clearance in the elderly.

A surgical airway may also be difficult in the geriatric population because the elderly have decreased cervical mobility; looser skin on the neck; and a stiffer, smaller cricothyroid membrane. Needle cricothyrotomies and bougie-assisted techniques may aid in securing the airway.

Mechanical ventilation can be a life-saving strategy in patients with acute respiratory failure. However, mechanical ventilation does have the potential to aggravate and precipitate lung injury. Once intubated, ventilator settings should be adjusted depending on the cause of respiratory failure. In the elderly there are data to suggest that low-volume, low-pressure ventilation (lung-protective ventilation) is associated with better outcomes.[19] Therefore, settings of 6 mL/kg and plateau pressure 30 cm $H_2O$ or less should be considered.

### Circulation

Circulation should be assessed by heart rate, blood pressure, skin perfusion, and mental status. Vital signs should be trended carefully instead of relying on just the initial triage vital signs. Blood pressure is often difficult to obtain in the very ill. It has been suggested that if a patient has peripheral pulses, then the pressure is about 60 mm Hg and if femoral pulses are palpable then they have a blood pressure of at east 40 mm Hg.[20] Failure to palpate a pulse does not automatically mean the patient is in arrest. There may be organized mechanical activity with an insufficient cardiac output to give meaningful circulation. The use of point-of-care ultrasound has allowed direct visualization of heart motion and can be used to guide therapy.

When determining how to resuscitate a geriatric patient, the goal is to optimize cardiac output while carefully monitoring cardiac activity. There are several physiologic changes that occur in the elderly that affect circulation during resuscitation. There is progressive stiffening of arteries and of the myocardium, which decreases cardiac output and can contribute to ventricular hypertrophy. In the geriatric patient when there is hemorrhage, infection, or pain, the normal response of tachycardia may be absent because the myocardium is less sensitive to catecholamines. Moreover, many of these patients take β-blockers and calcium channel blockers or other chronotropic drugs that further blunt the expected tachycardia that occurs with pain, hypovolemia, and shock. This in turn may lead to a delay in recognizing the severity of injury and therefore, the aggressive early treatment that may be necessary. Additionally, geriatric patients have relatively increased blood pressure in comparison with younger populations. When a physician gets a normal blood pressure in a geriatric patient they should consider the possibility that this may indicate hypoperfusion.

## DETECTING SHOCK

Shock is a life-threatening state where end-organ and tissue perfusion is insufficient and there is inadequate oxygen for normal metabolism. Advanced shock, regardless of cause, has a mortality of up to 40%.[21] Patients in shock who are sweating, tachycardic, and hypotensive are easy to spot. The geriatric population, for a variety of reasons, do not always manifest these obvious signs. Early signs and symptoms of shock including confusion, anxiety, and shortness of breath are often missed until they manifest as altered mental status, hypotension, tachycardia, oliguria, cool clammy skin, and metabolic acidosis.[22] In isolation these clinical features are neither sensitive nor specific for the diagnosis of shock. Factors that make the identification of shock more difficult in the geriatric population include changes in the cardiovascular reflexes, medication, comorbidities, and unknown baseline blood pressure. Baseline blood pressure increases with age, so a normal blood pressure in a patient who usually is hypertensive can represent a shock state.[23] The National Trauma Triage Protocol has recognized that systolic blood pressure less than 110 mm Hg may represent shock in those older than 65 years old. Automated blood pressure machines may overestimate the blood pressure in elderly patients because their arteries are stiff.

The elderly may also be less aware of their own illness because they have a 40% to 50% decreased perception of, and ventilatory response to, hypoxia and hypercapnia.[24] Because of physiologic changes and increased dead space, a normal respiratory rate in elderly patients may be as high as 25 breaths per minute. A rate of greater than 25 breaths per minute may be the first sign of a lower respiratory tract infection, heart failure, or other disorder.[25] Geriatric patients who have lost up to 35% of their intravascular volume are often not tachycardic, so the absence of tachycardia should not reassure the clinician about volume status or blood loss.[26] By the time there are vital sign changes, the patient may be in extremis. Skin turgor testing and capillary refill have been shown to have a specificity of around 10% and thus are not useful.[27] Orthostatic testing has been the subject of much debate. Studies measuring orthostatics from the supine to standing position showed reasonable specificity.[28] However, it should be noted that a lack of mobility can make standing difficult for the elderly. In patients who are healthy and are not on vasoactive medication a pulse increase of 20 beats per minute has specificity for hypovolemia of 98%. In addition, a decrease in systolic blood pressure of 20 mm Hg or greater has a specificity of 97%. A shock index (heart rate/systolic blood pressure) of greater than or equal to 0.7 has a specificity for hypovolemia of 99%.[29] Decreased urinary output should probably not be solely relied on as a sign of shock because it can be a late finding and may represent comorbid pathology instead of volume status.

Laboratory testing may aid in early identification of shock in the elderly. Point-of-care end tidal $CO_2$ has been shown to be an early predictor of metabolic acidosis and may be a way to quickly assess a patient's status.[30] Blood-urea-nitrogen and creatinine have been studied separately and as a ratio. Changes often reflect end-organ dysfunction, but in isolation do not always reliably predict shock or dehydration.[31] Studies have shown that an abnormal lactate, pH and $HCO3_3$ in sepsis and trauma correlate with increased morbidity and mortality.[32,33] Lactate in particular has been effectively used as a marker for shock. Lactate can be produced as a by-product of inadequate blood perfusion and as a marker of strained cellular metabolism. It can be used not only to help identify shock but also, with repeated levels, as a marker of the effectiveness of resuscitation. In septic shock, however, 10% to 15% of people are not lactate producers and acidosis is often a very late sign of shock. Ultrasound is being used more often as a rapid way to evaluate early shock. It aids in identification of shock and in categorizing the type of shock. Bedside assessment of the heart, inferior vena cava, Morison pouch, left upper quadrant, pelvis, aorta, and lungs is done quickly and effectively. The inferior vena cava can be evaluated to assess a patient's volume status. Specifically, the inferior vena cava can be visualized and the collapsibility estimated.[34] Patients can then be fluid resuscitated and their response seen in real time with repeat point-of-care ultrasound. Moreover, if the inferior vena cava is not collapsing with respiration it may indicate that the patient is not hypovolemic and that other treatments, such as inotropes, may need to be considered. In the end, there is no single test that perfectly predicts the development of shock, so a high index of suspicion should be maintained.

Even when shock is suspected, the type of shock can be cryptogenic. In any age group shock can be broken into hypovolemic, vasodilatory, cardiogenic, or obstructive (**Table 1**). In the elderly there is a tendency to assign hypotension to either septic or cardiogenic shock, even in the absence of supporting data. Many of the clinical manifestations provide clues to the underlying cause and are primarily used to narrow the differential diagnosis so that empiric therapies can be administered in a timely fashion. However, early assignment of the probable cause of shock may be wrong in up to 30% of cases.[35] A good history from family or review of nursing home records is essential. In the age of electronic medical records it is often possible to get a reasonable picture of a patient's past medical history, an old electrocardiogram, and a medication list that may become invaluable as resuscitation progresses. The physical examination that reveals a dialysis shunt or automatic implantable cardioverter-defibrillator often makes a significant difference in treatment. In the geriatric population there is more overlap between the four standard categories of shock, which may have additive effects. A patient, for example, with poor cardiac function that becomes septic has elements of both types of shock contributing to the overall clinical picture. Bedside ultrasound evaluation with protocols, such as the RUSH examination (**Fig. 1**), can reliably guide early therapy and assess improvement throughout the resuscitation.[35] By evaluating the inferior vena cava, the heart, the lungs, the abdomen, and the aorta, 80% of shock can be correctly identified and treatment begun in the first 15 minutes of care. Frequent repeat examinations can quickly and accurately gauge response to therapy and further guide resuscitation.

| Table 1 |
| Types of shock |

| Types of Shock | Obstructive | Cardiogenic | Hypovolemic | Distributive |
|---|---|---|---|---|
| Causes and special consideration in geriatrics | • Pulmonary embolus<br>• Pulmonic or triscupid valve obstruction<br>• Cardiac tamponade<br>• Tension pneuomothorax | • Arrhythmias (especially caused by hyperkalemia, digoxin toxicity, hypomagnesium)<br>• Valvular disease (especially aortic stenosis)<br>• Pericardial tamponade<br>• Myocardial infarction (especially with left ventricular failure)<br>• Myocarditis<br>• Cardiomyopathy<br>• Myocardial contusion | Hemorrhagic<br>• Trauma<br>• GI bleed (especially those on ASA, NSAIDS)<br>• AAA<br>• Major vascular damage<br>Nonhemorrhagic<br>• Inadequate intake<br>• GI losses: vomiting, diarrhea<br>• Losses from skin, respiratory, and renal<br>• Environmental exposures | Sepsis<br>• Equal frequency between gram-negative and gram-positive<br>• Fungal, viral, parasitic<br>Nonseptic<br>• Anaphylaxis<br>• Neurogenic<br>• Drugs (especially overdoses on medications) |

*Abbreviations:* AAA, abdominal aortic aneurysm; ASA, aspirin; NSAID, nonsteroidal anti-inflammatory drugs.

## *Hypovolemic/Vasodilatory*

These two types of shock are often linked because detection and treatment are similar. Both exhibit end-organ dysfunction in the setting of good cardiac function. The main difference is that vasodilatory shock states, such as sepsis and the rare neurogenic shock, are more responsive to vasoconstricting medication.

Once it can be determined that the major type of shock is hypovolemic/vasodilatory, treatment can be initiated even before the exact cause has been established. Rapid restoration of perfusion is predominantly achieved by the administration of intravenous (IV) crystalloids. There is often concern for fluid overload in the elderly, but this should not delay or prevent resuscitation. Using 250- to 500-mL boluses and frequent reassessment of the patient minimizes the risk of iatrogenic fluid overload.[36] Sepsis studies have consistently shown that clinicians tend to under resuscitate with fluids.[37] Patients may require 4 to 5 L in the initial resuscitation before tissue perfusion is restored. Monitoring input and output and keeping accurate records of fluids given is essential in the long-term care of these patients. Other interventions to restore perfusion, such as vasopressor therapy, inotropic therapy, and blood transfusion, can be added, depending on the response to fluid resuscitation, evidence for myocardial dysfunction, and presence of anemia.

The exact cause of the hypovolemia/vasodilation should be sought. Simple dehydration is common in the elderly. When assessing for dehydration or renal failure, the serum creatinine alone is not an appropriate marker on which to rely. As patients age they often have reduced muscle mass making their creatinine level a poor screening tool. Instead, when assessing for dehydration or renal function a patient's creatinine clearance should be calculated as it takes into consideration age and weight. Predisposing age-related changes to the kidney include decline in the renin-angiotensin system, lowered organ responsiveness to antidiuretic hormone, and

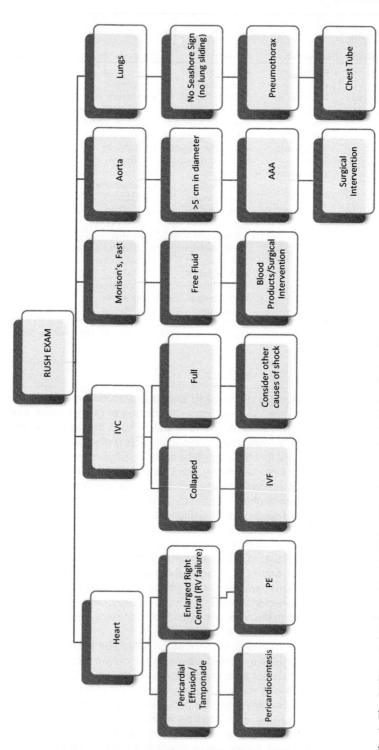

**Fig. 1.** The RUSH examination protocol. AAA, abdominal aortic aneurysm; IVC, inferior vena cava; IVF, intravenous fluids; PE, pulmonary embolism.

decreased ability to retain sodium in the distal tubules. This can be compounded by medications, such as diuretics, a decreased perception of thirst, and decreased mobility to access liquids. Hypernatremia is not uncommon in these situations. A high suspicion for sepsis must be maintained. The elderly do not always mount a fever or white blood cell count when infected. Geriatric patients may present with hypothermia as their only response to infection or no temperature alteration at all. Consider a rectal temperature on elderly patients because other readings may not be accurate. Medication and comorbidities can blunt the tachycardic response and hypotension is often a late finding. Therefore, the systemic inflammatory response syndrome, which is screened for in many emergency departments, is often absent.[38] Screen for infectious sources and consider initiating antibiotics in those cases where the cause of hypovolemia remains unclear. Hemorrhagic shock also presents as hypovolemia. One percent of patients 80 years old or older are hospitalized per year for GI bleeding.[39] Elderly patients are predisposed to bleeding mostly because they are often on aspirin, nonsteroidal anti-inflammatory drugs, and other antithrombotic and antiplatelet agents. Patients with liver disease are at risk because of portal hypertension, and renal patients have poorly adhering platelets. Geriatric patients with GI bleeding have higher rates of hospitalization, higher rates of rebleeding, and a higher mortality rate.[40] The presentation of GI bleeding can be as nonspecific as any form of shock. It is easy to assume that the hypovolemia is from dehydration or sepsis. The first hemoglobin and hematocrit value obtained may not obviously demonstrate bleeding if the patient has no prior values to work from. Looking at the mean corpuscular volume and the red blood cell distribution width may offer additional clues. Consider performing a rectal examination or checking for GI bleeding whenever a rectal temperature is performed.

Coagulopathy is a particular concern in the geriatric patient with hemorrhage. Coagulopathy and acidosis are worsened by hypothermia. If there is hypothermia, it should be addressed using warm fluids, warming devices, and warm blankets. The elderly have changes in their thermoregulation making it more important to warm these patients from the outset of treatment.

It is important to know what anticoagulants and antiplatelet medications the patient takes. Reversal of such medication may be necessary even before laboratory results are back, because they are at increased risk of hemorrhage after injury.[41] It is common for patients on antiplatelet medication to receive platelet transfusion when they have serious hemorrhage. Special care must be given to geriatric patients because transfusion-related acute lung injury is a serious complication. Patients with significant GI bleeding or who sustain intracranial bleeding and are on warfarin should be given vitamin K and fresh frozen plasma so that the international normalized ratio is less than 1.6.[42] The effects of vitamin K IV are seen within 12 to 24 hours. Although fresh frozen plasma is often dosed at 15 mL/kg, there is variability of the factor concentrations and the optimal dosing is still not known. Additionally, fresh frozen plasma can cause problems in geriatric patients with cardiovascular disease with regard to fluid overload. Prothrombin complex concentrates (PCCs) and recombinant activated factor VIIa can also be used in reversal of anticoagulation. Several nonrandomized studies showed that four factor PCC acts within minutes, when compared with fresh frozen plasma that takes hours, to reverse anticoagulation and decrease bleeding in patients with intracranial hemorrhage.[43] The three factor PCC may not reverse anticoagulation completely. Proof of improved clinical outcomes of one agent over another or the effectiveness of activated factor VIIa is still lacking. Rivaroxaban, dabigatran, and apixaban are new agents where reversal agents are only now being produced. Currently, the studies on the effectiveness in the clinical setting are not available.

For example, the reversal of dabigatran has only been demonstrated on mice.[44] It has been suggested that in severe situations hemodialysis may remove a certain amount of dabigatran and riveroxaban from the patient. There are also some preclinical trials and case reports that PCCs improve reversal in rivaroxaban and dabigatran.[45]

Trauma is predominantly a hypovolemic cause of shock but may have elements of other shock mechanisms. In the treatment of the elderly, there is no deviation from the guidelines of advanced trauma life support. In the traumatically injured patient, stressors that are usually tolerated by younger populations may cause serious negative effects in the elderly. Sources suggest that geriatric patients respond better when they are treated at designated trauma centers.[46] Trauma centers are best positioned to administer expedited and aggressive treatment.[47] Cryptogenic injury is more common in the geriatric population and altered mental status can be the only sign of injury. It should never be assumed that altered mental status is the patient's baseline, given the possibility of hypoxia, hypoglycemia, acute intracranial damage, or shock. Pulse oximetry, finger stick glucose, and naloxone are adjuncts that may be used in the patient suffering from altered mental status. Because the presentation of more severe illness may be difficult to recognize, the use of monitors and markers has been advocated. There has been a trend to move away from invasive hemodynamic monitoring, such as pulmonary artery catheterization. Instead there is increased use of noninvasive tests, such as base deficits and serum lactate. These two laboratory tests have been shown to be reliable in guiding resuscitation.[48] Lactate and base deficit are important and are used to evaluate severity of injury when vital signs may not be obviously abnormal. One study in the elderly noted that lactate and base deficit when elevated were linked to higher mortality in normotensive patients.[49] Moreover, the Eastern Association for Surgery of Trauma correlates a base deficit of $-6$ mEq/L or less to predict a 60% risk of mortality.[42] Serial lactates and base deficits may be drawn and followed. These can aid in the diagnosis of hypoperfusion and prevent imminent shock.[50] If they remain elevated, medical staff should be concerned that the resuscitation is not adequate.

The trend in trauma resuscitation is to decrease the use of IV fluids and focus instead on early interventions to control bleeding. When IV fluids are needed, crystalloids are the preferred starting choice. Blood products should be used when available. Do not hesitate to give blood to geriatric patients with severe trauma. Significant improvement to hospital discharge has been demonstrated in elderly patients receiving massive transfusions posttrauma, even in the presence of multiple risk factors for mortality.[51] Restrictive resuscitation or transfusion based on age alone cannot be supported. Early aggressive resuscitation of elderly trauma patients along specific guidelines directed at the geriatric population is justified and may further improve outcomes.[51]

One specific injury worth mentioning is cardiac contusion. In general, cardiac contusion is a poorly characterized entity with varied presentations. Arrhythmias are relatively common as is some degree of cardiac dysfunction with diminished contractility in the absence of arrhythmia or hemorrhage. In younger populations cardiac contusion usually requires very little alteration in care. In the geriatric population, with their diminished reserve, the addition of a cardiac contusion to even relatively minor injuries can be disastrous.[10] Echocardiography is warranted in patients with suspected cardiac contusion for any clinical findings suggestive of hypotension or acute heart failure.[52] Identified injuries should be managed appropriately; patients without identifiable injury but with evidence of dysfunction should be admitted for cardiac monitoring. Some authors advocate admitting geriatric patients with cardiac contusion to a higher level of care.[53]

## Cardiogenic

Cardiogenic shock includes patients in arrest, those with significant arrhythmias, and those with decreased cardiac output. Most of the studies used for advanced cardiac life support are data collected from geriatric populations, so they can be applied without alteration. Cardiopulmonary resuscitation has been studied in the geriatric population and is still believed to be an effective treatment regardless of varying factors, such as where the arrest took place, initial rhythm, length of downtime, and comorbidities.[54] Hyperkalemia should be suspected and treated in those with evidence of hemodialysis or worsening renal failure. Patients on digoxin are always at risk for toxicity with an alteration in their renal function. Patients suffering chest pain who take sildenafil citrate or tadalafil should not be given nitroglycerin. Diuretics predispose patients to electrolyte disturbances. Hypomagnesemia in particular should be considered. Magnesium therapy should be used for torsades de pointes and should be considered in patients with biventricular failure presenting with malignant arrhythmias.[55]

MI with left ventricular failure remains the most common cause of cardiogenic shock. It is critical to exclude complicating factors that may cause shock in patients with MI. Chief among these are the mechanical complications: ventricular septal rupture, contained free wall rupture, and papillary muscle rupture. In the setting of cardiogenic shock the decision to slow the rate and allow better filling and cardiac output must be weighed against the negative inotropic effect of the medications used to achieve this. Bedside ultrasound evaluation with even a rough evaluation of cardiac output may guide therapy. When needed, use pharmacologic support including inotropic and vasopressor agents. Unfortunately, inotropes increase myocardial ATP consumption such that short-term hemodynamic improvement occurs at the cost of increased oxygen demand when the heart is already failing and supply is already limited. These drugs should be used in the lowest possible doses because higher vasopressor doses are associated with poorer survival.[56] Currently, the American College of Cardiology/American Heart Association guidelines recommend norepinephrine for more severe cardiogenic shock.[57] Depending on the stability of the patient there are data to support the use of percutaneous coronary intervention in geriatric patients with MI complicated by cardiogenic shock. Data suggest that survival is improved among patients referred for angiography. In this population, 56% of patients survived to be discharged from the hospital, and of the hospital survivors, 75% were alive at 1 year.[58] Hypothermia has been advocated in the post–cardiac arrest patient especially those whose initial rhythm is ventricular fibrillation. Although some hypothermia protocols exclude older patients, one study found up to 27% of patients older than 75 had a good functional outcome at 6 months, and functional outcomes of elderly survivors were similar to younger patients.[59]

## Obstructive

Causes of obstructive shock include pulmonary emboli, pneumothorax, aortic stenosis, and cardiac tamponade. All of these in turn cause circulatory insufficiency and hypotension. A good history sometimes points toward the diagnosis. The classic findings of pulmonary embolism or tamponade are not always present. A distended right ventricle or unsuspected pericardial fluid (**Fig. 2**) are part of the reasons for considering bedside ultrasound in undifferentiated shock patients. The diagnosis of this cause of shock is confounded by preexisting conditions. Pulmonary hypertension from any cause or congestive heart failure may elevate right-sided pressures and chronically give findings that mimic these shock states. Once discovered these states can be appropriately treated. The general treatment of obstructive shock includes

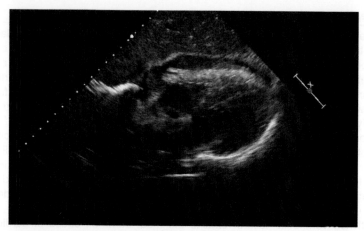

**Fig. 2.** Echocardiogram demonstrating pericardial fluid.

maintaining right-sided filling pressure so the cardiac output is preserved until efforts to relieve the obstruction are initiated. Fluid therapy is vitally important to improve filling and thus cardiac output, whereas inotropic support likely provides only mild temporary benefit. Treatment of massive pulmonary embolism in the elderly has been studied. One study showed that clinical symptoms at admission were similar in the elderly and younger populations. The mean absolute improvement in the lung scan perfusion defect, the rate of major bleeding, and the long-term evolution were not statistically different between older and younger patients when treated with recombinant tissue plasminogen activator.[60] Old age should not preclude thrombolytic therapy in massive pulmonary embolism, provided there is no other contraindication for thrombolytic treatment.

## SUMMARY

Resuscitating the elderly is a complex and difficult task. Respecting their wishes when available should guide the resuscitation decisions. Overall mortality is high for geriatric patients in shock, but outcomes may be good especially in those with a high functioning premorbid state. The clinician should be aware of the patient's past medical history and medications, and tailor therapy based on these factors. It is important to use adjunctive tests and reassessment to adjust resuscitation whenever available. Aggressive treatment should not be withheld just because a patient is older.

## REFERENCES

1. United States Census Bureau. An aging nation: the older population in the United States population estimates and projections estimates and projections. Available at: https://www.census.gov/prod/2014pubs/p25-1140.pdf. Accessed May 20, 2016.

2. Mueller PS, Hook CC, Fleming KC. Ethical issues in geriatrics: a guide for clinicians. Mayo Clin Proc 2004;79:554–62.

3. Banks SE, Lewis MC. Trauma in the elderly consideration for anesthetic management. Anesthesiolo Clin 2012;11:1.

4. Angus D, Wax RS. Epidemiology of sepsis: an update. Crit Care Med 2001; 29(Suppl 7):109–16.
5. Brown BA. The history of advance directives. A literature review. J Gerontol Nurs 2003;29(9):4–14.
6. Emanuel LL, Barry MJ, Stoeckle JD, et al. Advance directives for medical care–a case for greater use. N Engl J Med 1991;324(13):889–95.
7. Gasner MR. Financial penalties for failing to honor patient wishes to refuse treatment. St Louis Univ Public Law Rev 1992;11:499–520.
8. Schears RM. Emergency physicians' role in end-of-life care. Emerg Med Clin North Am 1999;17:539–59.
9. Nonbeneficial Emergency Medical Interventions (Policy Statement) (Dallas TX: American College of Emergency Physicians. 1998. Available at: https://www. acep.org/Clinical—Practice-Management/Non-Beneficial-(-Futile-)-Emergency-Medical-Interventions/. Accessed May 20, 2016.
10. Scalea T, Simon H, Duncan AO, et al. Geriatric blunt multiple trauma: improved survival with early invasive monitoring. J Trauma 1990;30(2):129–36.
11. Orlando Hung MM, editor. Management of the difficult and failed airway. 1st edition. New York: McGraw-Hill; 2008.
12. Alvis B, Hughes C. Physiology considerations in geriatric patients. Anesthesiolo Clin 2015;33:447–56.
13. Sprung J, Gajic O, Warner DO. Review article: age related alterations in respiratory function—anesthetic considerations. Can J Anaesth 2006;53:1244–57.
14. Law AJ, Broemling N, Cooper RM, et al. The difficult airway with recommendations for management. Part 2: the anticipated difficult airway. Can J Anaesth 2013;60:1119–38.
15. Sharma G, Goodwin J. Effect of aging on respiratory system physiology and immunology. Clin Interv Aging 2006;1(3):253–60.
16. Ma OJ, Edwards JH, Meldon SW. Geriatric trauma in Tintinalli's. Emerg Med 1992;1684–6.
17. Ram FSF, Picot J, Lightowler J, et al. Non-invasive positive pressure ventilation for treatment of respiratory failure due to exacerbations of chronic obstructive pulmonary disease. Cochrane Database Syst Rev 2004;(1):CD004104.
18. Gray A, Goodacre S, Newby DE, et al. Noninvasive ventilation in acute cardiogenic pulmonary edema. N Engl J Med 2008;359:142–51.
19. Serpa Neto A, Cardoso S, Manetta J, et al. Association between use of lung-protective ventilation with lower tidal volumes and clinical outcomes among patients without acute respiratory distress syndrome: a meta-analysis. JAMA 2012;308(16):1651–9.
20. Deakin CD, Low JL. Accuracy of the advanced trauma life support guidelines for predicting systolic blood pressure using carotid, femoral, and radial pulses: observational study. BMJ 2000;321(7262):673–4.
21. Martin GS. Sepsis, severe sepsis and septic shock: changes in incidence, pathogens and outcomes. Expert Rev Anti Infect Ther 2012;10:701–6.
22. Rivers E, Nguyen B, Havstad S, et al. Early goal-directed therapy in the treatment of severe sepsis and septic shock. N Engl J Med 2001;345(19):1368–77.
23. Hefferan DS, Thakkar RK, Monaghan SF, et al. Normal presenting vital signs are unreliable in geriatric blunt trauma victims. J Trauma 2010;69:813.
24. Wahba WM. Influence of aging on lung function: clinical significance of changes from age twenty. Anesth Analg 1983;62:764–76.
25. McFadden JP, Price RC, Eastwood HD, et al. Raised respiratory rate in elderly patients: a valuable physical sig. Br Med J (Clin Res Ed) 1982;284(6316):626–7.

26. Jones AE, Tayal VS, Sullivan DM, et al. Randomized, controlled trial of immediate versus delayed goal-directed ultrasound to identify the cause of nontraumatic hypotension in emergency department patients. Crit Care Med 2004;32(8):1703–8.
27. Schriger DL, Baraff LJ. Capillary refill: is it a useful predictor of hypovolemic status? Ann Emerg Med 1991;20:601–5.
28. Baraff LJ, Schriger DL. Orthostatic vital signs: variation with age, specificity, and sensitivity in detecting a 450-mL blood loss. Am J Emerg Med 1992;10(2):99–103.
29. Gregory P, Victorino MD, Wisner DH. Does tachycardia correlate with hypotension after trauma? [Retrospective study]. J Am Coll Surg 2003;196:679–84.
30. Kartal M, Eray O, Rinnert S, et al. EtCO$_2$: a predictive tool for excluding metabolic disturbances in nonintubated patients. Am J Emerg Med 2011;29(1):65–9.
31. Feinfeld DA, Bargouthi H, Niaz Q, et al. Massive and disproportionate elevation of blood urea nitrogen in acute azotemia. Int Urol Nephrol 2002;34(1):143–5.
32. Tiruvoipati R, Ong K, Gangopadhyay H, et al. Hypothermia predicts mortality in critically ill elderly patients with sepsis. BMC Geriatr 2010;10:70.
33. Andersen LW, Mackenhauer J, Roberts JC, et al. Etiology and therapeutic approach to elevated lactate. Mayo Clin Proc 2013;88(10):1127–40.
34. Nagdev A, Merchant R, Tirado-Gonzalez A, et al. Emergency department bedside ultrasonographic measurement of the caval index for noninvasive determination of low central venous pressure. Ann Emerg Med 2010;55(3):290–5.
35. Perera P, Mailhot T, Riley D, et al. The RUSH exam: rapid ultrasound in SHock in the evaluation of the critically ill. Emerg Med Clin North Am 2010;28(1):29–56.
36. Milzman D, Rothenhaus T. Resuscitation of the geriatric patient. Emerg Med Clin North Am 1996;14:233–44.
37. Sehgal V, Bajwa SJ, Sehgal R, et al. Clinical conundrums in management of sepsis in the elderly. J Trans Intern Med 2015;3.3:106–12.
38. Kaukonen KM, Bailey M, Pilcher D, et al. Systemic inflammatory response syndrome criteria in defining severe sepsis. N Engl J Med 2015;372:1629–38.
39. Kaplan RC, Heckbert SR, Koepsell TD, et al. Risk factors for hospitalized gastrointestinal bleeding among older persons. J Am Geriatr Soc 2001;49:126–33.
40. Farrell JJ, Friedman LS. Gastrointestinal bleeding in older people. Gastroenterol Clin North Am 2000;29:1–36.
41. Mina AA, Bair HA, Howells GA, et al. Complications of preinjury warfarin use in the trauma patient. J Trauma 2003;54:842–7.
42. Calland JF, Ingraham AM, Martin N, et al. Evaluation and management of geriatric trauma: an eastern association for the surgery of trauma practice management guideline. J Trauma 2012;73:S348.
43. Demeyere R, Gillardin S, Arnout J, et al. Comparison of fresh frozen plasma and prothrombin complex concentrate for the reversal of oral anticoagulants in patients undergoing cardiopulmonary bypass surgery: a randomized study. Vox Sang 2010;99(3):251–60.
44. Wahl WL, Miller JT. Geriatric Trauma and Critical Care. Vol. 1. Pharmacology. New York: Springer; 2014. p. 345–52.
45. Marlu R, Hodaj E. Effect of non-specific reversal agents on anticoagulant activity of dabigatran and rivaroxaban: a randomised crossover ex vivo study in healthy volunteers. Thromb Haemost 2012;108(2):217.
46. Celso B, Tepas J, Langland-Orban B, et al. A systematic review and meta-analysis comparing outcome of severely injured patients treated in trauma centers following the establishment of trauma systems. J Trauma Acute Care Surg 2006;60.2:371–8.

47. Demetriades D, Sava J, Alo K, et al. Old age as criterion for trauma team activation. J Trauma 2001;51(4):754–6.
48. Brown CV, Shoemaker WC, Wo CC, et al. Is noninvasive hemodynamic monitoring appropriate for the elderly critically injured patient. J Trauma 2005;58: 102–7.
49. Callaway DW, Shapiro NI, Donnino MW, et al. Serum lactate and base deficit as predictors of mortality in normotensive elderly blunt trauma patients. J Trauma 2009;66:1040–4.
50. Husain FA, Martin MJ, Mullenix PS, et al. Serum lactate and base deficits as predictors of mortality and morbidity. Am J Surg 2003;185:485.
51. Mitra B, Olaussen A, Cameron PA, et al. Massive blood transfusions post trauma in the elderly compared to younger patients. Injury 2014;45(9):1296–300.
52. Clancy K, Velopulos C, Bilaniuk JW, et al. Screening for blunt cardiac injury: an Eastern Association for the Surgery of Trauma practice management guideline. J Trauma Acute Care Surg 2012;73:S301.
53. Sybrandy K, Cramer M, Burgersdijk C. Diagnosing cardiac contusion: old wisdom and new insights. Heart 2003;89(5):485–9.
54. Tresch DD, Heudebert G, Kutty K, et al. Cardiopulmonary resuscitation in elderly patients hospitalized in the 1990s: a favorable outcome. J Am Geriatr Soc 1994; 42:137–41.
55. Kaye P, O'Sullivan I. The role of magnesium in the emergency department. Emerg Med J 2002;19(4):288–91.
56. Valente S, Lazzeri C, Vecchio S, et al. Predictors of in-hospital mortality after percutaneous coronary intervention for cardiogenic shock. Int J Cardiol 2007; 114:176–82.
57. Antman EM, Anbe DT, Armstrong PW, et al. ACC/AHA guidelines for the management of patients with ST-elevation myocardial infarction: executive summary: a report of the American College of Cardiology/American Heart Association Task Force on Practice Guidelines (Writing Committee to Revise the 1999 Guidelines for the Management of Patients With Acute Myocardial Infarction). Circulation 2004;110:588–636.
58. Prasad A, Lennon RJ, Rihal CS, et al. Outcomes of elderly patients with cardiogenic shock treated with early percutaneous revascularization. Am Heart J 2004;147(6):1066–70.
59. Seder DB, Patel N, McPherson J, et al. Geriatric experience following cardiac arrest at six interventional cardiology centers in the United States 2006-2011: interplay of age, do-not-resuscitate order, and outcomes. Crit Care Med 2014; 42(2):289–95.
60. Gisselbrecht M, Diehl JL, Meyer G, et al. Clinical presentation and results of thrombolytic therapy in older patients with massive pulmonary embolism: a comparison with non-elderly patients. J Am Geriatr Soc 1996;44(2):189–93.

# Pharmacology in the Geriatric Patient

Katherine Louise Welker, MD, MPH*, Mark B. Mycyk, MD

## KEYWORDS

• Aging • Polypharmacy • Drug interactions • Clinical pharmacists

## KEY POINTS

• A higher proportion of emergency department patients in the future will be elderly.
• Elderly patients are often prescribed multiple medications by multiple providers.
• Physiological changes with age affect drug metabolism, effect, and elimination.
• Drug interactions are more common in elderly patients.
• Involving clinical pharmacists can avoid drug interactions and polypharmacy and improve resource utilization.

## INTRODUCTION

According to the US Census Bureau, from 2012 to 2050 the country will undergo significant aging, wherein the proportion of persons 65 years and older (defined as "older population") will increase at a more rapid pace when compared with persons younger than 65 years.[1] As technology and medical knowledge continue to advance, a growing number of older patients will survive previously fatal disease processes, such as cancer, organ transplantation, and human immunodeficiency virus. With this increasing proportion of elderly patients, pharmacologic issues specific to this patient population will become more pronounced because the need for long-term medication use naturally increases with age.[2]

Although medication reconciliation in the emergency department (ED) has been an important national priority, understanding the long-term implications of polypharmacy has only recently received close attention. Recent data confirm that most front-line caregivers have seen increased rates of prescription drug use in all ages in the United States (from 51% in 1999–2000 to 59% in 2011–2012).[2] More importantly, during that same time period, the rate of polypharmacy in the United States doubled. Simply being on a few medications when younger significantly increases the risk for polypharmacy as one gets older.[3] The problem of polypharmacy is not limited to the United States,

Disclosure: None.
Department of Emergency Medicine, Cook County Health and Hospitals System, 1900 West Polk Street, Chicago, IL 60612, USA
* Corresponding author.
E-mail address: welkerk@gmail.com

Emerg Med Clin N Am 34 (2016) 469–481
http://dx.doi.org/10.1016/j.emc.2016.04.003                    emed.theclinics.com
0733-8627/16/$ – see front matter © 2016 Elsevier Inc. All rights reserved.

but instead is a worldwide phenomenon. A Scottish study demonstrated patients prescribed 10 or more medications increased from 4.9% in 1995 to 17.2% in 2010.[4] Polypharmacy in the elderly is particularly important to recognize in the ED, because with increased age comes increased frailty, defined here as decreased function of multiple organs, loss of physiologic reserve, and increased risk of disease and death.

The definition of "polypharmacy" is controversial. It is important to note 2 themes, which emerge consistently in most published works on polypharmacy: either too many medications are prescribed or medications that are not clinically indicated are administered.[5,6] Definitions of polypharmacy in published studies have ranged from 2 to 10 prescribed medications. Today, the most commonly accepted definition for polypharmacy by scholars in current use of 5 or more prescribed, because that number of medications is associated with poor mental and physical health.[7]

## PATIENT EVALUATION OVERVIEW

Complications from medications should always be considered in the emergency physician's (EP) differential diagnosis.[8] Medication overuse and polypharmacy are only recently being recognized as common reasons for ED evaluation, and the number of cases will continue to increase as the population gets older and more patients are prescribed even more medications.[9,10] Acute delirium from pharmaceuticals is underrecognized in the elderly, but should always be considered near the top of the EP's differential.[11,12] Elderly patients undergoing ED evaluation for altered mental status or delirium could result from using too many medications prescribed by too many providers, in cases when a patient unintentionally uses leftover medications that were discontinued but not discarded appropriately, in cases when they have visual impairment and take the wrong medications, in cases where they use another household member's medications in place of their own, or in cases when they use their pets' medications in addition to their own.[13]

Evaluation of medications should happen at multiple stages during the ED visit, from the time of initial triage until final disposition to home or to the inpatient unit. It should include currently prescribed medications, previously prescribed medications, access to other household member or pet medications, and use of over-the-counter and herbal products. Despite progress in medical reconciliation with the introduction of electronic health records (EHRs), problems specific to this system include incomplete lists of medications when a patient uses multiple health facilities, historical medications not being verified, but remaining in the record, and lack of universal participation in medical record sharing, such as Care Everywhere. Use of an ED pharmacist can assist with rapid assessment of drug-drug interactions, adverse drug reactions, and other pharmaceutical-related complications. In fact, American College of Emergency Physicians recognizes the importance of ED pharmacists in a 2015 position statement: "The emergency medicine pharmacist should serve as a well-integrated member of the ED multidisciplinary team who actively participates in patient care decisions, including resuscitations, transitions of care, and medication reconciliation to optimize pharmacotherapy for ED patients."[14]

Several tools have been developed to prevent polypharmacy or inappropriate medication use in elderly patients; although not ED-friendly, it is important for the EP to be familiar with them. The Beers Criteria, developed by geriatricians and updated in 2015, are the most widely used tool for evaluating appropriate medication use in the elderly.[15] The utility of the Beers Criteria is easily illustrated by comparing the difference between nursing home residents cared for by family medicine physicians and those cared for by geriatricians. Those cared for by family medicine physicians had

13.15 greater odds of being prescribed 9 or more medications and 6.25 greater odds of being prescribed one or more potentially inappropriate medications when compared with those cared for by geriatricians.[16] This difference is especially notable, because patients cared for by geriatricians were found to be more complex with more comorbid diseases.

Beers Criteria include identifying medications in the following categories:

- Potentially inappropriate medication use in older adults
- Potentially inappropriate medication use in older adults due to drug-disease or drug-syndrome interactions that may exacerbate the disease or syndrome
- Potentially inappropriate medications to be used with caution in older adults
- Potentially clinically important non-anti-infective drug-drug interactions that should be avoided in older adults
- Non-anti-infective medications that should be avoided or have their dosage reduced with varying levels of kidney function in older adults

Beers Criteria identify patients at higher risk for admission to the hospital from medication complications.[17]

The Norwegian General Practice (NORGEP) Criteria are another tool for optimizing prescriptions in the elderly. The NORGEP criteria include 2 tables of 21 single medications and 15 drug combinations considered by an expert panel to be potentially pharmacologically inappropriate for patients aged 70 years or older.[18]

Both the Beers and the NORGEP Criteria are extensive, and although partially subjective, are grounded in common sense and include references for their decisions in their respective populations. Although the Beers Criteria focus mostly on potentially inappropriate *individual* medications, the NORGEP criteria also identify potentially dangerous *combinations* of drugs. They are the most commonly used tools by specialists outside of the ED.

Tools more adaptable to the ED environment include checklist or judgment-based tools. The Screening Tool of Older Person's Prescriptions and Screening Tool to Alert doctors to Right Treatment are examples of checklist tools created to identify medications that should be avoided and "irrational prescribing omissions."[19] An example of a judgment-based tool is the Medication Appropriateness Index.[20] These tools were developed by literature review and expert opinion but have not been externally validated.

Another tool to assess inappropriate medication use is the Anticholinergic Risk Scale. The elderly are especially sensitive to anticholinergics because of decreased function of multiple organs and loss of physiologic reserve.[21] This tool is well recognized by clinical pharmacists and is useful in the ED setting where anticholinergics such as diphenhydramine are commonly used.[22]

Another potentially useful tool for identifying at-risk patients greater than 80 years old is the 80+ score.[19] Using this internally validated tool, patients at high risk for either death or rehospitalization within 1 year are those with current or history of malignancy, current pulmonary disease, impaired renal function, residing in nursing home, or current prescription for opioid or proton pump inhibitor (PPI).[19]

Based on these definitions, criteria, and risk factors for pharmaceutical complications in the elderly, the EP should always perform the steps in **Box 1** when caring for an elderly patient.

Performing each of these steps takes time, especially in geriatric patients; thus, assistance from clinical pharmacists and other midlevel providers is important to optimize the outcome in these patients.[14]

---

**Box 1**
**Thoughtful emergency care for elderly patients**

1. Confirm age, sex

2. Obtain complete medical history

3. Obtain social history

4. Confirm correct, up-to-date medication list
   a. Compare medications with those listed in a tool (of your choice) for potentially inappropriate medication
   b. Review list for historical or unnecessary medications
   c. Review list of other accessible pharmaceuticals in the household

5. Consult with the primary medical provider and pharmacist for appropriate medication reconciliation at time of disposition

6. Check baseline laboratory test results before starting new medications

---

## PHARMACOLOGIC TREATMENT OPTIONS
### Pathophysiology

#### Cardiovascular system
Elderly people commonly have cardiovascular disease and require medications for this organ system. They also have decreased cardiac reserve, increased blood pressure partly due to decreased compliance of vasculature, loss of overall myocardial contractility, decreased vagal tone, and left ventricular hypertrophy.[23] All of these factors are exacerbated by decreased sensitivity to catecholamines, causing elderly patients to be even more sensitive to cardiac medications.[24]

#### Respiratory system
Aging is associated with loss of lung elasticity, decreased functional volume (despite maintained total lung capacity), and decreased vital capacity, all leading to decreased ability to eliminate carbon dioxide. Furthermore, forced exhaled volume decreases, increasing work of breathing.

#### Gastrointestinal system
In addition to decreased blood flow and liver function that changes with age, as countless medications are metabolized by the liver, this is an important consideration in medication administration and reconciliation. Decreased liver mass and decreased hepatic and biliary uptake and transport also contribute to deranged drug metabolism.[25]

#### Urinary system
Kidneys are the primary means for elimination of medications. With age, renal mass decreases and glomerular filtration rate decreases for several reasons even in healthy elderly patients. Some of these reasons include decreased blood flow, decreased vascular compliance, and decreased muscle mass. Decreased muscle mass complicates evaluation of kidney function, because serum creatinine may not be as reliable a measure of kidney dysfunction, because it reflects muscle mass, which is frequently decreased in elderly people.

#### Endocrine system
Elderly patients experience decreased insulin secretion and insulin sensitivity, leading to decreased glucose tolerance; also complicating diabetes management in this population is deranged glucose counterregulation.[26]

## Nervous system

Like total body mass and liver mass, brain weight decreases by 20% with age, with a comparable loss of neurons.[26] Although the synapse itself is not thought to change, elderly patients are more sensitive to analgesic and sedative/hypnotic medications, requiring dose reductions even before metabolism is considered. Possible explanations are alterations in calcium homeostasis or even structural changes in receptors, such as γ-aminobutyric acid A and N-methyl-D-aspartate receptors (**Box 2**).[27]

## Pharmacology

There are a countless number of medications available in the United States, and more are being developed and marketed daily. Elderly patients frequently require multiple medications because they often have multiple medical problems. However, before prescribing medications to the elderly, it is important to consider how metabolism and elimination are different when compared with younger patients. Dosing a medication based on age alone is not sufficient, because organ function reserve and specific, age-related derangements in metabolism of drugs as well as normal compensatory mechanisms vary by individual. Relying on the expertise of a clinical pharmacist can help optimize dosing.

Generally speaking, total body water decreases with age because of decreased muscle mass and increased body fat,[27] affecting the distribution of hydrophilic and lipophilic drugs and resulting in higher peak drug concentrations after a bolus or rapid infusion.[28] It also leads to larger volume of distribution and can affect the duration of

---

**Box 2**
**Pathophysiologic changes in elderly**

*Cardiovascular*
- Decreased cardiac reserve
- Decreased cardiac contractility
- Decreased sensitivity to catecholamines

*Respiratory*
- Decreased elasticity
- Decreased functional volume and vital capacity

*Gastrointestinal*
- Decreased hepatic mass
- Decreased hepatic blood flow

*Urinary*
- Decreased renal mass
- Decreased glomerular filtration rate

*Endocrine*
- Decreased insulin secretion
- Decreased glucose tolerance

*Nervous system*
- Decreased brain mass
- Loss of neurons

---

drug effect. Furthermore, albumin concentration decreases, increasing the free fraction of protein-bound xenobiotics.[28]

Aging can affect absorption of xenobiotics, with decreased secretion of gastric acid, decreased rate of gastric emptying, reduced splanchnic blood flow, and decreased mucosal surface area, decreasing overall absorption.[24] Conversely, drugs that undergo first-pass metabolism will be more bioavailable in elderly patients, because hepatic flow and mucosal absorption are decreased. Decreased hepatic function and metabolism are some of the most pertinent factors in geriatric pharmacology.

Decreased renal function is the most recognized factor in geriatric pharmacology. Renal function is reduced in the elderly because of a reduced number of functioning nephrons, decreased glomerular filtration rate, and decreased renal blood flow (**Box 3**).[24]

Each medication class is associated with specific potential adverse effects because of the metabolic changes that occur in the elderly.

*Cardiac medications*
Cardiac medications are among the most commonly used medications in the elderly. With decreased elimination leading to increased half-life, as well as reliance of these medications on existing physiologic responses, cardiac medications are easily the most dangerous class of medications in the elderly.[29] There are many classes of drugs, but those most pertinent for the EP are antiarrhythmics, antihypertensives, anticoagulants, and ionotropic agents. When considering treating an elderly patient with these medications, a common mantra, "start low, go slow," is key. The elderly will have decreased responses to some medications, creating possibly delayed effects, with a prolonged half-life. For instance, medications requiring endogenous compensatory homeostatic response for effect, such as some cardiovascular medications, will not produce the intended effect as quickly as with a younger patient because of the blunted physiologic response that naturally comes with age. Further complicating matters is that cardiovascular medications have been shown to be associated with acute kidney injury, and that each addition of a cardiac medication increases an elderly patient's risk of having acute kidney injury by 30% when evaluating prehospitalization and posthospitalization serum creatinine measurements in patients taking any number of cardiovascular medications, such as antihypertensives, antiarrhythmics, diuretics, lipid-lowering agents, and antiplatelet agents.[30]

*Analgesics*
Analgesics can be divided into opioids and nonopioids, although tramadol does not fit wholly into either category because of its multiple effects at various receptors. Opioids are medications such as fentanyl, hydromorphone, morphine, oxycodone, hydrocodone, and codeine. There has been a dramatic increase in prescribing of opioids in US EDs, but responsible opioid prescribing requires all providers to remember that

---

**Box 3**
**Metabolic factors affecting pharmacologic therapy in elderly**

- Decreased total body water
- Increased body fat
- Decreased albumin concentration
- Decreased gastric acid secretion
- Decreased mucosal surface area

elderly patients are more sensitive to these medications and usually require decreased dosing[31]; this should prompt all prescribers, especially EPs, to have a lower threshold for offering naloxone rescue prescriptions to elderly patients or their family members when opioids are being prescribed.

Nonopioid analgesics are led by nonsteroidal anti-inflammatory drugs (NSAIDs). As a class, NSAIDs have proven to be safe and effective analgesics that are normally well tolerated as long as used at the right doses. In 2000, 70% of elderly people reported taking NSAIDs at least once weekly.[32] NSAIDs work by inhibiting prostaglandins, which, mediated by cyclo-oxygenase 1 and 2, are partially responsible for renal hemostasis. Renal dysfunction, therefore, a relatively common finding in elderly patients, is a contraindication to therapy with NSAIDs. Care must be taken when prescribing these medications in all elderly patients, specifically because of decreased renal blood flow.[32] Gastrointestinal (GI) irritation is also more common with NSAIDs in the elderly, so antacids and other GI medications are often subsequently prescribed to relieve GI symptoms. However, according to the 80+ risk stratification score, caution is warranted in prescribing PPIs because use of PPIs in the elderly is associated with an increased risk of rehospitalization or death. Possible explanations include the association of PPI use with an increased risk of *Clostridium difficile* and pneumonia; PPIs are also a proxy for gastric disease.[19]

*Neurologic medications*
Elderly patients are at an increased risk of delirium, falls, and other adverse effects from polypharmacy with neurologically acting medications, such as antiepileptics or anti-Parkinson agents. Dopamine content and the number of dopamine receptors decrease with age, leading to more frequent and severe extrapyramidal symptoms when elderly patients are treated with dopamine blocking agents such as neuroleptics and metoclopramide. Similarly, decreased acetylcholine increases the risk of anticholinergic effects of neuroleptics and tricyclic antidepressants.[22] Long-term antipsychotic therapy in geriatrics is associated with a high incidence of tardive dyskinesia, akathisia, and parkinsonian symptoms. Other nonneurologic adverse effects with antiepileptics, such as cardiac and hematologic adverse effects, are also seen more commonly in elderly patients.[26]

More obvious adverse effects seen in the ED from psychotropic medications are injuries from falls. Administration of psychotropics, benzodiazepines, neuroleptics, and other tranquilizers in older people were associated with increased odds of falling when compared with those not on these medications.[33,34]

*Endocrine medications*
Elderly patients experience decreased glucose tolerance and counterregulation. This fact is important for the EP to be aware of, because this causes increased risk of hypoglycemia from sulfonylureas even when dosing does not change. Hypoglycemia is also a complication from unintentional overdoses of insulin when administered at an incorrect dose because of poor eyesight. Other physiologic changes that occur with age result in increased risk of adverse effects from treatment with metformin, such as lactic acidosis (**Table 1**).

## NONPHARMACOLOGIC TREATMENT OPTIONS

Medical management of many disease processes has improved over the years. Too often in the ED, pharmacologic treatment is relied on. Especially in the geriatric population, avoiding polypharmacy or potential new drug-drug interactions whenever possible should be a priority. Rather than adding another medication to their current

**Table 1**
**Common overdoses in elderly patients**

| Medication Class | Medication | Symptoms | Treatment |
|---|---|---|---|
| Cardiovascular | Digoxin | Altered mental status, weakness, bradycardia, arrhythmias | Digoxin immune Fab |
| | β-Blockers | Hypotension, bradycardia | Glucagon |
| | Calcium channel blockers | Hypotension, bradycardia[a] | High-dose insulin |
| Analgesics | Opioids | Respiratory depression, sedation | Naloxone |
| | Acetaminophen | Nausea, vomiting, abdominal pain | N-acetylcysteine |
| | Aspirin | Altered mental status, tinnitus | Urinary alkalinization, hemodialysis |
| Neurologic | Benzodiazepines | Sedation, respiratory depression | Supportive care |
| | Antidepressants | Altered mental status, arrhythmias | Supportive care |
| | Antipsychotics | Altered mental status, gait changes, arrhythmias | Supportive care |
| Endocrine | Insulin | Altered mental status, sedation | Glucose |
| | Sulfonylureas | Altered mental status, sedation | Octreotide |

[a] Reflex tachycardia can sometimes predominate.

list of medications, the EP should first ask if other nonpharmacologic treatment options are available (**Table 2**).

One of the more problematic complaints in elderly patients is pain, whether it is acute pain from a new injury or chronic pain from worsening arthritis. The elderly are more sensitive to many analgesics, and the risks of commonly prescribed medications in these patient needs to be remembered. Worsening renal dysfunction can occur with chronic NSAID therapy; increased risk of falls, sedation, constipation, and respiratory depression can occur from prescribed opioids. Therefore, it is important to recommend other therapies for pain. These other pain therapies include referring patients to their primary doctors for physical and occupational therapy and recommending massage and heat therapy for muscular pain or stiffness. Chronic pain from a variety of physical ailments is particularly challenging in the elderly, because chronic pain is not driven by nociception, but is related to emotional and psychosocial factors, making it even more amenable to nonpharmacologic treatment, such as addressing social stressors, substance abuse, mental health, and providing social support.[35] These management regimens are infrequently recommended in the ED, but are important tools for providers to avoid polypharmacy.

For disease processes such as diabetes and hypertension, patient education surrounding lifestyle and diet modifications, such as exercise plans and pill boxes, can

**Table 2**
**Nonpharmacologic treatment options**

| Indication | Therapy |
|---|---|
| Pain | Massage, heat, physical therapy, exercise, social support, coping tools |
| Hypertension | Diet modification, exercise |
| Diabetes | Diet and lifestyle modification, exercise, nutritionist involvement |
| Psychiatric disorder | Behavioral therapy, counseling, social support |

⊃e used in conjunction with, or in lieu of, pharmacologic therapy. Multidisciplinary ᴛeams, including physicians, nurses, pharmacists, and dieticians, have been shown ᴛo be effective in treating hypertension.[36]

Nonpharmacologic interventions as simple as discontinuing possibly inappropriate ᴍedications have been shown to improve outcome. In one study of 75 elderly patients ⊃resenting to a hospital with behavioral disturbances, anxiety, depression, or delu- realsions and/or hallucinations, those patients in whom benzodiazepines (prescribed as ᴅcheduled treatment) were discontinued had shorter length of stay and decreased ᴨeed for antidepressant or antipsychotic use.[37]

Too often, EPs are focused on inappropriate medications instead of inappropriate ᴛreatment: this includes inappropriate doses, duration of therapy, and drug ᴎnteractions.[38]

The EP should prevent polypharmacy whenever possible. Many tools are now avail-aᴘble to help the EP's medical decision making, including electronic prescribing ser-vices, a national prescription database, educational initiatives, institution (or primary ᴄcare physician) imposed limits on the number of prescribers, as well as other medica-tion reviews and prescription checklists.

## COMBINATION THERAPIES

Drug interactions are common. In one study of 1600 elderly, nonhospitalized patients, 46% had at least one potentially significant adverse drug combination prescribed, and 10% were severe.[20] Theoretically, in an elderly patient prescribed 5 or more medica-tions, probability of drug-drug interaction is 50%; this becomes 100% at 7 or more prescriptions.[39] These interactions are often overlooked by prescribing providers, especially in an ED setting. EHR warnings can aid with avoiding potential deleterious interactions, but cannot catch all possible drug interactions because of alarm fatigue or overrides built in to these EHR systems.[40] Dangerous interactions include drug-drug, drug-disease, drug-food, drug-alcohol, drug-supplements, and drug-nutritional status interactions. Drug-drug interactions are the only potential interac-tions an electronic medical record can reliably find, but this system is not perfect, because it assumes that a patient's medications are all accurately recorded, that the patient is getting all of their medications only from one source, and that the pro-vider is not experiencing alarm fatigue or automatically overriding the alarm.[41]

Identifying possible drug interactions without the aid of a tool, such as the NORGEP criteria or the EHR, requires better understanding of possible causes of drug interac-tions. Cause is either pharmacokinetic (eg, hepatic cytochrome P450 isoenzymes) or pharmacodynamic, which depends on the pharmacologic activity of both drugs.[20] Some drug interactions are less common but important to note. Examples include metoclopramide for gastric dysmotility in a patient with Parkinson disease (PD), causing worsening PD (drug-disease); methadone in a patient concomitantly drinking grapefruit juice, leading to decreased metabolism of methadone and possible toxicity (drug-food); benzodiazepines in a patient who regularly uses alcohol, causing increased falls (drug-alcohol); ginkgo as a supplement in someone taking aspirin daily, leading to deranged platelet function and bleeding (drug-supplement); phenytoin for seizures in a patient with low albumin, causing increased free phenytoin and toxicity (drug-nutritional status).[20]

Another important factor contributing to drug interactions in the elderly is multiple prescribers. In one study, 37% of medications taken by elderly patients were not prescribed by their primary doctor, and 6% of medications were not on their physi-cian's list.[42]

---

**Box 4**
**Recommendations for emergency department pharmacology in geriatrics**

- Detailed medical reconciliation with assistance of clinical pharmacist
- Obtain social history with assistance of social worker
  - Living situation
  - Activities of daily living
  - Eyesight, medication administration
  - Substance abuse
  - Psychiatric complaints

- Nonpharmacologic treatment whenever possible
  - Consider physiologic changes when prescribing medication

- Discussion with primary doctor

- Speak with family regarding accountability with assistance of ancillary staff

---

## TREATMENT RESISTANCE/COMPLICATIONS

Geriatric patients are at increased risk for adverse drug effects and drug interactions and also at risk for treatment complications particular to comorbid conditions. For example, with age come dementia and other cognitive decline, causing confusion and the real possibility of mistakenly taking incorrect medications or multiple doses of one medication, either by redundant prescriptions from multiple prescribers or simply by forgetting they already took a daily dose. Age is also associated with worsening eyesight, making reading medication labels difficult.

An EP can be proactive when evaluating elderly patients with negative ED workups for weakness and dizziness by recommending these patients keep a medication diary with doses and time of administration to avoid medication complications that may have resulted in that ED visit.

## INTEGRATING CLINICAL PHARMACISTS IN THE EMERGENCY DEPARTMENT

EPs have been shown to neglect potential adverse drug interactions in elderly people. In 2001, a study demonstrated 4% of elderly people presented to an ED for an adverse drug-related event not recognized by the EP, and that number has been estimated to be much higher today.[8,43]

Involvement of clinical pharmacists in patient care teams has been shown to reduce all visits to hospitals, EDs, and drug-related readmissions by 16%, 47%, and 80%, respectively.[44] Pharmacist involvement in patient care of elderly people was also shown to decrease the number of potentially inappropriate medications prescribed and the number of necessary medications omitted,[45] translating not only to better patient care but also to decreased costs.

Another study showed decreased inappropriate prescribing scores (24% vs 6%) and decreased adverse drug events (30% vs 40%) in elderly Veterans Affairs patients who met with a clinical pharmacist during all outpatient clinic visits to evaluate their medication regimens and to make recommendations.[46] These results were sustained at 12 months and provide more support for the involvement of clinical pharmacists in the ED to reduce polypharmacy in older patients (**Box 4**).

## SUMMARY

Elderly patients are an increasing proportion of patients emergency providers will be encountering. They often have decreased renal and hepatic function, leading to decreased metabolism and elimination. Polypharmacy, and consequently, drug-drug interactions are important risk factors to consider in elderly patients. Multiple tools are available to help with appropriate medication use in the elderly and reduce pharmaceutical complications. Using clinical pharmacists as integrated members of the multidisciplinary ED team is one of the most useful strategies to improve outcomes of the elderly.

## REFERENCES

1. Ortman JM, Velkoff VA, Hogan H. An aging nation: the older population in the United States. US Department of Commerce Economics and Statistics Administration. Washington, DC: US Census Bureau; 2014. p. 25–1140.
2. Kantor ED, Rehm CD, Haas JS, et al. Trends in prescription drug use among adults in the United States from 1999-2012. JAMA 2015;314(17):1818–31.
3. Veehof L, Stewart R, Haaijer-Ruskamp F, et al. The development of polypharmacy. A longitudinal study. Fam Pract 2000;17(3):261–7.
4. Guthrie B, Makubate B, Hernandez-Santiago V, et al. The rising tide of polypharmacy and drug-drug interactions: population database analysis 1995-2010. BMC Med 2015;13:74.
5. Moen J, Antonov K, Larsson CA, et al. Factors associated with multiple medication use in different age groups. Ann Pharmacother 2009;43(12):1978–85.
6. Linjakumpu T, Hartikainen S, Klaukka T, et al. Use of medications and polypharmacy are increasing among the elderly. J Clin Epidemiol 2002;55(8):809–17.
7. Gnjidic D, Hilmer SN, Blyth FM, et al. Polypharmacy cutoff and outcomes: five or more medicines were used to identify community-dwelling older men at risk of different adverse outcomes. J Clin Epidemiol 2012;65(9):989–95.
8. Hohl CM, Zed PJ, Brubacjer JR, et al. Do emergency physicians attribute drug-related emergency department visits to medication-related problems? Ann Emerg Med 2010;55(6):493–502.
9. Samaras N, Chevalley T, Samaras D, et al. Older patients in the emergency department: a review. Ann Emerg Med 2010;56(3):261–9.
10. Scheffer AC, van Hensbroek PB, van Dijk N, et al. Risk factors associated with visiting or not visiting the accident & emergency department after a fall. BMC Health Serv Res 2013;13:286.
11. Rosen T, Connors S, Clark S, et al. Assessment and management of delirium in older adults in the emergency department: literature review to inform development of a novel clinical protocol. Adv Emerg Nurs J 2015;37(3):183–96.
12. Hein C, Forgues A, Piau A, et al. Impact of polypharmacy on occurrence of delirium in elderly emergency patients. J Am Med Dir Assoc 2014;15(11):850.e11–5.
13. Ashawesh K, Abdulqawi R, Ahmad S. Self-poisoning with pet medications. South Med J 2007;100(8):854.
14. American College of Emergency Physicians. Clinical pharmacist services in the ED. Ann Emerg Med 2015;66(4):444–5.
15. American Geriatrics Society 2015 Beers Criteria Update Expert Panel. American Geriatrics Society 2015 updated Beers Criteria for potentially inappropriate medication use in older adults. J Am Geriatr Soc 2015;63(11):2227–46.
16. Monroe T, Carter M, Parish A. A case study using the Beers List Criteria to compare prescribing by family practitioners and geriatric specialists in a rural nursing home. Geriatr Nurs 2011;32(5):350–6.

17. Lu WH, Wen YW, Chen LK, et al. Effect of polypharmacy, potentially inappropriate medications and anticholinergic burden on clinical outcomes: a retrospective cohort study. CMAJ 2015;187(4):E130–7.

18. Rognstad S, Brekke M, Fetveit A, et al. The Norwegian General Practice (NORGEP) criteria for assessing potentially inappropriate prescriptions to elderly patients. A modified Delphi study. Scand J Prim Health Care 2009;27(3):153–9.

19. Alassaad A, Melhus H, Hammarlund-Udenaes M, et al. A tool for prediction of risk of rehospitalisation and mortality in the hospitalized elderly: secondary analysis of clinical trial data. BMJ Open 2015;5:e007259.

20. Mallet L, Spinewine A, Huang A. The challenge of managing drug interactions in elderly people. Lancet 2007;370(9582):185–91.

21. Naja M, Zmudka J, Hannat S, et al. In geriatric patients, delirium symptoms are related to the anticholinergic burden. Geriatr Gerontol Int 2016;16:424–31.

22. Rudolph JL, Salow MJ, Angelini MC, et al. The anticholinergic risk scale and anticholinergic adverse effects in older persons. Arch Intern Med 2008;168(5):508–13.

23. Tonner PH, Kampen J, Scholz J. Pathophysiological changes in the elderly. Best Pract Res Clin Anaesthesiol 2003;17(2):163–77.

24. Aronow WS, Frishman WH, Cheng-Lai A. Cardiovascular drug therapy in the elderly. Cardiol Rev 2007;15(4):195–215.

25. Herrlinger C, Klotz U. Drug metabolism and drug interactions in the elderly. Best Pract Res Clin Gastroenterol 2001;15(6):897–918.

26. Turnheim K. Drug therapy in the elderly. Exp Gerontol 2004;39(11–12):1731–8.

27. Vuyk J. Pharmacodynamics in the elderly. Best Pract Res Clin Anaesthesiol 2003;17(2):207–18.

28. Sadean MR, Glass PS. Pharmacokinetics in the elderly. Best Pract Res Clin Anaesthesiol 2003;17(2):191–205.

29. Mowry JB, Spyker DA, Brooks DE, et al. 2014 Annual Report of the American Association of Poison Control Centers' National Poison Data System (NPDS): 32nd Annual Report. Clin Toxicol (Phila) 2015;53(10):962–1147.

30. Chao CT, Tsai HB, Wu CY, et al. Cumulative cardiovascular polypharmacy is associated with the risk of acute kidney injury in elderly patients. Medicine (Baltimore) 2015;94(31):e1251.

31. Mazer-Amirshahi M, Mullins PM, Rasooly I, et al. Rising opioid prescribing in adult U.S. emergency department visits: 2001-2010. Acad Emerg Med 2014;21(3):236–43.

32. Stillman MJ, Stillman MT. Choosing nonselective NSAIDs and selective COX-2 inhibitors in the elderly. A clinical use pathway. Geriatrics 2007;62(2):26–34.

33. Marra EM, Mazer-Amirshahi M, Brooks G, et al. Benzodiazepine prescribing in older adults in U.S. ambulatory clinics and emergency departments (2001-10). J Am Geriatr Soc 2015;63(10):2074–81.

34. Bloch F, Thibaud M, Dugué B, et al. Psychotropic drugs and falls in elderly people: updated literature review and meta-analysis. J Aging Health 2011;23(2):329–46.

35. Ballantyne JC, Sullivan MD. Intensity of chronic pain–the wrong metric. N Engl J Med 2015;373(22):2098–9.

36. Corrigan MV, Pallaki M. General principles of hypertension management in the elderly. Clin Geriatr Med 2009;25(2):207–12.

37. Yokoi Y, Misal M, Oh E, et al. Benzodiazepine discontinuation and patient outcome in a chronic geriatric medical/psychiatric unit: a retrospective chart review. Geriatr Gerontol Int 2014;14(2):388–94.

38. Laroche ML, Charmes JP, Bouthier F, et al. Inappropriate medications in the elderly. Clin Pharmacol Ther 2009;85(1):94–7.
39. Delafuente JC. Understanding and preventing drug interactions in elderly patients. Crit Rev Oncol Hematol 2003;48(2):133–43.
40. Grizzle AJ, Mahmood MH, Ko Y, et al. Reasons provided by prescribers when overriding drug-drug interaction alerts. Am J Manag Care 2007;13(10):573–8.
41. Weingart SN, Toth M, Sands DZ, et al. Physicians' decisions to override computerized drug alerts in primary care. Arch Intern Med 2003;163(21):2625–31.
42. Frank C, Godwin M, Verma S, et al. What drugs are our frail elderly patients taking? Do drugs they take or fail to take put them at increased risk of interactions and inappropriate medication use? Can Fam Physician 2001;47:1198–204.
43. Hohl CM, Dankoff J, Colacone A, et al. Polypharmacy, adverse drug-related events, and potential adverse drug interactions in elderly patients presenting to an emergency department. Ann Emerg Med 2001;38(6):666–71.
44. Gillespie U, Alassaad A, Henrohn D, et al. A comprehensive pharmacist intervention to reduce morbidity in patients 80 years or older: a randomized controlled trial. Arch Intern Med 2009;169(9):894–900.
45. Gillespie U, Alassaad A, Hammarlund-Udenaes M, et al. Effects of pharmacists' interventions on appropriateness of prescribing and evaluation of the instruments' (MAI, STOPP and STARTs') ability to predict hospitalization—analyses from a randomized controlled trial. PLoS One 2013;8(5):e62401.
46. Hanlon JT, Weinberger M, Samsa GP, et al. A randomized, controlled trial of a clinical pharmacist intervention to improve inappropriate prescribing in elderly outpatients with polypharmacy. Am J Med 1996;100(4):428–37.

# Geriatric Trauma

Casper Reske-Nielsen, MD, Ron Medzon, MD*

## KEYWORDS

- Geriatric • Trauma • Injury • Aging

## KEY POINTS

- Geriatric trauma patients are a unique patient population that require individualized assessment and management strategies.
- Changing pathophysiology, increased incidence of co-morbid conditions and the use of anticoagulant medications augment the impact of trauma on geriatric patients.
- Geriatric trauma patients are often under triaged therefore a high index of suspicion should be maintained even with seemingly minor mechanisms of injury.
- Use of diagnostic imaging for geriatric trauma patients should be liberal.
- Elderly patients are at high risk of suicide and elder abuse.

## INTRODUCTION
### Epidemiology

The population of the United States is aging. By 2030, 1 in 5 Americans will be more than 65 years old[1] and by 2050 the US Census projects that the population aged 65 years and older will double and approximately 4.5% of the population will be more than 85 years old.[2] By then, geriatric patients will make up nearly 40% of all trauma cases.[3,4]

In 2013, unintentional injury was the eighth leading of cause of death in older patients, with an estimated 25,000 deaths related to falls.[5,6] Trauma in the elderly costs more than $34 billion in direct medical costs every year. Approximately three-quarters of the total cost is related to traumatic brain injury (TBI) and injuries to the lower extremities, including hip fractures.[7]

The care of elderly patients with trauma presents a unique set of challenges. The combination of comorbid health conditions, prescribed medications, and frailty makes older patients more vulnerable to trauma and subsequent complications, including infections, pneumonia, venous thromboembolism, and multisystem organ failure. Patients more than 65 years old are twice as likely to die compared with younger patients with similar injury severity score (ISS). Studies suggest that mortality increases 6.8% for every year beyond age 65 years.[3,8] Elderly patients are undertriaged a significant

Disclosures: None.
Emergency Medicine, Boston Medical Center, Dowling 1 South, One Boston Medical Center Place, Boston, MA 02118, USA
* Corresponding author.
E-mail address: ron.medzon@bmc.org

Emerg Med Clin N Am 34 (2016) 483–500
http://dx.doi.org/10.1016/j.emc.2016.04.004
0733-8627/16/$ – see front matter © 2016 Elsevier Inc. All rights reserved.

portion of the time and are more likely to go to a nontrauma center than younger patients. Some investigators recommend that any patient older than 70 years with trauma should be transported to a trauma center regardless of their ISS.[9,10]

This article addresses the challenge of treating geriatric patients with trauma, covering differences in anatomy and physiology, triage and resuscitations, as well as addressing some special situations, including elder abuse, hypothermia, and suicide.

## Geriatric Anatomy and Physiology

### Frailty, aging versus underlying disease

Mortality after trauma increases with age starting as young as age 40 years. However, chronologic age has been shown to be less important in trauma than frailty. Frailty is defined as impairment of function of multiple systems that increases the susceptibility to physical and physiologic stressors.[3,11,12] Frailty is difficult to quantify because the index tools are long and time consuming, making them difficult to apply in the emergency setting.[13] The patient's baseline functional status and evidence of sarcopenia may be considered as surrogate markers of frailty.[13,14] Frail patients with poor functional status and multiple comorbidities have been shown to have worse outcomes after trauma.

### Head and neck

Traumatic brain injury is the leading cause of traumatic death in the elderly. The brain shrinks over time. Decreasing brain volume causes stretching of the bridging veins, making them more susceptible to tearing and bleeding from the shearing forces in trauma. Furthermore, cerebrovascular autoregulation and free radical clearance are impaired with age. This process contributes not only to worsened brain injury in elderly patients but to delayed recovery.[15,16] Elderly patients are at higher risk for significant intracranial injury in minor head trauma, and have more frequent bleeds and severity of intracranial hemorrhage (ICH) if taking oral anticoagulants.[17] It is important to note that the clinical decision rules designed to decrease the use of computed tomography (CT) brain in minor head trauma have all found increased significant findings on CT in the elderly. Therefore, although use of clinical judgment is advised in determining the need for advanced imaging in patients more than 65 years old with minor head injury, the clinician should have a lower threshold to CT scan this population.[18,19] Similarly, the same 2 research groups (NEXUS II c-spine, Canadian c-spine) excluded elderly patients from the low-risk decision rule because of higher numbers of significant fractures in this population.

### Chest

**Cardiac** Heart disease may affect outcomes of elderly patients with trauma through diminished cardiac reserve. Patients with a history of congestive heart failure (CHF), and those on warfarin or β-blockers are at higher risk of poor outcomes after trauma.[20] The exact mechanism and physiology related to worse outcomes in CHF are not entirely understood and there are no clear studies to guide management in the emergency department (ED). It is thought that the decreased reserve is related to structural and functional cardiac changes of aging and a significant reduction in cardiac function during the stress of trauma. During evaluation of a geriatric patient with trauma the clinician should take a careful cardiac and medication history. Hypotension and poor cardiac output should be treated with inotropic and chronotropic medications and consideration of balloon pump in severe cases.[20]

### Pulmonary

The mechanics and physiology of breathing change with age. Increased chest wall rigidity and worsening kyphosis may lead to impaired respiratory muscle insertion mechanics, and when combined with a weakened diaphragm may lead to decreased fraction of expiratory volume in 1 second ($FEV_1$) and decreased vital capacity, and result in an overall decline in respiratory reserve. Elderly patients may also have impaired lung function from underlying chronic obstructive pulmonary disease, pulmonary fibrosis, or scarring. In addition, geriatric patients have a significantly lower diffusing lung capacity for carbon monoxide and decreased partial pressure of oxygen, which may explain why elderly patients can have significant hypoxia at lower levels of physiologic stress.[21] These physiologic changes make elderly patients with trauma more susceptible to the stresses of acute blood loss and fluid resuscitation.

## Abdomen

**Liver and kidney disease** Underlying hepatic and renal disease increase mortality in elderly patients with trauma. The ability of the liver to withstand injury decreases with age. Furthermore, cirrhosis increases the susceptibility to ischemic and reperfusion injuries, the risk of hemorrhage, posttrauma complications, and mortality.[21–23] Elderly patients also have an increased incidence of kidney disease, which may make them more prone to contrast-induced nephropathy (CIN). A recent study suggests that elderly patients with normal renal function are not at increased risk of CIN compared with younger patients.[24] Oral hypoglycemic medications can increase the risk of CIN, so it is important to communicate this with radiology, and to limit scans with contrast to only those patients who need them, to avoid iatrogenic harm. A normal creatinine level should be interpreted with caution because elderly patients typically have less muscle mass, therefore a high normal value may reflect acute kidney injury or chronic kidney disease.[24]

## Musculoskeletal

**Fragile bones and skin** Aging causes several normal, expected physiologic changes to both muscle and bone, making elderly patients more susceptible to fractures even in the absence of underlying osteoporosis. Aging bones are more easily fractured with minor trauma, for example in falls from standing. In addition to weaker bones, older patients have a loss of muscle mass leading to sarcopenia and a subsequently decreased structural support that protects younger patients from injury. Sarcopenia is one of the defining characteristics of frailty syndrome. As frailty increases, functional decline ensues, leading to decreased mobility and deconditioning, increasing the risk of falls and injury.[25] Given the increased risk of musculoskeletal injury in the elderly, emergency practitioners should have a low threshold of obtaining plain film radiographs. Elderly patients who are unable to walk after the trauma should undergo advanced imaging such as CT or magnetic resonance imaging (MRI) of the hip even with normal radiographs. MRI is more sensitive (100%) for occult fracture but is more time consuming and expensive than CT (sensitivity 87%).[25,26] One group of investigators suggests an algorithm whereby patients with an initial negative radiograph who have a low-energy mechanism of injury and who are at high risk of osteoporosis undergo MRI, and others CT.[27]

## History: Mechanism of Injury

### Falls

Falls are the leading cause of trauma-related mortality in the elderly, and the rate of falls is increasing.[13,28,29] Women and white people are most likely to fall.[30] Elderly patients who fall are more likely to have complications of the fall, be hospitalized, be admitted to the intensive care unit, and subsequently require discharge to a rehabilitation facility.

**Mortality** The overall estimated mortality of geriatric patients after a fall is between 7% and 11%. The strongest predictor of mortality is increased age. After admission for a fall, the 1-year mortality may be as high as 33% with a 44% 1-year readmission rate.[31] The elderly are less likely to die as a direct result of the trauma and more likely to die from secondary complications. TBI is the most common direct cause of death from a fall.[32]

**Risk factors**   Frailty and comorbidities both contribute to the risk of falling and the subsequent sequelae of the fall. The pattern of injury is directly related to the mechanism. Falls are often multifactorial and the exact cause may be difficult to determine in an emergency setting. Recent data suggest that many of these patients may have occult infections.[33]

   Several risk factors for falling have been identified in the geriatric population (**Table 1**). Older women who have had previous falls are at the greatest risk. Slowed gait and reaction times contribute significantly to falling. Decreased reaction times may be a consequence of underlying arthritis, poor vision, sarcopenia, and chronic medication use.[13] Pain is also a contributor because it may lead to a fear of moving. Muscles weaken from subsequent lack of physical activity, leading to poor gait and deconditioning. Interventions to treat pain, to address the fear of falling, and improve balance have been shown to decrease the risk of falls.[34,35]

## Motor vehicle collision

As the population ages there will be more elderly drivers on the roads, with an estimated 25 million drivers more than 65 years of age in 2012. Geriatric patients account for 17% of all motor vehicle crash (MVC) fatalities. Emergency providers can expect to see an increased proportion of geriatric patients with MVC injuries in the future. Older patients are more likely to have more severe injuries at low speeds and to be admitted to the intensive care unit. Elderly patients have a higher mortality, higher cost of admission, and higher use of acute rehabilitation facilities after an MVC.[36]

## Pedestrian struck

Geriatric patients account for approximately 20% to 30% of pedestrians struck and killed by a motor vehicle. Decreased visual acuity, decreased reaction times, difficulty ambulating, as well as impaired judgment place elderly patients at increased risk of

**Table 1**
**Contributing factors to injuries in elderly patients**

| Acute Illness | Chronic Medical Condition | Environmental Factors | Other |
|---|---|---|---|
| New medications | Osteoporosis | Rugs | Older age |
| Syncope | Osteoarthritis | Lighting | Female |
| Dysrhythmias | CVA | Stairs | Alcohol or drug use |
| CVA, TIA | Ischemic heart disease | Bathtubs/showers | Elder abuse |
| Acute MI | Anemia | Footwear | |
| Seizure | DM | Walking aids | |
| Acute renal failure | HTN | Uneven ground | |
| Infection | Gait or balance impairment | Weather | |
| Hypoglycemia | Visual impairment | Pets | |
| AAA | Depression | | |
| Dehydration | Polypharmacy | | |
| Acute fractures | Parkinson disease | | |
| | Dementia | | |

*Abbreviations:* AAA, abdominal aortic aneurysm; CVA, cerebral vascular accident; DM, diabetes mellitus; HTN, hypertension; MI, myocardial infarct; TIA, transient ischemic attack.
*Adapted from* Aschkenasy MT, Rothenhaus TC. Trauma and falls in the elderly. Emerg Med Clin North Am 2006;24(2):413–32, vii; and Sattin RW. Falls among older persons a public health perspective. Annu Rev Public Health 1992;13:489–508.

being struck. Older pedestrians who are hit by a motor vehicle have a higher incidence of severe injury and death compared with younger patients.[37,38] Even with seemingly minor or low-energy trauma, the concern for serious injury in elderly patients should remain high.

## Clinical work-up

### Triage/history of present illness

Geriatric patients with trauma are frequently undertriaged both in the prehospital setting and in the ED.[39] The literature suggests that general prehospital triage guidelines are ineffective for elderly patients.[40] Vital signs are unreliable, underlying comorbidities are common, and the use of certain medications can mask the physiologic effect of the trauma or exacerbate it.[41] Certain risk factors may lead to undertriage, including age, female sex, and a fall-related injury.[13,39] Even minor deviations from normal vital signs are associated with increased risk of death. Tachycardia with a heart rate (HR) greater than 150 beats per minute has a mortality of almost 70%. Similarly, a systolic blood pressure of 90 mm Hg carries a 30% mortality.[39,42] Even small changes in mental status are associated with worse outcomes. Studies have shown that geriatric patients with a Glasgow Coma Scale (GCS) score of 14 have a significantly higher mortality and are at higher risk of TBI compared with younger adults with a similar GCS.[43] Elderly patients with trauma should be evaluated at a trauma center and the trauma team should be activated.

**Injury severity score: is it helpful in trauma evaluation?** Use of the ISS in the triage of patients with trauma is common practice. However, its applicability to elderly patients is debated. One recent study supporting its use found that an ISS greater than or equal to 16 and specific injury patterns including brain, chest, and abdomen-pelvic injuries were associated with a significant increase in mortality.[44,45]

It is important to take a careful history. Certain underlying disease processes affect clinical outcomes in geriatric patients with multitrauma.[3,8] These factors include heart disease, peripheral arterial disease, coagulation disorders, malignancy, and obesity.[46]

### Past medical history/medications and reversal agents

When taking the history, it is important to note any conditions that uniquely affect the geriatric patient with trauma, as discussed earlier. Elderly patients are more likely to be on medications before their traumatic event. β-Blocker and oral anticoagulant (OAC) use is common. The effect of β-blockers on posttraumatic vital signs is debated. Isolated use of β-blockers did not have a significant impact on presenting vital signs.[40] Only patients taking a combination of β-blockers, calcium channel blockers, and an angiotensin-converting enzyme inhibitor or angiotensin receptor binding agent showed blunted hemodynamic responses to trauma.[31] Medications, especially antihypertensive and sedatives, may also increase the risk of trauma, in particular falls.[31]

Oral anticoagulants are prescribed for many common conditions, including atrial fibrillation, stroke, thromboembolism, and medical management after cardiac revascularization. Some of the more common agents include warfarin, rivaroxaban, apixaban, dabigatran, clopidogrel, and aspirin.

Patients who are on OACs and subsequently fall are at greater risk of dying. This effect is most significant in patients with head injuries, specifically skull fractures, and intracranial hemorrhage, but is also higher with intra-abdominal injuries. The mortality effect of OAC seems to increase after age 70 years and is irrespective of different anticoagulation regimens.[21,22,47–51] Rapid reversal of international normalized ratio (INR) in the setting of intracranial hemorrhage slows progression of the bleed and reduces mortality.[50]

## Initial Management and Resuscitation

Initial resuscitation should begin with the basic ABCs (airway, breathing, and circulation) as in any other patient with trauma. All patients with trauma should be placed on supplemental oxygen to preoxygenate and for apneic oxygenation should endotracheal intubation become necessary.[52,53] Geriatric patients have higher Mallampati scores, increased rigidity of the cervical spine, and poor dentition, all of which may make bag-valve mask ventilation and endotracheal intubation more difficult.[51] The changes associated with decreased functional reserve also affect intubation and mechanical ventilation.

Furthermore, elderly patients may have associated degenerative changes of the jaw, which may make complete opening of the mouth difficult. If intubation is required, rapid sequence intubation medicine doses should be adjusted accordingly. Benzodiazepines and etomidate doses should be reduced by approximately 20% to 40% to decrease their hemodynamic effects.[54] Ketamine is less prone to cause hypotension but should be used with caution in patients with ischemic heart disease because it increases myocardial oxygen demand.[55] The secondary survey should include complete exposure of the patient and a quick neurologic assessment. The physical examination may be more difficult in elderly patients. The abdominal examination may be unreliable because of decreased pain perception, cognitive decline, or minimization by the patient.[56] In addition, their neurologic examination may be complicated by underlying dementia or altered mental status from other causes, such as infection or stroke, all of which may have contributed to the trauma. Given the risk of serious injury even with minor trauma, liberal use of CT scans is appropriate.

### Do-not-resuscitate status

During resuscitation it is critical to consider the patient's wishes for resuscitation and to consider the possible futility of such resuscitation. Certain risk factors, including hypotension, age greater than 74 years, and higher ISS, increase the risk of mortality but do not predict mortality. Age alone should never be used as the sole determinant to limit care.[4,57–59]

### Assessment for unstable patients

Aggressive resuscitation should be initiated in all unstable patients with trauma. Any patient with persistently abnormal vital signs or not responsive to resuscitation efforts, and those who have evidence of active hemorrhage or deteriorating mental status, should be considered unstable.[60] Seemingly stable geriatric patients with trauma should be thoroughly evaluated for occult life-threatening injuries. A serum lactate level and base deficit should be obtained in elderly patients with trauma because abnormal values indicate impending deterioration and may predict mortality.[61] However, normal values should not be used to rule out serious injury. Serum lactate and base deficit values should be repeated after initial resuscitation and persistently abnormal values should be investigated further.[61]

Hemodynamic monitoring in elderly patients with trauma is essential. Slight changes in HR or blood pressure may signify unrecognized injury and should be investigated thoroughly. Pulmonary artery catheters are being replaced by ultrasonography and echocardiography and studies suggest that the data obtained from the two are comparable.[62]

### Reversing anticoagulants

Current guidelines recommend assessing the patient's INR and activated partial thromboplastin time and prothrombin time and to rapidly reverse any abnormalities.

Patients with increased INR may benefit from rapid reversal with fresh frozen plasma (FFP) or prothrombin complex concentrate (PCC) and vitamin K. Note that normalization of prothrombin time or INR does not always correlate with decreased bleeding. The newer anticoagulants rivaroxaban, apixaban, and dabigatran do not yet have proven reversal agents; however, some studies show that PCC may be a reasonable choice with life-threatening bleeding (**Table 2**). Clinical trials are ongoing, investigating the use of monoclonal antibody reversal agents for rivaroxaban, apixaban, and edoxaban. The US Food and Drug Administration recently approved idarucizumab, a monoclonal antibody, for reversal of dabigatran in the setting of an acute bleed.[63,64]

## Diagnostic Evaluation

A thorough assessment of whether the fall was related to a neurologic or cardiac event is critical, because these events are more common in the elderly population. The circumstances surrounding the event, including environmental factors, substance use, acute or chronic medical conditions, medications, and the patient's baseline functional capacity, should also be investigated.[65] Determining the events surrounding the fall or trauma can help with appropriate disposition of the patient. An electrocardiogram should be done in all elderly patients with trauma. Use of plain films or CT scanning of the affected organ systems should be liberal. Long bones easily fracture, and older patients do not always experience the same degree of pain relative to the severity of injury. A FAST (focused abdominal sonogram in trauma) examination is quick and easy to perform and should be performed in elderly patients with trauma with moderate to severe mechanisms.

Geriatric patients presenting with multisystem trauma pose a challenge to emergency department providers. As discussed previously, vital signs can be unreliable in the elderly and their physiologic response to trauma variable. In addition, plain film radiography has poor sensitivity to rule out serious injury in patients with multisystem trauma. When there is evidence of multisystem involvement patients should undergo whole-body CT.[66] Other studies advocate the use of whole-body CT in older patients with any concerning mechanism of injury or for those who present with a distracting injury.[67]

## Head injuries

TBI is the fifth leading cause of death in the elderly. Most TBIs are the result of low-impact, ground-level falls.[68] Geriatric patients are more likely to have more severe TBI and longer hospital admissions, and are more likely to die or be discharged to subacute nursing facilities after a head injury compared with young patients.[69,70] Patients more than 65 years of age with a GCS of 14 have a mortality of 10% to 15% compared with zero in younger patients with similar injuries.[71] The American College of Emergency Physicians recommends that any patients more than 60 years of age with

| Table 2 | | |
|---|---|---|
| **Anticoagulants and potential reversal agents** | | |
| **Anticoagulant Agent** | **Mechanism of Action** | **Potential Reversal Agent** |
| Warfarin | Vitamin K antagonist | FFP, PCC, vitamin K |
| Dabigatran | Direct thrombin inhibitor | Idarucizumab |
| Rivaroxaban | Factor Xa direct inhibitor | PCC |
| Apixaban | Factor Xa direct inhibitor | PCC |
| Enoxaparin | Anti–thrombin III inhibitor | Protamine (partially effective) |
| Heparin | Anti–thrombin III inhibitor | Protamine |

loss of consciousness or who are taking an OAC should undergo brain CT. Repeat brain CT imaging should be reserved for patients with a change in their neurologic examination or for those patients who cannot reliably be examined.[72] Patients taking oral anticoagulants who have minor trauma and a normal brain CT may be safely discharged because the risk of delayed bleeding is low. Patients should be given clear return instructions.[73]

### Cervical spine injuries

Similarly, elderly patients are at a significantly increased risk of cervical spine fractures after trauma. Those more than 64 years of age are twice as likely to have a cervical spine injury (CSI) as younger patients with the same mechanism of injury. As a result of degenerative changes and stiffening of the lower cervical spine, elderly patients are at increased risk of higher CSI (C1–C2 and odontoid fractures vs C6–C7).[74] Application of the NEXUS decision rule in the elderly has been debated because geriatric patients may have CSI with lower-energy mechanisms of injury. Several studies have shown that the NEXUS criteria perform equally well in patients more than 80 years old.[72,75] However, given the increased risk of CSI, it is recommend that a CT scan of the cervical spine be obtained if CT brain is ordered because the risk of concomitant CSI is about 5%.[74–76] Other studies recommend obtaining a CT scan of the cervical spine and brain regardless of the mechanism of injury in geriatric patients.[77]

### Thoracic trauma

Blunt thoracic trauma in the elderly carries a significant risk of complications and mortality, even with isolated rib fractures.[78] The most common complications include pneumonia and pulmonary contusions. The risk of mortality after a rib fracture is proportional to the number of fractured ribs and may serve as a predictor of trauma severity and risk of complications.[70,79] Age more than 85 years; initial systolic blood pressure of less than 90 mm Hg; 3 or more unilateral rib fractures; or the presence of pneumothorax, hemothorax, or pulmonary contusion may be helpful in predicting adverse outcomes. However, these factors have not yet been validated.[80] Elderly patients with 1 or more rib fractures are at high risk of mortality and therefore their dispositions should be carefully considered.

### Musculoskeletal injuries

Musculoskeletal injuries are very common in elderly patients with trauma. The risk of osteoporosis and subsequent fractures increases with age. There are an estimated 9 million osteoporotic fractures worldwide every year, which significantly contribute to the disease burden in North America. Women are more affected than men.[81,82] Overall, fractures in the geriatric patient population carry a high morbidity and mortality and negatively affect both the patients' quality of life and society at large.[83]

Forearm fractures are the most common, with hip fractures a close second. It is estimated that hip fractures will cost approximately $35 billion per year by 2040. Geriatric patients have a high mortality following a hip fracture and it is crucial that these patients receive expedient and coordinated care. Early surgical repair, balanced with medical optimization, has been shown to significantly reduce mortality and improve the chance of patients returning to their previous functional states.[84] Evidence suggests that a dedicated orthogeriatric team approach to these patients may improve outcomes, including mortality and quality of life.[83]

Pelvic fractures are less common but carry an equally high mortality of 5% to 20%.[85,86] Elderly patients who sustain pelvic fractures are at increased risk of hemorrhage, are more likely to require angiography and blood transfusion, and are 4 times more likely to die as a result of their injuries. Lateral compression fractures are more common and more likely to require blood transfusion in geriatric patients compared with younger patients.[87] A recent large study of stable pelvic fractures found that age more than 70 years, higher ISS, altered mental status, and need for blood transfusion predicted mortality.[68] Older patients with pelvic fractures should be aggressively resuscitated because evidence suggests that, even with appropriate treatment and disposition, mortality remains high.[85,86]

## Disposition

Whether discharging or admitting patients, a multidisciplinary approach should be taken, including involvement of social work, case management, family members, and the patient's primary care physician, because the risk of recurrent falls is very high in the elderly population. Certain factors increase the risk of a recurrent fall, including a history of multiple falls, impaired mobility, poor strength, and depression.[87] Questions to consider before discharge include whether the patient has an acute underlying condition that requires further evaluation.

Can the patient walk?

Can the patient perform activities of daily living?

What resources does the patient have at home?

Is a home safety visit available?

Given the increased risk of complications and mortality, most elderly patients with trauma need admission to the hospital. As previously discussed, a significant percentage of elderly patients with trauma are under-triaged. Evidence supports direct triage or transfer to a dedicated trauma center if there is concern for any significant injury and certainly if there is a need for surgical, neurosurgical, orthopedic, or burn care. Transfer should not be delayed to obtain diagnostic tests that will not change management or disposition. Studies have shown that delays in care may affect morbidity and mortality in elderly patients with trauma, but the data are limited and more research is needed to definitively conclude that transfer improves outcomes.[88,89]

Patients with a minor isolated injuries may be considered for discharge. Careful consideration should be given to patients with isolated rib fractures. If there is suspicion for potential respiratory compromise, then the patient should be admitted. If there is concern for concomitant injury, such as head injury, or if the patient's history is limited by underlying medical conditions such as dementia or altered mental status, strong consideration should be given to admission.

Several factors must be considered before discharge, including the cause of the injury, what the patient's home environment is like, who will be able assist the patient at home if needed, and who will follow-up with the patient. If a definitive discharge plan is not available, admission should be considered to facilitate coordination of an appropriate care plan.

## Summary

As the population ages, geriatric patients with trauma will become increasingly common. The elderly are a unique population with respect to mechanism of injury, injury types, morbidity, and mortality. They are vulnerable to minor traumatic events and are likely to have poor outcomes if not treated aggressively. Physicians, particularly emergency medicine physicians and trauma surgeons, should be familiar with the physiologic changes of aging, understand the potential underlying comorbidities that affect elderly patients with trauma, and maintain a high index of suspicion for serious injury for all geriatric patients with trauma. Use of laboratory and diagnostic imaging studies should be liberal and physicians should have a low threshold to admit elderly patients with trauma.

## Special Situations

### Elder abuse

Elder mistreatment or abuse can be defined as intentional actions that cause harm or create a serious risk of harm, whether or not this is intended, to a vulnerable elder by that person's caregiver or a person who holds a trusted position in relation to that elder.[90] It can also include the failure of the caregiver to satisfy the elder's basic needs or to protect that person from harm. Looking at the magnitude of the problem epidemiologically, nearly 25% of elders have reported psychological abuse. Six percent of older people in one study reported abuse within 1 month of the survey, and 5.6% of couples reported violence in their relationship. Five percent of family members surveyed in this study reported physical abuse toward care recipients with dementia in a 1-year period.[91] When studying the literature on recorded rates of elder abuse using objective data, the incidence is significantly lower.[92,93] There is a disconnect between what is being reported objectively and what elders are saying when asked directly. It is thought that a reasonably safe estimate is that 1 in 4 elders have experienced some form of abuse.[90] ED clinicians should recognize the importance of asking about potential abuse of elderly patients, because they often report it if asked.

**Risk factors and types of elder abuse** Elder abuse is an international problem. Studies from Asia to Europe and North America all report similar data. The greatest risk factor seems to be dementia.[94] Close to half of individuals in America more than 85 years of age have some degree of dementia, and up to one-half of these people are abused. Institutionalized individuals with disabilities, especially women older than 65 years, are at significant risk for interpersonal violence (>50%) compared with only 21% of women without disabilities.[92,95] Other types of elder abuse, in order of prevalence include, financial (5.2%), emotional and both physical neglect and to a lesser extent sexual abuse (0.6%).

**Health impact of elder abuse** Elders who experience even modest abuse have a 300% increase in risk of death compared with nonabused cohorts. They have a higher incidence of bone and joint disorders, digestive problems, depression, anxiety, chronic pain, increased blood pressure, and heart problems. There is an estimated cost of $5.3 billion in extra health care costs related to elders who are abused.

### Management principles

**Assessment** Assessing elderly patients should include screening questions about how they are managing their daily lives and whether they are experiencing any psychosocial stress, because this is a risk factor for abuse. Ideally the patient should be interviewed alone. Caregivers should also be interviewed and assessed for caregiver fatigue because this can increase the risk of elder abuse. The patient's cognitive and functional status must be assessed, and, if there is any concern by the clinician, this should be addressed before discharging the patient.

**Capacity** In the end, it is up to the ED clinician to make a judgment on the elder's capacity for decision making if there is suspicion or evidence for abuse. Taking into account the risk factors mentioned earlier, there should be a low threshold for admitting these patients to get them out of their potentially abusive environments, at least until a preliminary investigation into the patient's safety is conducted.

**Disposition** If it is determined that the patient is experiencing abuse, then discharge must be coordinated with home health services. If available, a social worker should be involved, the case should be reported, and a safe environment should be established.

If there is family, they must be appropriately involved in this process. Also, clinicians must try to facilitate treatment of the underlying disease. For example, a physical limitation by a treatable illness may be causing anxiety and depression, causing the patient to act out, and putting the patient at risk for abuse by caregivers.

**Reporting** All states mandate reporting for probable suspicion of elder abuse. Adult Protective Services should be notified. They will take a report and start an investigation. If the patient is in a licensed long-term care facility, there are long-term care ambassadors who are charged with investigating alleged incidents.

### Hypothermia in the elderly

There are almost no studies on hypothermia in the elderly. By definition, hypothermia is the unintentional decline of body temperature less than 35°C. The coordinated systems of thermoregulation fail because the compensatory responses to minimize heat loss through radiation, conduction, convection, respiration, and evaporation are limited. A longitudinal study of patients noted an age-related decline in thermoregulatory capacity in aging individuals. Those people at risk for hypothermia seem to have a low resting peripheral blood flow, and a nonconstrictive pattern of vasomotor response to cold. They also have a higher incidence of orthostatic hypotension.[96-98]

**Survival of elderly with hypothermia** Case reports of elderly patients surviving after presenting with core temperatures of less than 28°C (82°Fahrenheit) have been published. Slow active external rewarming was used in those cases. The prognosis worsens as the patient's age increases. Passive and active rewarming techniques are equally effective in elderly patients and have similar associated risks.[99-101]

**Rewarming techniques** Passive rewarming techniques include warm blankets, heating lamps, and warm humidified air. Patients may also be actively warmed using intravenous warm saline or cavitary lavage. Thoracic lavage has been studied in populations including patients as old as 72 years with a mean core temperature of 24°C (75° Fahrenheit).[102] Most patients had no blood pressure or pulse on presentation. Patients either had tube thoracostomies done with lavage with warm fluids, or thoracotomies with lavage of warm fluids. They achieved a rewarming rate of 2.95°C per hour. Median time to sinus rhythm was 120 minutes, and median hospital stay was 2 weeks. Twenty-eight percent died, 85% had pulmonary complications, and 80% of survivors had full neurologic recovery. More recently cardiopulmonary bypass (CPB) and extracorporeal membrane oxygenation (ECMO) have been used for active rewarming of severely hypothermic patients.[103-105] CPB confers significantly lower mortality (15.5% vs 53.3% standard rewarming in one study), with up to 60% surviving and 80% returning to previous level of activity. Patients receiving ECMO faired even better than the CPB patients. No data exist for survival and neurologic outcome in the elderly. At this time, patients who present with accidental hypothermia and in cardiac arrest should be strongly considered for CPB or ECMO, and it seems that thoracotomy or tube thoracostomy with warm irrigation before this confers a superior survival rate.

### Suicide in the elderly

In North America, approximately 12 per 100,000 individuals 65 years of age and older die by suicide. Older white men have the highest prevalence. Risk factors include suicidal ideation (SI), suicidal behavior, mental illness, medical illness, losses and poor social supports, functional impairment, and low resiliency.[106,107] In a Danish study, in addition to these risk factors, the investigators found homelessness, alcohol and drug dependence, institutionalized elders, prisoners, and other socially excluded people to be at highest risk for suicide. In the Netherlands, one-third of all suicides are attempted by elderly individuals.[108,109]

**Observations in suicidal elders** Certain patterns can be seen in elders with SI that lead to peers, loved ones, and caregivers missing the signs. Because many elderly patients survive major life events, loved ones assume that they are capable of coping with another major life event, loss, or threatening condition. Depression may not be apparent to relatives or may be assumed to be a natural reaction to aging. If relatives suspect depression, they may not know that it is a treatable condition or where they can seek treatment. The elderly depressed may not share their depressed thoughts about death and dying. They may not admit SI. Their symptoms of depression may be confused with the normal aging process.[110–112]

**Detecting suicidal ideation in the elderly** Few older adults who die by suicide have seen a mental health specialist in the days or weeks leading up their deaths. However, many have seen some type of caregiver, typically a primary care doctor. As a result, ED clinicians have an obligation to screen for depression and SI in elders, because its detection could save the patient's life. Any of the patient's social supports, friends, family, spouses, and institutional caregivers should be asked about the patient's mood and any concern for depression and SI. Studies have shown a strong correlation between the social support/proxy having a strong impression of the patient's risk for depression and active SI and actual depression and SI in the patient.[110] It is therefore incumbent on ED clinicians to ask the supports whether they think the patient is depressed or suicidal, and, if so, to act aggressively on that information.

**Treatment** Treatment is multifactorial. If acute severe clinical depression is detected in an elderly ED patient, then it is appropriate for the clinician to request an emergent psychiatric consult in the ED. Improving the severity of a patient's active illness may improve the patient's mood and depression, so clearly finding and treating all ongoing medical issues is important. Ensuring strong social supports and close psychiatric follow-up if necessary is also indicated. In addition, a Danish study found that limiting access for violent means of death reduced the rate of suicide. Be certain that the family removes any firearms in the household and takes away heavily sedating medications such as barbiturates, benzodiazepines, and narcotics. They should also limit contact with carbon monoxide gas produced by domestic gas furnaces or automobiles. The job of ED clinicians is primarily one of detection, prevention, and referral. Detection only occurs when the questions are asked, and the questions are only asked if the clinician is aware of the magnitude of the problem and keeps this in mind when evaluating the elderly patient.

## REFERENCES

1. Colby SJ, Ortman J. Projections of the size and composition of the U.S. population: 2014 to 2060. 2015. Available at: https://www.census.gov/content/dam/Census/library/publications/2015/demo/p25-1143.pdf. Accessed May 9, 2016.
2. Ortman JM, Velkoff VA, Hogan H. An aging nation: the older population in the United States. U.S. Department of Commerce Economics and Statistics Administration U.S. CENSUS BUREAU; 2014. Available at: census.gov. Accessed May 9, 2016.
3. Hildebrand F, Pape HC, Horst K, et al. Impact of age on the clinical outcomes of major trauma. Eur J Trauma Emerg Surg 2015;1–16.

4. Hashmi A, Ibrahim-Zada I, Rhee P, et al. Predictors of mortality in geriatric trauma patients: a systematic review and meta-analysis. J Trauma Acute Care Surg 2014;76(3):894–901.
5. Centers for Disease Control and Prevention – leading cause of death. Available at: http://www.cdc.gov/nchs/data/hus/hus15.pdf#019. Accessed May 9, 2016.
6. Center for Disease Control and Prevention – unintentional injury deaths. Available at: http://www.cdc.gov/injury/wisqars/leadingcauses.html. Accessed May 9, 2016.
7. Center for Disease Control and Prevention – costs of falls among older adults. Available at: http://www.cdc.gov/homeandrecreationalsafety/falls/fallcost.html. Accessed May 9, 2016.
8. Tornetta P 3rd, Mostafavi H, Riina J, et al. Morbidity and mortality in elderly trauma patients. J Trauma 1999;46(4):702–6.
9. Goodmanson NW, Rosengart MR, Barnato AE, et al. Defining geriatric trauma: when does age make a difference? Surgery 2012;152(4):668–74 [discussion: 674–5].
10. Zafar SN, Shah AA, Zogg CK, et al. Morbidity or mortality? Variations in trauma centres in the rescue of older injured patients. Injury 2016;47(5):1091–7.
11. Dodds R, Sayer AA. Sarcopenia and frailty: new challenges for clinical practice. Clin Med (Lond) 2015;15(Suppl 6):s88–91.
12. Joseph B, Pandit V, Zangbar B, et al. Superiority of frailty over age in predicting outcomes among geriatric trauma patients: a prospective analysis. JAMA Surg 2014;149(8):766–72.
13. Kozar RA, Arbabi S, Stein DM, et al. Injury in the aged: geriatric trauma care at the crossroads. J Trauma Acute Care Surg 2015;78(6):1197–209.
14. Searle SD, Mitnitski A, Gahbauer EA, et al. A standard procedure for creating a frailty index. BMC Geriatr 2008;8:24.
15. Thompson HJ, McCormick WC, Kagan SH. Traumatic brain injury in older adults: epidemiology, outcomes, and future implications. J Am Geriatr Soc 2006;54(10):1590–5.
16. Czosnyka M, Balestreri M, Steiner L, et al. Age, intracranial pressure, autoregulation, and outcome after brain trauma. J Neurosurg 2005;102(3):450–4.
17. Medzon R, Rothenhaus T, Bono CM, et al. Stability of cervical spine fractures after gunshot wounds to the head and neck. Spine (Phila Pa 1976) 2005;30(20):2274–9.
18. Hoffman JR, Wolfson AB, Todd K, et al. Selective cervical spine radiography in blunt trauma: methodology of the National Emergency X-Radiography Utilization Study (NEXUS). Ann Emerg Med 1998;32(4):461–9.
19. Stiell IG, Wells GA, Vandemheen KL, et al. The Canadian C-spine rule for radiography in alert and stable trauma patients. JAMA 2001;286(15):1841–8.
20. Ferraris VA, Ferraris SP, Saha SP. The relationship between mortality and preexisting cardiac disease in 5,971 trauma patients. J Trauma 2010;69(3):645–52.
21. Grossman MD, Miller D, Scaff DW, et al. When is an elder old? Effect of preexisting conditions on mortality in geriatric trauma. J Trauma 2002;52(2):242–6.
22. Poulose N, Raju R. Aging and injury: alterations in cellular energetics and organ function. Aging Dis 2014;5(2):101–8.
23. Talving P, Lustenberger T, Okoye OT, et al. The impact of liver cirrhosis on outcomes in trauma patients: a prospective study. J Trauma Acute Care Surg 2013;75(4):699–703.
24. McGillicuddy EA, Schuster KM, Kaplan LJ, et al. Contrast-induced nephropathy in elderly trauma patients. J Trauma 2010;68(2):294–7.
25. Milte R, Crotty M. Musculoskeletal health, frailty and functional decline. Best Pract Res Clin Rheumatol 2014;28(3):395–410.

26. Haubro M, Stougaard C, Torfing T, et al. Sensitivity and specificity of CT- and MRI-scanning in evaluation of occult fracture of the proximal femur. Injury 2015;46(8):1557–61.

27. Cannon J, Silvestri S, Munro M. Imaging choices in occult hip fracture. J Emerg Med 2009;37(2):144–52.

28. Kharrazi RJ, Nash D, Mielenz TJ. Increasing trend of fatal falls in older adults in the United States, 1992 to 2005: coding practice or reporting quality? J Am Geriatr Soc 2015;63(9):1913–7.

29. Cigolle CT, Ha J, Min LC, et al. The epidemiologic data on falls, 1998-2010: more older Americans report falling. JAMA Intern Med 2015;175(3):443–5.

30. Nordell E, Jarnlo GB, Jetsén C, et al. Accidental falls and related fractures in 65-74 year olds: a retrospective study of 332 patients. Acta Orthop Scand 2000;71(2):175–9.

31. Carpenter CR, Avidan MS, Wildes T, et al. Predicting geriatric falls following an episode of emergency department care: a systematic review. Acad Emerg Med 2014;21(10):1069–82.

32. Allen CJ, Hannay WM, Murray CR, et al. Causes of death differ between elderly and adult falls. J Trauma Acute Care Surg 2015;79(4):617–21.

33. Blair AJ, Manian FA. Coexisting systemic infections (CSIs) in patients presenting with a fall: tripped by objects or pathogens? Abstract 813. Presented at IDWeek. San Diego, October 7–11, 2015.

34. Patel KV, Phelan EA, Leveille SG, et al. High prevalence of falls, fear of falling, and impaired balance in older adults with pain in the United States: findings from the 2011 National Health and Aging Trends Study. J Am Geriatr Soc 2014;62(10):1844–52.

35. Sattin RW. Falls among older persons a public health perspective. Annu Rev Public Health 1992;13:489–508.

36. Vogel JA, Ginde AA, Lowenstein SR, et al. Emergency department visits by older adults for motor vehicle collisions. West J Emerg Med 2013;14(6):576–81.

37. Reith G, Lefering R, Wafaisade A, et al. Injury pattern, outcome and characteristics of severely injured pedestrian. Scand J Trauma Resusc Emerg Med 2015;23:56.

38. O'Hern S, Oxley J, Logan D. Older adults at increased risk as pedestrians in Victoria, Australia: an examination of crash characteristics and injury outcomes. Traffic Inj Prev 2015;16(Suppl 2):S161–7.

39. Kodadek LM, Selvarajah S, Velopulos CG, et al. Undertriage of older trauma patients: is this a national phenomenon? J Surg Res 2015;199(1):220–9.

40. Rehn M. Improving adjustments for older age in pre-hospital assessment and care. Scand J Trauma Resusc Emerg Med 2013;21:4.

41. Evans DC, Khoo KM, Radulescu A, et al. Pre-injury beta blocker use does not affect the hyperdynamic response in older trauma patients. J Emerg Trauma Shock 2014;7(4):305–9.

42. Heffernan DS, Thakkar RK, Monaghan SF, et al. Normal presenting vital signs are unreliable in geriatric blunt trauma victims. J Trauma 2010;69(4):813–20.

43. Caterino JM, Raubenolt A, Cudnik MT. Modification of Glasgow Coma Scale criteria for injured elders. Acad Emerg Med 2011;18(10):1014–21.

44. Newgard CD, Holmes JF, Haukoos JS, et al. Improving early identification of the high-risk elderly trauma patient by emergency medical services. Injury 2016;47(1):19–25.

45. Bolorunduro OB, Villegas C, Oyetunji TA, et al. Validating the Injury Severity Score (ISS) in different populations: ISS predicts mortality better among Hispanics and females. J Surg Res 2011;166(1):40–4.

46. Wutzler S, Maegele M, Marzi I, et al. Trauma registry of the German Society for Trauma Surgery. Association of preexisting medical conditions with in-hospital mortality in multiple-trauma patients. J Am Coll Surg 2009;209(1):75–81.

47. Boltz MM, Podany AB, Hollenbeak CS, et al. Injuries and outcomes associated with traumatic falls in the elderly population on oral anticoagulant therapy. Injury 2015;46(9):1765–71.

48. Ivascu FA, Howells GA, Junn FS, et al. Predictors of mortality in trauma patients with intracranial hemorrhage on preinjury aspirin or clopidogrel. J Trauma 2008; 65(4):785–8.

49. Pieracci FM, Eachempati SR, Shou J, et al. Use of long-term anticoagulation is associated with traumatic intracranial hemorrhage and subsequent mortality in elderly patients hospitalized after falls: analysis of the New York state administrative database. J Trauma 2007;63(3):519–24.

50. Ivascu FA, Howells GA, Junn FS, et al. Rapid warfarin reversal in anticoagulated patients with traumatic intracranial hemorrhage reduces hemorrhage progression and mortality. J Trauma 2005;59(5):1131–7 [discussion: 1137–9].

51. Ramly E, Kaafarani HM, Velmahos GC. The effect of aging on pulmonary function: implications for monitoring and support of the surgical and trauma patient. Surg Clin North Am 2015;95(1):53–69.

52. Adjusted Weingart SD. Preoxygenation, reoxygenation, and delayed sequence intubation in the emergency department. J Emerg Med 2011;40(6):661–7.

53. Weingart SD, Levitan RM. Preoxygenation and prevention of desaturation during emergency airway management. Ann Emerg Med 2012;59(3):165–75.e1.

54. Narang AT, Sikka R. Resuscitation of the elderly. Emerg Med Clin North Am 2006;24(2):261–72, v.

55. Craven R. Ketamine. Anaesthesia 2007;62(Suppl 1):48–53.

56. Marco CA, Schoenfeld CN, Keyl PM, et al. Abdominal pain in geriatric emergency patients: variables associated with adverse outcomes. Acad Emerg Med 1998;5(12):1163–8.

57. Duvall DB, Zhu X, Elliott AC, et al. Injury severity and comorbidities alone do not predict futility of care after geriatric trauma. J Palliat Med 2015;18(3):246–50.

58. Calland JF, Ingraham AM, Martin N, et al. Evaluation and management of geriatric trauma: an Eastern Association for the Surgery of Trauma practice management guideline. J Trauma Acute Care Surg 2012;73(5 Suppl 4):S345–50.

59. Zhao FZ, Wolf SE, Nakonezny PA, et al. Estimating geriatric mortality after injury using age, injury severity, and performance of a transfusion: the geriatric trauma outcome score. J Palliat Med 2015;18(8):677–81.

60. Kirkpatrick AW, Ball CG, D'Amours SK, et al. Acute resuscitation of the unstable adult trauma patient: bedside diagnosis and therapy. Can J Surg 2008;51(1): 57–69.

61. Davis JW, Kaups KL. Base deficit in the elderly: a marker of severe injury and death. J Trauma 1998;45(5):873–7.

62. Tchorz KM, Chandra MS, Markert RJ, et al. Comparison of hemodynamic measurements from invasive and noninvasive monitoring during early resuscitation. J Trauma Acute Care Surg 2012;72(4):852–60.

63. Das A, Liu D. Novel antidotes for target specific oral anticoagulants. Exp Hematol Oncol 2015;4:25.

64. FDA. FDA approves Praxbind, the first reversal agent for the anticoagulant Pradaxa. 2015. Available at: http://www.fda.gov/NewsEvents/Newsroom/PressAnnouncements/ucm467300.htm. Accessed May 9, 2016.

65. Aschkenasy MT, Rothenhaus TC. Trauma and falls in the elderly. Emerg Med Clin North Am 2006;24(2):413–32, vii.

66. Sampson MA, Colquhoun KB, Hennessy NL. Computed tomography whole body imaging in multi-trauma: 7 years experience. Clin Radiol 2006;61(4): 365–9.

67. Shannon L, Peachey T, Skipper N, et al. Comparison of clinically suspected injuries with injuries detected at whole-body CT in suspected multi-trauma victims. Clin Radiol 2015;70(11):1205–11.

68. Wang H, Phillips JL, Robinson RD, et al. Predictors of mortality among initially stable adult pelvic trauma patients in the US: data analysis from the National Trauma Data Bank. Injury 2015;46(11):2113–7.

69. Dams-O'Connor K, Cuthbert JP, Whyte J, et al. Traumatic brain injury among older adults at level I and II trauma centers. J Neurotrauma 2013;30(24): 2001–13.

70. Gowing R, Jain MK. Injury patterns and outcomes associated with elderly trauma victims in Kingston, Ontario. Can J Surg 2007;50(6):437–44.

71. Bouras T, Stranjalis G, Korfias S, et al. Head injury mortality in a geriatric population: differentiating an "edge" age group with better potential for benefit than older poor-prognosis patients. J Neurotrauma 2007;24(8):1355–61.

72. Haider AA, Rhee P, Orouji T, et al. A second look at the utility of serial routine repeat computed tomographic scans in patients with traumatic brain injury. Am J Surg 2015;210(6):1088–94.

73. Nishijima DK, Offerman SR, Ballard DW, et al. Immediate and delayed traumatic intracranial hemorrhage in patients with head trauma and preinjury warfarin or clopidogrel use. Ann Emerg Med 2012;59(6):460–8.e1–7.

74. Touger M, Gennis P, Nathanson N, et al. Validity of a decision rule to reduce cervical spine radiography in elderly patients with blunt trauma. Ann Emerg Med 2002;40(3):287–93.

75. Bub LD, Blackmore CC, Mann FA, et al. Cervical spine fractures in patients 65 years and older: a clinical prediction rule for blunt trauma. Radiology 2005; 234(1):143–9.

76. Ngo B, Hoffman JR, Mower WR. Cervical spine injury in the very elderly. Emerg Radiol 2000;7:287–91.

77. Wang H, Coppola M, Robinson RD, et al. Geriatric trauma patients with cervical spine fractures due to ground level fall: five years experience in a level one trauma center. J Clin Med Res 2013;5(2):75–83.

78. Elmistekawy EM, Hammad AA. Isolated rib fractures in geriatric patients. Ann Thorac Med 2007;2(4):166–8.

79. Stawicki SP, Grossman MD, Hoey BA, et al. Rib fractures in the elderly: a marker of injury severity. J Am Geriatr Soc 2004;52(5):805–8.

80. Lotfipour S, Kaku SK, Vaca FE, et al. Factors associated with complications in older adults with isolated blunt chest trauma. West J Emerg Med 2009;10(2): 79–84.

81. Johnell O, Kanis JA. An estimate of the worldwide prevalence and disability associated with osteoporotic fractures. Osteoporos Int 2006;17(12):1726–33.

82. O'Malley NT, Blauth M, Suhm N, et al. Hip fracture management, before and beyond surgery and medication: a synthesis of the evidence. Arch Orthop Trauma Surg 2011;131(11):1519–27.

83. Roth T, Kammerlander C, Gosch M, et al. Outcome in geriatric fracture patients and how it can be improved. Osteoporos Int 2010;21(Suppl 4):S615–9.

84. Della Rocca GJ, Crist BD. Hip fracture protocols: what have we changed? Orthop Clin North Am 2013;44(2):163–82.

85. O'brien DP, Luchette FA, Pereira SJ, et al. Pelvic fracture in the elderly is associated with increased mortality. Surgery 2002;132(4):710–4 [discussion: 714–5].

86. Henry SM, Pollak AN, Jones AL, et al. Pelvic fracture in geriatric patients: a distinct clinical entity. J Trauma 2002;53(1):15–20.

87. Stalenhoef PA, Diederiks JP, Knottnerus JA, et al. A risk model for the prediction of recurrent falls in community-dwelling elderly: a prospective cohort study. J Clin Epidemiol 2002;55(11):1088–94.

88. Garwe T, Roberts ZV, Albrecht RM, et al. Direct transport of geriatric trauma patients with pelvic fractures to a level I trauma center within an organized trauma system: impact on two-week incidence of in-hospital complications. Am J Surg 2012;204(6):921–5 [discussion: 925–6].

89. Hill AD, Fowler RA, Nathens AB. Impact of interhospital transfer on outcomes for trauma patients: a systematic review. J Trauma 2011;71(6):1885–900 [discussion: 1901].

90. National center on elder abuse. Administration on aging. Available at: http://www.ncea.aoa.gov/library/data/. Accessed May 9, 2016.

91. Dong X. Elder abuse: research, practice, and health policy. The 2012 GSA Maxwell Pollack Award Lecture. Gerontologist 2014;54(2):153–62.

92. Amstadter AB, Cisler JM, McCauley JL, et al. Do incident and perpetrator characteristics of elder mistreatment differ by gender of the victim? Results from the National Elder Mistreatment Study. J Elder Abuse Negl 2011;23(1): 43–57.

93. J.A. Teresi, M. Ramirez, J. Ellis. A staff intervention targeting resident-to-resident elder mistreatment (R-REM) in long-term care increased staff knowledge, recognition and reporting: results from a cluster randomized trial. Int J Nurs Stud 2013;50(5):644–56.

94. Cooper C, Lodwick R, Walters K, et al. Observational cohort study: deprivation and access to anti-dementia drugs in the UK. Age Ageing 2016;45(1):148–54.

95. Acierno R, Hernandez MA, Amstadter AB. Prevalence and correlates of emotional, physical, sexual, and financial abuse and potential neglect in the United States: the National Elder Mistreatment Study. Am J Public Health 2010;100(2):292–7.

96. Ranhoff AH. Accidental hypothermia in the elderly. Tidsskr Nor Laegeforen 2002;122(7):715–7 [in Norwegian].

97. Ranhoff AH. Accidental hypothermia in the elderly. Int J Circumpolar Health 2000;59(3–4):255–9.

98. Scalise PJ, Mann MC, Votto JJ, et al. Severe hypothermia in the elderly. Conn Med 1995;59(9):515–7.

99. Soteras Martínez I, Subirats Bayego E, Reisten O. Accidental hypothermia. Med Clin (Barc) 2011;137(4):171–7 [in Spanish].

100. Incagnoli P, Bourgeois B, Teboul A, et al. Resuscitation from accidental hypothermia of 22 degrees C with circulatory arrest: importance of prehospital management. Ann Fr Anesth Reanim 2006;25(5):535–8 [in French].

101. Clift J, Munro-Davies L. Best evidence topic report. Is defibrillation effective in accidental severe hypothermia in adults? Emerg Med J 2007;24(1):50–1.

102. Plaisier BR. Thoracic lavage in accidental hypothermia with cardiac arrest–report of a case and review of the literature. Resuscitation 2005;66(1):99–104.

103. Sepehripour AH, Gupta S, Lall KS. When should cardiopulmonary bypass be used in the setting of severe hypothermic cardiac arrest? Interact Cardiovasc Thorac Surg 2013;17(3):564–9.

104. Cortés J, Galván C, Sierra J, et al. Severe accidental hypothermia: rewarming by total cardiopulmonary bypass. Rev Esp Anestesiol Reanim 1994;41(2): 109–12 [in Spanish].

105. Splittgerber FH, Talbert JG, Sweezer WP, et al. Partial cardiopulmonary bypass for core rewarming in profound accidental hypothermia. Am Surg 1986;52(8): 407–12.

106. Heisel MJ, Conwell Y, Pisani AR, et al. Concordance of self- and proxy-reported suicide ideation in depressed adults 50 years of age or older. Can J Psychiatry 2011;56(4):219–26.

107. Heisel MJ. Suicide and its prevention among older adults. Can J Psychiatry 2006;51(3):143–54.

108. Nordentoft M. Prevention of suicide and attempted suicide in Denmark. Epidemiological studies of suicide and intervention studies in selected risk groups. Dan Med Bull 2007;54(4):306–69.

109. McIntosh JL. Suicide prevention in the elderly (age 65-99). Suicide Life Threat Behav 1995;25(1):180–92.

110. Kerkhof AJ, Visser AP, Diekstra RF, et al. The prevention of suicide among older people in The Netherlands: interventions in community mental health care. Crisis 1991;12(2):59–72.

111. Awata S. Prevention of suicide in the elderly. Seishin Shinkeigaku Zasshi 2005; 107(10):1099–109 [in Japanese].

112. Awata S, Seki T, Koizumi Y, et al. Factors associated with suicidal ideation in an elderly urban Japanese population: a community-based, cross-sectional study. Psychiatry Clin Neurosci 2005;59(3):327–36.

# Sepsis and Other Infectious Disease Emergencies in the Elderly

Stephen Y. Liang, MD, MPHS[a,b,*]

## KEYWORDS

- Infections • Sepsis • Pneumonia • Urinary tract infection • Meningitis
- Skin and soft tissue infection • Elderly

## KEY POINTS

- Infectious diseases are responsible for significant morbidity and mortality among elders.
- Immunosenescence, declining physical barriers to pathogens, and mounting medical co-morbidities increase an elder's vulnerability to a wide range of infections.
- Atypical clinical presentations of infection are common in the elderly.
- Timely recognition and appropriate empirical antimicrobial therapy for infectious disease can increase survival and optimize clinical outcomes.

## INTRODUCTION

The world is aging. The number of individuals aged 60 years and older is expected to increase globally from 841 million in 2013 to more than 2 billion by 2050.[1] In the United States, persons aged 65 years and older are anticipated to double in number from 43.1 million in 2012 to 83.7 million by 2050.[2] Fueled by a generation of baby boomers born between 1946 and 1964, more than a fifth of the US population will surpass 65 years of age by 2030. From 2009 to 2010, elders accounted for more than 19 million visits made to US emergency department (ED) visits, representing 15% of all ED visits

Disclosures: S.Y. Liang reports no conflicts of interest in this work. S.Y. Liang is the recipient of a KM1 Comparative Effectiveness Research Career Development Award (KM1CA156708-01) and received support through the Clinical and Translational Science Award (CTSA) program (UL1RR024992) of the National Center for Advancing Translational Sciences (NCATS) as well as the Barnes-Jewish Patient Safety and Quality Career Development Program, which is funded by the Foundation for Barnes-Jewish Hospital.
[a] Division of Emergency Medicine, Washington University School of Medicine, 660 South Euclid Avenue, Campus Box 8072, St Louis, MO 63110, USA; [b] Division of Infectious Diseases, Washington University School of Medicine, 660 South Euclid Avenue, Campus Box 8051, St Louis, MO 63110, USA
* Division of Infectious Diseases, Washington University School of Medicine, 660 South Euclid Avenue, Campus Box 8051, St Louis, MO 63110.
E-mail address: syliang@wustl.edu

Emerg Med Clin N Am 34 (2016) 501–522
http://dx.doi.org/10.1016/j.emc.2016.04.005
0733-8627/16/$ – see front matter © 2016 Elsevier Inc. All rights reserved.
emed.theclinics.com

nationally.[3] More than a third of these visits warranted hospital admission for further care. As new advances in medicine and improved access to health care continue to extend the envelope of life expectancy worldwide, emergency physicians must be well versed in the timely, comprehensive, and compassionate care of our elders.

Infectious diseases account for widespread morbidity and mortality among the elderly. In 2012 alone, infectious diseases accounted for 13.5% (3.1 million) of all visits made by elders to US EDs.[4] Hospitalization rates for infectious diseases in this segment of our population have steadily risen over the past 2 decades.[5,6] Although respiratory tract infections, primarily pneumonia, account for most of these admissions, hospitalization rates for sepsis and urinary tract infections (UTIs) have dramatically increased since 2000, particularly in those aged 85 years and older.[7] From 1998 to 2004, infectious diseases accounted for almost 14% of all hospitalizations of older adults in the United States, with total charges in excess of $261 billion.[8] Not surprisingly, pneumonia and sepsis accounted for almost 60% of those charges. In a large retrospective study of 323 acute-care hospitals in California from 2009 to 2011, infection-related readmissions comprised more than a quarter of 30-day all-cause readmissions.[9] Although mortality from heart disease, malignancy, chronic pulmonary disease, and cerebrovascular disease far outpaces mortality from infectious diseases in persons aged 65 years and older, pneumonia, influenza, and sepsis remain significant causes of death among elders in the United States.[10]

The spectrum of infectious diseases in the elderly is wide ranging. This review examines the unique risk factors that render the elderly vulnerable to infection and focuses on the diagnosis and emergent management of severe sepsis and septic shock, pneumonia, urinary tract infections, central nervous system infections, and skin and soft tissue infections.

## AGING AND INFECTION

The aging immune system creates a natural state of immunosuppression in the elderly, predisposing to infection. Immunosenescence is characterized prominently by a decline in adaptive immunity. Although circulating memory T cells increase over time in response to continued antigenic stimulation, the pool of naïve T cells is depleted through age-related thymic involution, compromising the primary T-cell response to new antigens.[11,12] Loss of T-cell receptor repertoire diversity and intrinsic age-related naïve T-cell defects further impair the effectiveness of this cell-mediated immune response. As the pool of antigen-experienced memory B cells expands with age displacing naïve B cells necessary for new antibody formation, humoral immunity is likewise blunted. Reduced B-cell repertoire diversity, devolution of critical T-cell interactions needed for B-cell activation and differentiation, and decreased antibody affinity dampen the humoral response to infection and vaccines alike.[12] Immunosenescence is also marked by the dysregulation of innate immunity.[13,14] Polymorphonuclear neutrophils exhibit reduced chemotaxis, phagocytosis, and intracellular killing of pathogens, due in part to reduced toll-like receptor expression and activation. Similarly, age-associated decreases in macrophage, natural killer, and dendritic cell function are apparent. Impaired immune responses to new pathogens may also arise from basal activation of the innate immune system with increasing age, evidenced by increased levels of proinflammatory cytokines (eg, interleukin 6, tumor necrosis factor-$\alpha$), clotting factors, and acute phase reactants (eg, C-reactive protein). Attributed to chronic viral infections (eg, cytomegalovirus) and cellular damage as well as age-related hormonal and metabolic changes, such dysregulated inflammatory responses may likewise contribute to the development of noninfectious diseases, such as atherosclerosis and Alzheimer disease.[14] The aging immune system is a complex phenomenon that we have yet to fully comprehend. Physical barriers to infection, such as the skin, wane with age, hastened in the setting of immobility. Weakening of the gag and cough reflexes, incomplete urinary bladder emptying, and other age-related changes allow pathogens to access and establish infection in previously protected compartments. Surgical wounds and medical devices (eg, central venous catheters, urinary catheters, endotracheal tubes) commonly used in health care circumvent these natural defenses altogether. Prosthetic joints, heart valves, cardiac pacemaker-defibrillators, and other implanted hardware can serve as a nidus for infection. Dementia, impaired coordination, and frequent falls and injuries further predispose the elder to infection. Malnutrition and peripheral vascular disease can impede wound healing. Other comorbid conditions, including diabetes mellitus, chronic obstructive pulmonary disease (COPD), chronic kidney disease, and malignancy, may also increase an elder's overall risk of infection. Those receiving immunosuppression for solid organ or bone marrow transplants, malignancy, or a host of inflammatory conditions are at even greater risk of infection involving a broad range of pathogens.

Atypical presentations are a hallmark of most diseases in the elder, often rendering the diagnosis of infection challenging. Nonspecific symptoms associated with acute functional decline are common including confusion, frequent falls, difficulty ambulating, reduced food intake, dysphagia, incontinence, weight loss, and failure to thrive, all of which can also be seen in a wide range of noninfectious processes in the elderly. Age-related dementia and polypharmacy can further limit the clinician's ability to obtain a reliable history of symptoms from patients. Underreporting or downplaying of symptoms by patients can delay presentation to care for significant infections.

Fever, traditionally defined as a body temperature greater than 38°C (100.4°F), is absent or blunted in up to a third of elderly patients with an acute infection.[15] Diminished thermoregulatory capacity and abnormal production and response to endogenous pyrogens with aging may be partly to blame. In patients hospitalized with moderate to severe pneumonia, the average temperature during the first 3 days of illness decreases by 0.15°C (0.3°F) with each decade increase in age, equating to a 1°C (1.8°F) difference in temperature between a 20-year-old and an 80-year-old patient with pneumonia.[16] Healthy elders are also likely to have lower baseline body temperatures than younger adults.[17] Febrile response may be delayed in many instances. In view of this, fever in older long-term care residents has been defined as (1) a single oral temperature greater than 37.8°C (>100.0°F), (2) repeated oral temperatures greater than 37.2°C (>99.0°F) or rectal temperatures greater than 37.5°C (>99.5°F), or (3) more than a 1.1°C (>2.0°F) increase in temperature greater than baseline; it may be reasonable to apply this definition to the elderly population as a whole.[18] Tympanic thermometry is comparable in diagnostic accuracy with rectal thermometry for identifying infection when a lower fever cutoff of 37.3°C (99.1°F) is used; temporal artery thermometry is significantly less accurate.[19] However, body temperatures greater than 38°C (100.4°F) generally equate with serious illness in elders presenting to the ED.[20] Likewise, hypothermia relative to baseline body temperatures may also signal life-threatening infection, particularly in sepsis.[21]

## SEVERE SEPSIS AND SEPTIC SHOCK

Sepsis is a clinical syndrome that is characterized by a dysregulated inflammatory response to severe infection (**Table 1**). Severe sepsis is defined as sepsis-induced organ hypoperfusion and dysfunction, outwardly manifesting as acute kidney injury,

**Table 1**
**Sepsis definitions**

| | |
|---|---|
| Sepsis | Infection (documented or suspected) plus some of the following SIRS criteria[a]:<br>• Fever (>38.3°C or 100.4°F) or hypothermia (<36°C or 96.8°F)<br>• Tachycardia (heart rate >90/min)<br>• Tachypnea (>20 breaths/min)<br>• Leukocytosis (WBC count >12 × 10$^3$/μL), leukopenia (WBC count <4 × 10$^3$/μL), or bandemia (>10%) |
| Severe sepsis | Sepsis-induced tissue hypoperfusion or organ dysfunction as evidenced by any of the following:<br>• Sepsis-induced hypotension<br>  ○ SBP <90 mm Hg<br>  ○ MAP <70 mm Hg<br>  ○ SBP decrease >40 mm Hg or <2 standard deviations less than normal for age in the absence of other causes of hypotension<br>• Lactate greater than upper limits of normal<br>• Urine output <0.5 mL/kg/h for more than 2 h despite adequate fluid resuscitation<br>• Acute lung injury with Pao$_2$/Fio$_2$ <250 in the absence of pneumonia<br>• Acute lung injury with Pao$_2$/Fio$_2$ <200 in the presence of pneumonia<br>• Creatinine >2.0 mg/dL<br>• Bilirubin >2.0 mg/dL<br>• Platelet count <100 × 10$^3$/μL<br>• Coagulopathy (international normalized ratio >1.5) |
| Septic shock | Severe sepsis plus sepsis-induced hypotension unresponsive to fluid resuscitation (30 mL/kg of crystalloid) |

*Abbreviations:* Fio$_2$, fraction of inspired oxygen; MAP, mean arterial pressure; SBP, systolic blood pressure; SIRS, systemic inflammatory response syndrome; WBC, white blood cell.

[a] Additional general, inflammatory, hemodynamic, organ dysfunction, and tissue perfusion variables used as diagnostic criteria for systemic inflammatory response syndrome can be found in the most recent update of the Surviving Sepsis Campaign guidelines.[38]

*Data from* Dellinger RP, Levy MM, Rhodes A, et al. Surviving Sepsis Campaign: international guidelines for management of severe sepsis and septic shock: 2012. Crit Care Med 2013;41(2):580–637.

coagulopathy, encephalopathy, acute respiratory distress syndrome, and hypotension due to vasodilation, increased endothelial permeability, and functional adrenal insufficiency. Septic shock is distinguished by sepsis-induced hypotension that is refractory to adequate fluid resuscitation. More than half of all cases of sepsis in the United States occur in adults older than 65 years.[22,23] The relative risk (RR) for developing sepsis is 13.1 times greater in elders (95% confidence interval [CI], 12.6–13.6) compared with those less than 65 years of age, and elders are 1.56 times more likely to die of sepsis (95% CI, 1.52–1.61).[22] The incidence, disease severity, and mortality associated with sepsis are disproportionately high among the elderly in part because of immunosenescence, prolonged host inflammatory responses, a tendency toward coagulation activation and impaired fibrinolysis, and an increased susceptibility to microbial mediators, including endotoxin leading to profound and persistent hypotension.[24,25] This hyperinflammatory state is followed by profound immunosuppression as a result of T-cell exhaustion in elderly patients, further increasing mortality and morbidity through secondary infections.[26,27] Although significant advances have been made in emergency and critical care, mortality can range anywhere from 12.1% to 25.6% in severe sepsis to 30% to 50% in septic shock.[28–30] Increasing age is an independent risk factor for severe sepsis and related mortality.[31] Nursing home residence, a likely marker of frailty and multiple comorbidities, has also been associated with an increased risk of severe sepsis and death in elders.[32]

Respiratory infections, bloodstream infections, and genitourinary infections are the most common underlying causes of sepsis in the elderly.[22,23,31,32] Elders are more likely to develop sepsis due to gram-negative infections, particularly in the setting of pneumonia, and fungal infections compared with those less than 65 years of age.[22] Those residing in long-term care facilities or with frequent health care contact may be at risk for infection with multidrug-resistant organisms. Clinical presentations of sepsis in the elderly can be muted until overwhelming infection devolves into septic shock. Severe infections, including those involving the bloodstream, are heralded predominantly by atypical symptoms, such as confusion, falls, malaise, incontinence, immobility, and syncope, rather than classic presentations of subjective fever, chills, cough, dysuria, or other symptoms of localized infection.[33–35] Elders with severe bloodstream infections are often febrile, but this may be less common with advanced age (>85 years).[34] Compared with younger adults, elders are less likely to be tachycardic and more prone to tachypnea and acute respiratory distress with severe infection.[34–36] Most elders mount a significant leukocytosis in the setting of sepsis and bloodstream infection.[34,35,37]

The initial management of severe sepsis and septic shock in elderly patients should focus on timely empirical antimicrobial therapy and aggressive volume resuscitation in accordance with current established international guidelines.[38] Although several paradigms have been proposed to explain the role of infection in triggering and sustaining the immunologic cascade leading to cellular injury, irreversible organ damage, and death in severe sepsis and septic shock, appropriate antimicrobial therapy is critical to rapidly reducing pathogen load and improving mortality.[39,40] Empirical antimicrobial therapy is considered appropriate if it has in vitro activity against a causative pathogen before it has been identified in the laboratory workup (eg, microbiologic culture, rapid molecular diagnostics). In a retrospective study of 5715 patients with septic shock, inappropriate initial antimicrobial therapy occurred in almost 20% of patients and was associated with a 5-fold reduction in survival.[28] For this reason, empirical antimicrobial therapy should cover both gram-positive and gram-negative bacteria. When available, hospital antibiograms can help inform empirical therapy by highlighting regional and patient population–specific differences in antimicrobial susceptibilities for common bacteria. The most likely anatomic source of infection should also guide antimicrobial selection so that therapeutic drug levels are achievable in infected tissue and fluid (eg, lung, urine, cerebrospinal fluid [CSF]). Recent hospitalization, residence in a long-term care facility, antimicrobial exposure, and prior colonization or infection with a resistant organism should prompt expansion of empirical therapy to include organisms such as methicillin-resistant *Staphylococcus aureus* (MRSA), vancomycin-resistant *Enterococcus*, and multidrug-resistant gram-negative bacilli. Antifungal therapy is warranted in the setting of immunosuppression (eg, human immunodeficiency virus infection, hematologic malignancy, solid organ or hematologic stem cell transplant), neutropenia, prior extensive antimicrobial exposure, or extensive colonization with *Candida*. Empirical antimicrobial therapy should be initiated within the first hour of recognition of severe sepsis or septic shock. In a major retrospective study of septic shock, administration of appropriate antimicrobial therapy within the first hour of hypotension was associated with a 79.9% survival to hospital discharge.[41] Survival declined by 7.6% with each subsequent hour, with a survival rate of 42% at a median delay of 6 hours. Early and appropriate antimicrobial therapy is essential to survival in severe sepsis and septic shock.[42–44] Microbiologic cultures (eg, blood cultures) should be obtained before administering antimicrobials to help tailor pathogen-specific therapy but should not significantly delay treatment (>45 minutes), particularly in septic shock.

Pharmacokinetic and pharmacodynamic optimization of antimicrobial therapy to rapidly achieve therapeutic serum drug concentrations further enhances the clearance of pathogens in severe sepsis and septic shock.[39] Initial antimicrobial therapy should start at the maximum recommended dose while taking into account baseline renal or hepatic insufficiency that may predispose an elder to drug toxicity. Age-related changes in body composition, total body water, and serum albumin all impact drug concentrations. Interstitial third spacing due to increased capillary permeability in sepsis can lead to subtherapeutic drug concentrations for many antimicrobials. Clinical pharmacists can play an invaluable role in selecting dosing strategies that maximize antimicrobial effect in severe sepsis, septic shock, and other severe infections in the ED.[45] In addition to antimicrobial therapy, adequate source control (eg, abscess drainage, removal of an infected central venous catheter) is also integral to decreasing pathogen burden.

Protocolized, quantitative resuscitation strategies using intravenous fluids, vasopressors, inotropes, and blood transfusions seek to correct the circulatory dysfunction that results from the intense inflammatory response in severe sepsis and septic shock. Early goal-directed therapy using invasive hemodynamic monitoring has been shown to significantly reduce mortality in a landmark study.[46] However, several recent randomized, multicenter studies have failed to recreate the success of this strategy, likely because of improved awareness, timely diagnosis, and early treatment of severe sepsis and septic shock over the past decade.[47–49] Current guidelines support an initial minimum fluid challenge of 30 mL/kg of crystalloid in patients with sepsis-induced organ hypoperfusion, hypovolemia, or hyperlactatemia ($\geq 4$ mmol/L).[38] Additional fluid challenges may be administered based on dynamic or static measures of fluid responsiveness. Elders with congestive heart failure, chronic renal insufficiency, or end-stage renal disease may benefit from guarded resuscitation with smaller fluid boluses to avoid volume overload. Vasopressors are recommended in the setting of hypotension that has not responded to initial volume resuscitation, with norepinephrine being the preferred agent. Although many sepsis intervention trials include elderly patients, those with significant medical comorbidities at risk of death are often excluded.[50] Trials targeting high-risk elderly patients with severe sepsis or septic shock are greatly needed to better inform specific recommendations taking into account the altered physiology of aging. Nevertheless, standardized resuscitation protocols for severe sepsis and septic shock improve mortality in the elderly, likely through earlier recognition, empirical antimicrobial therapy, and aggressive volume resuscitation.[37]

Indicators of poor prognosis in elderly patients with severe sepsis include the presence of shock, elevated serum lactate levels, and organ failure (particularly respiratory or cardiac). When present, hypothermia is an independent predictor of increased mortality in elderly patients with sepsis.[21] Leukemoid reactions (white blood cell count >30.0 $\times$ 10$^3$/$\mu$L) carry a grave prognosis in elderly patients with sepsis.[51] There is evidence to suggest that Predisposition Insult Response and Organ failure (PIRO), Sequential Organ Failure Assessment (SOFA), and Mortality in Emergency Department Sepsis (MEDS) scores may be useful in predicting mortality in elderly patients with sepsis presenting to the ED.[52,53] Biomarkers, including cardiac troponin I and N-terminal probrain natriuretic peptide, may also have a role in predicting mortality in elders with severe sepsis or septic shock.[54,55]

Elderly survivors of sepsis incur significant morbidity, frequently requiring skilled nursing and rehabilitative care after their acute hospitalization.[22] Severe sepsis exacts a considerable toll on elderly survivors in the form of long-term functional disability and moderate to severe cognitive impairment.[56,57] Controlling for individual presepsis levels and trajectories of geriatric comorbid conditions (eg, cachexia, incontinence, injurious falls), higher rates of low body mass index (<18.5 kg/m$^2$) have also been demonstrated in elderly survivors of severe sepsis, suggesting that severe sepsis increases sarcopenia, the age-related loss of skeletal muscle mass.[58] Such changes in brain function and body composition contribute to frailty, increasing elders' need for assistance with activities of daily living and threatening their independence. Survivors of severe sepsis and other critical illness often require significant additional health care compared with their premorbid state, frequently in inpatient settings.[59] From the vantage point of both the patients and the health care system, the early recognition and treatment of infectious diseases commonly encountered in elderly patients presenting to the ED must, therefore, assume an added urgency in order to prevent progression to severe sepsis and septic shock. Likewise, candid discussions with patients, family, and other care providers in the ED centered on patient preferences, goals of care, and anticipated clinical outcomes in severe sepsis and septic shock are particularly important given the high mortality and morbidity associated with this disease.

## PNEUMONIA AND INFLUENZA

Sir William Osler[60] penned, "pneumonia may well be called the friend of the aged." Furthermore, "a knowledge that the onset of pneumonia is insidious and that the symptoms are ill-defined and latent, should put the practitioner on his guard."[60] A century later, this characterization of pneumonia in the elderly holds true. More than 900,000 cases of community-acquired pneumonia (CAP) occur annually among US seniors, and approximately 1 in 20 adults older than 85 years develop CAP each year.[61] Pneumonia is the most common infectious disease indication for hospitalization among adults more than 65 years of age.[5,6] In 2013, influenza and pneumonia resulted in more than 48,000 deaths among elders in the United States.[10] Elders are at increased risk for CAP because of impaired mucociliary clearance and diminished protective cough reflexes, which allow inhaled or aspirated pathogens to gain access to the lower respiratory tract. Increased lung compliance and reduced vital capacity contribute to decreased functional reserve in old age, rendering the elder less able to compensate for serious pulmonary infection. These vulnerabilities are further compounded by chronic pulmonary disease (eg, COPD), asthma, and tobacco dependence, all well-established risk factors for CAP.[61] Congestive heart failure, diabetes mellitus, poor functional status, low body weight, and recent weight loss also place elders at risk for developing pneumonia.[61,62]

A combination of cough, fever, and dyspnea was absent in two-thirds of elders diagnosed with CAP in one study, whereas almost half presented with delirium or acute confusion.[63] Fever was absent in more than a third of elders. Other symptoms, including chills, sweats, pleuritic chest pain, headache, and myalgias, are also less common in the elders with CAP compared with changes in mental status.[64,65] This characterization holds true as well for elders residing in long-term care facilities, even in those with severe pneumonia.[66,67] The presence of tachypnea with CAP increases with age.

In the United States, *Streptococcus pneumoniae* is the most common cause of CAP in community-dwelling elders.[65,68,69] *Haemophilus influenzae, Legionella pneumophila, Chlamydia pneumoniae, Mycoplasma pneumoniae,* and less commonly gram-negative bacilli are also causative pathogens. Elders residing in long-term care facilities are susceptible to pneumonia from the same organisms but also to *S aureus*, gram-negative bacilli including *Klebsiella pneumoniae* and *Pseudomonas aeruginosa*, and anaerobes, the last category of organisms occurring in the context of aspiration.[66,67] Pneumonia due to multidrug-resistant organisms, such as MRSA and gram-negative bacilli, varies among elderly long-term care facility populations.[66,67,70] Elders older than 75 years have a 15-fold higher incidence of pneumonia due to influenza than young adults.[68] Other respiratory viruses commonly associated with pneumonia in the elderly include human metapneumovirus, parainfluenza virus, respiratory syncytial virus, and rhinovirus.[69]

Elders presenting to the ED with fever, tachypnea, or any clinical suspicion for pneumonia should undergo chest radiography. However, the accuracy of radiography may be limited in the face of poor functional status, early pneumonia, or immunocompromised states; computed tomography of the chest may have increased utility.[71] In addition to standard laboratory tests, patients requiring hospitalization, particularly to an intensive care unit, should have 2 blood cultures drawn before the administration of antimicrobials to guide definitive therapy.[72] Pneumococcal and *Legionella* urinary antigen testing can further aid in determining the cause of pneumonia. Severity-of-illness scores taking into account epidemiologic, clinical, and diagnostic factors can help identify elders at high risk for mortality with CAP and inform admission decisions. The Pneumonia Severity Index (PSI) has been evaluated in elders and in EDs as a strategy for identifying low risk patients with CAP who can be safely treated as outpatients (**Table 2**).[73–76] The CURB-65 score (Confusion, Uremia, blood urea nitrogen >7 mmol/L or 20 mg/dL; Respiratory rate $\geq$30 breaths per minutes; Blood pressure, systolic <90 mm Hg or diastolic $\leq$60 mm Hg; Age $\geq$65 years) has also been validated in older adults presenting with CAP (**Table 3**).[77,78] No difference in overall test performance has been identified between PSI, CURB-65, or CRB-65 (which excludes laboratory testing to assess for uremia).[79] These scores incorporate age as a primary variable; therefore, increasing age translates to greater predicted mortality risk. In the end, clinical judgment taking into account comorbid illness, new supplemental oxygen requirements, the inability to take oral medications, patient safety, and other social considerations also factor into ED decision-making regarding hospitalization for CAP.[80]

In accordance with current guidelines, empirical outpatient antimicrobial therapy for CAP in healthy elders should consist of a macrolide (eg, azithromycin, clarithromycin) for a minimum of 5 days, although doxycycline is also acceptable.[72] Those with comorbidities, including chronic cardiac, pulmonary, hepatic or renal disease, diabetes mellitus, malignancy, or immunosuppression, should be treated with a respiratory fluoroquinolone (eg, levofloxacin) or a combination of a β-lactam (high-dose amoxicillin or amoxicillin-clavulanate) and a macrolide. Patients should be afebrile for 48 to 72 hours and demonstrate signs of clinical improvement before antimicrobials are discontinued. Elders requiring hospital admission should receive an intravenous β-lactam (eg, ceftriaxone, cefotaxime) and a macrolide. Empirical antimicrobial coverage for critically ill patients should be expanded to cover *Pseudomonas* infection using a combination of an antipneumococcal, antipseudomonal β-lactam (eg, cefepime, piperacillin-tazobactam, meropenem), and either azithromycin or a fluoroquinolone. Additional coverage for MRSA may consist of either vancomycin or linezolid. The decision to empirically treat for multidrug-resistant organisms, such as MRSA or gram-negative bacilli, should take into account the severity of disease and individual risk factors, including prior antibiotic treatment and recent hospitalization. Much debate surrounds the concept of health care–associated pneumonia (which includes elders residing in long-term care facilities, those hospitalized $\geq$2 days in the preceding 3 months, those receiving home infusion therapy or domiciliary wound care, and those who have received hemodialysis in the past month) and its ability to

**Table 2**
**Pneumonia severity index**

| Characteristic | Points |
|---|---|
| Demographic factors | |
| Age (y) | |
| Men | Age |
| Women | Age −10 |
| Nursing home residence | +10 |
| Coexisting illness | |
| Malignancy (active) | +30 |
| Liver disease | +20 |
| Congestive heart failure | +10 |
| Cerebrovascular disease | +10 |
| Chronic kidney disease | +10 |
| Physical examination findings | |
| Altered mental status | +20 |
| Respiratory rate ≥30 breaths/min | +20 |
| SBP <90 mm Hg | +20 |
| Temperature <35°C (95°F) or ≥40°C (104°F) | +15 |
| Pulse ≥125 beats/min | +10 |
| Laboratory and radiographic findings | |
| Arterial pH <7.35 | +30 |
| BUN ≥11 mmol/L or 30 mg/dL | +20 |
| Sodium <130 mmol/L | +20 |
| Glucose ≥14 mmol/L or 250 mg/dL | +10 |
| Hematocrit <30% | +10 |
| $Pao_2$ <60 mm Hg | +10 |
| Pleural effusion on chest radiograph | +10 |

| Total Points | Risk Class | Treatment Options |
|---|---|---|
| No comorbidities | I | Outpatient therapy |
| ≤70 | II | Outpatient therapy or brief hospitalization |
| 71–90 | III | |
| 91–130 | IV | Hospitalization |
| >130 | V | |

Abbreviations: BUN, blood urea nitrogen; SBP, systolic blood pressure.
Adapted from Fine MJ, Auble TE, Ycaly DM, et al. A prediction rule to identify low-risk patients with community-acquired pneumonia. N Engl J Med 1997;336(4):247.

identify patients at risk for CAP due to multidrug-resistant organisms.[81] Timely administration of antimicrobials (within 4 hours of hospital arrival) for CAP has been associated with reduced in-hospital mortality, 30-day mortality, and length of stay among Medicare patients older than 65 years.[82]

The 30-day mortality for elders with CAP ranges from 0.4% to 2.0% in outpatients to 12.5% to 15% in those requiring hospitalization.[61,83] Mortality may be higher in nursing home residents because of advanced age, multiple comorbidities, and poor functional status compared with community-dwelling elders.[66] Predictors of mortality include advanced age (≥90 years), impaired consciousness, anemia, pleural effusion,

| Table 3 |
| --- |
| **CURB-65 score** |

Assign 1 point for each of the following elements present:
- Confusion (new disorientation to person, place, or time or based on specific mental status test)
- *U*remia (BUN >7 mmol/L or 20 mg/dL)
- *R*espiratory rate ($\geq$30 breaths/min)
- *B*lood pressure (SBP <90 mm Hg or DBP <60 mm Hg)
- Age >*65* years

| Total | 30-d Mortality Risk | Treatment Options |
| --- | --- | --- |
| 0 or 1 | Low | Outpatient therapy appropriate |
| 2 | Moderate | Consider hospitalization |
| $\geq$3 | High | Hospitalization, consider intensive care unit |

*Abbreviations:* BUN, blood urea nitrogen; DBP, diastolic blood pressure; SBP, systolic blood pressure.
*Adapted from* Lim WS, van der Eerden MM, Laing R, et al. Defining community acquired pneumonia severity on presentation to hospital: an international derivation and validation study. Thorax 2003;58(5):377–82.

and multilobar infiltrates.[84] Specific comorbid illnesses, including hip fracture, COPD, and cerebrovascular disease, also adversely impact 30-day mortality.[85] Elders diagnosed with CAP often have a prolonged recovery, particularly if a history of COPD is present.[86] Given the significant burden of pneumonia among the elderly, pneumococcal and influenza vaccination are important disease prevention strategies in this high-risk population.

## URINARY TRACT INFECTION

UTIs including cystitis and pyelonephritis comprise almost 5% of all ED visits made annually by adults older than 65 years in the United States.[87] In a cohort of community-dwelling elderly women, the prevalence of UTI was 16.5%.[88] Among the women more than 85 years of age, almost 30% had been diagnosed with a UTI in the preceding year and 60% in the preceding 5 years.[89] In community-dwelling elderly men, the incidence of UTI increases significantly with each decade after 60 years of age but remains less than half that of women through the eighth decade of life.[90,91] After pneumonia, UTI is the second most common infectious disease for which elders are hospitalized.[5,6] Increased postvoid residual volume, decreased average and peak urinary flow rates, and a reduction in voided urine predispose the elder to urinary stasis, setting up conditions conducive to bacterial colonization, multiplication, and infection of the aging urinary tract. Neurogenic bladder resulting from stroke, Alzheimer disease, and Parkinson disease as well as urinary outlet obstruction due to prostatic hypertrophy in men can further impair effective bladder emptying. Periurethral bacterial colonization in postmenopausal women, chronic prostatitis in men, and infected renal or bladder calculi can serve as reservoirs for triggering recurrent UTIs. Among elders more than 85 years of age, recent UTI, urinary incontinence, frequent falls, cognitive impairment, the inability to perform activities of daily living, and recent delirium are all predictors of UTI.[89,92]

Elders with UTI are more likely to present to the ED with altered mental status rather than fever or classic urinary symptoms, such as dysuria, frequency, or urgency.[93] However, when present, acute dysuria is more specific for UTI than urinary frequency or urgency.[94] In a retrospective study, more than a quarter of elders older than 70 years eventually diagnosed with bacteremic UTI initially presented with confusion.[95] Nearly as many presented with cough or shortness of breath. Compared with younger women, postmenopausal women more frequently endorse nonspecific symptoms, including urinary incontinence, lower abdominal pain, lower back pain, chills, constipation, or diarrhea, rather than voiding symptoms.[96] Other nonlocalizing symptoms may include loss of appetite, nausea, vomiting, or falls. Atypical presentations, including altered mental status and gastrointestinal symptoms, also abound in elders with pyelonephritis; but fever and chills are more consistently present.[97] Up to a third of elders with pyelonephritis may complain of flank pain, and half may have costovertebral angle tenderness on examination.

*Escherichia coli* remains the most common cause for UTI in the elderly, followed by *Enterococcus*, *Proteus mirabilis*, and *K pneumoniae*.[88,96,98,99] Group B streptococcus (*Streptococcus agalactiae*), *Staphylococcus saprophyticus*, *Providencia stuartii*, and *Pseudomonas aeruginosa* are also more frequent causes of UTI in the elderly than younger adults. Laboratory evaluation of UTI in the ED should consist of a urinalysis performed on a clean-catch urine specimen followed by urine culture if positive. Urine tests can be challenging to interpret because of contamination by periurethral flora and the increased prevalence of asymptomatic bacteriuria in elders. For this reason, urine tests are most helpful in ruling out rather than establishing the diagnosis of UTI in the ED. A negative leukocyte esterase and nitrite test has a negative predictive value of 100% for UTI in nursing home residents suspected to have this diagnosis.[100] In elderly women, the presence of pyuria ($\geq$10 white blood cells per high power field) in combination with a positive leukocyte esterase and/or nitrite test has been shown to have a sensitivity of 84.8%, specificity of 81.6%, and positive predictive value of 47.2% for UTI.[88] Catheterized urine specimens yielded a lower proportion of false-positive urinalyses (31%) compared with clean catch (48%) in one study of elderly women treated in the ED.[101] Urine cultures can also be problematic to interpret as infected elders may exhibit lower bacterial colony counts ($10^2$ to $10^3$ colony forming units [CFU] per mL) compared with the traditional cutoff for younger adults ($10^5$ CFU/mL).[102]

One approach to deciding when to start antimicrobial therapy for UTI in elderly women in outpatient settings hinges on the presence of at least 2 of the following: fever (>38°C), clinical symptoms (acute dysuria, frequency, dysuria, suprapubic pain, costovertebral angle tenderness), pyuria, or a positive urine culture.[103] Asymptomatic bacteriuria should not be treated with antimicrobials. Although not intended specifically to address postmenopausal women, current guidelines for the management of UTI in adult women recommend trimethoprim-sulfamethoxazole (TMP-SMX) as first-line empirical therapy if local resistance rates for pathogens causing cystitis are less than 20%.[104] Nitrofurantoin has also been endorsed for the treatment of cystitis in women and can be used in elders depending on creatinine clearance and their capacity to recognize signs of pulmonary toxicity.[103] Fluoroquinolones should be reserved for complicated infections (eg, pyelonephritis). For men, either TMP-SMX or a fluoroquinolone should be used to treat UTI. A short course of antimicrobial therapy (3–6 days) is appropriate for treating uncomplicated cystitis in elderly women.[105] Longer durations totaling 7 to 14 days are recommended to treat pyelonephritis and any UTI in an elderly man.[104] Significant resistance to fluoroquinolones and other antimicrobials have been documented in elderly community-dwelling and long-term care facility populations alike, due in part to widespread and sometimes lax use of antimicrobials.[87,91,98,99,106,107] Antibiograms detailing local antimicrobial resistance patterns for common urinary pathogens can help inform appropriate empirical therapy in the ED. Likewise, close outpatient follow-up to assess for clinical improvement and review of the appropriateness of empirical antimicrobial therapy based on urine culture results can help tailor further management.

Although most elders with UTI will be treated as outpatients, those with severe UTI including associated bloodstream infection will require hospitalization and intravenous antimicrobial therapy. Predictors of severe UTI include the presence of fever, altered mental status, hemodynamic instability, leukocytosis, and end-organ dysfunction.[108,109] In-hospital mortality among elders with bacteremic UTI may be as high as 30%.[109] Therefore, hospitalized elders with severe UTI and emerging sepsis should receive broad-spectrum antimicrobial therapy pending urine and blood cultures.

## CENTRAL NERVOUS SYSTEM INFECTION

Although the incidence of bacterial meningitis among adults in the United States has declined since the introduction of the H influenzae type B and pneumococcal conjugate vaccines over the past quarter century, mortality associated with this disease remains more than 20% in those aged 65 years and older.[110] Streptococcus pneumoniae is the leading cause of bacterial meningitis in elders, whereas meningitis due to Neisseria meningitidis or H influenzae is relatively uncommon. Listeria monocytogenes, group B Streptococcus, and gram-negative bacteria (eg, E coli, K pneumoniae) can be causative pathogens in this population.[110–115] Predisposing conditions, such as otitis, sinusitis, or pneumonia, may be present and sepsis may complicate up to a third of cases.[112,114–116] Elders may have fever, headache, or neck stiffness but more commonly exhibit altered mental status, seizure, stupor, or coma.[111–117] Abnormal neurologic findings are often present, including focal motor deficits, cranial nerve abnormalities, and aphasia.[115,117] Kernig and Brudzinski signs may be absent or unreliable as osteoarthritis, degenerative disc disease, and movement disorders (eg, Parkinson disease) can render such maneuvers difficult to execute, much less interpret. Lumbar puncture should be strongly considered as part of the standard evaluation for mental status change in the elderly, even if patients are afebrile. Computed tomography of the head before lumbar puncture is a prudent step in evaluating the elder with fever and altered mental status given the risk for an intracranial mass lesion (eg, brain abscess, malignancy, or hematoma). CSF analysis generally reveals a pleocytosis (>10 white blood cells/mm$^3$), and a culture of the CSF should be obtained. Empirical antibiotic therapy for bacterial meningitis in the elderly should consist of intravenous vancomycin and a third-generation cephalosporin (eg, ceftriaxone) with expanded coverage for L monocytogenes, usually intravenous ampicillin, pending finalization of the CSF culture.[118] If a lumbar puncture cannot be performed expediently, empirical antimicrobial therapy should be initiated without further delay given the high mortality associated with bacterial meningitis. Adjuvant corticosteroid therapy has been associated with fewer neurologic sequelae across all types of bacterial meningitis (RR, 0.83; 95% CI, 0.69–1.0) and reduced mortality in S pneumoniae meningitis (RR, 0.84; 95% CI, 0.72–0.98) based on analyses of existing randomized controlled trials.[119]

Viral encephalitis should be a part of the differential diagnosis of any elder presenting with altered mental status or behavioral change. Herpes simplex encephalitis (HSE) due predominantly to herpes simplex virus (HSV) type 1 is one of the most common forms of sporadic fatal encephalitis worldwide, accounting for 10% to 15% of all viral encephalitis cases.[120] Often encountered in the elderly,[121,122] HSE can manifest with fever, headache, language difficulties, memory impairment, behavioral or personality changes, psychosis, or seizures. CSF analysis may reveal pleocytosis or hemorrhage but can also be acellular in up to 15% of patients early in the course of disease.[123–125] Although polymerase chain reaction (PCR) of the CSF is highly sensitive (>95%) and specific (>99%) for HSV,[120] it too can be negative in the early stages of disease.[123,126] In situations whereby the clinical suspicion for HSE is high, repeat lumbar puncture in 3 to 7 days to obtain CSF for HSV PCR may be warranted to safely exclude the diagnosis.[120] Temporal and/or inferior frontal lobe edema and hemorrhage characteristic of HSE is best visualized with MRI of the brain; bilateral temporal lobe involvement is a late but pathognomonic finding. Advanced age, depressed level of consciousness, prolonged duration of symptoms before presentation, extensive brain involvement on MRI, and delayed antiviral therapy (>2 days) have all been associated with poor outcomes in HSE.[123,127,128] Without appropriate antiviral therapy, mortality from HSE historically approaches 70%.[129] Therefore, empirical intravenous acyclovir should be initiated in an elder with suspected encephalitis while awaiting the results of the HSV PCR to evaluate for HSE.[120] Adjusted dosing may be necessary in the setting of renal insufficiency to prevent acyclovir-induced crystalluria and nephrotoxicity.

## SKIN AND SOFT TISSUE INFECTIONS

Atrophy and reduced elasticity, turgor, and perfusion render aging skin prone to tears and pressure ulcer formation, particularly in the setting of comorbid diabetes mellitus, peripheral vascular disease, and impaired mobility. Decreased skin turnover and malnutrition contribute to delayed wound healing. Compromised skin serves as a portal of entry for S aureus, Streptococcus species, and other bacteria leading to infections of the skin and soft tissues. Venous stasis and lymphedema, often following surgical disruption of the lymphatics during saphenous vein harvesting or axillary node dissection, can also increase the risk for cellulitis and erysipelas. The incidence of lower extremity cellulitis has been shown to increase by 43.8% per 10-year increment in age, and up to a fifth of patients will experience a recurrence of cellulitis within 2 years.[130] Skin and soft tissue infections (SSTIs) are particularly common in elderly long-term care facility populations.[131] The presence of skin erythema, induration, fluctuance, and purulent wound drainage help distinguish between purulent (furuncles, carbuncles, abscess) and nonpurulent (cellulitis, erysipelas, necrotizing infection) SSTIs.[132] In patients with a chronic wound, increasing pain may be a helpful sign of infection; but its absence does not rule it out.[133] Pain out of proportion to physical findings has long been a hallmark of necrotizing infection. Systemic toxicity manifests as fever, confusion, functional decline, and hypotension and may indicate severe infection as well.

Current guidelines recommend treatment of mild purulent infections with incision and drainage alone. In moderate infections, this should be accompanied by empirical antimicrobial therapy with either TMP-SMX or doxycycline to cover S aureus, particularly MRSA, for 5 to 7 days.[132] In moderate to severe infections requiring hospitalization, empirical intravenous vancomycin, daptomycin, linezolid, telavancin, or ceftaroline can be substituted instead. For nonpurulent infections, typically attributable to Streptococcus, oral antimicrobial therapy for mild cases can consist of penicillin V potassium, a cephalosporin (eg, cephalexin), dicloxacillin, or clindamycin for at least 5 days. Moderate infections should be treated with intravenous penicillin, ceftriaxone, cefazolin, or clindamycin. Severe infections warrant emergent surgical evaluation for potential necrotizing disease in tandem with empirical intravenous vancomycin and either piperacillin/tazobactam or a carbapenem. Infected pressure ulcers are a source of increased mortality among elders.[134] Necrotizing soft tissue infections involving the fascia and muscle likewise bear high mortality, particularly in those who develop early organ dysfunction.[135]

## EXPANDING INFECTIOUS DISEASE CONSIDERATIONS IN THE ELDERLY

Elders are at risk for a remarkable diversity of infection beyond the major disease entities discussed in this review. From endocarditis involving native and prosthetic heart valves to musculoskeletal infections, including septic arthritis and prosthetic joint infections, advances in medicine have not only extended life but also increased opportunities and expanded niches for infections to take root. Pressure ulcers and diabetic foot wounds can progress to debilitating osteomyelitis. Vertebral osteomyelitis, often masquerading as chronic back pain, can simmer undiagnosed until neurologic compromise. Repetitive antimicrobial exposure can predispose to devastating and recurrent *Clostridium difficile* infection and increases the potential for colonization and future infection with multidrug-resistant organisms. Immunocompromised states, whether from human immunodeficiency virus infection or intentional immunosuppression for malignancy, transplantation, or autoimmune disease, significantly expand the differential diagnosis in the elder presenting with fever to the ED to include a long list of unusual bacterial, viral, fungal, and parasitic diseases. Healthy as well as chronically ill elders returning from holiday abroad can bring back a wide range of tropical and vector-borne diseases in a world that has become increasingly smaller thanks to commercial air travel. Although traditionally regarded as inpatient consultants, infectious disease specialists can be a valuable resource to emergency physicians charged with the care of the infected elder not only in expanding the diagnostic evaluation but also assisting with appropriate selection of empirical antimicrobial therapy.

## SUMMARY

Aging sets the stage for an increased predisposition to infection through waning immunity and declining anatomic and physiologic defenses against pathogens. Atypical presentations for infectious diseases are commonplace, even in severe infection. As our population ages, elders will increasingly turn to the ED for timely and comprehensive care of acute illness. With increased vigilance and armed with a deeper understanding of the unique aspects of infection in this complex patient population, emergency physicians can play an integral part in the early recognition and appropriate management of a wide spectrum of infectious diseases in the elderly, including sepsis, pneumonia, UTI, central nervous system infections, and SSTIs, thereby reducing morbidity and mortality and optimizing patient outcomes.

## REFERENCES

1. United Nations, Department of economic and social affairs, population division (2013). New York: World Population Ageing; 2013. ST/ESA/SER.A/348.
2. Ortman JM, Velkoff VA, Hogan H. An aging nation: the older population in the United States, current population reports, P25–1140. Washington, DC: U.S. Census Bureau; 2014.
3. Albert M, McCaig LF, Ashman JJ. Emergency department visits by persons aged 65 and over: United States, 2009-2010. NCHS Data Brief, No. 130. Hyattsville (MD): National Center for Health Statistics; 2013.
4. Goto T, Yoshida K, Tsugawa Y, et al. Infectious disease-related emergency department visits of elderly adults in the United States, 2011-2012. J Am Geriatr Soc 2016;64(1):31–6.
5. Curns AT, Holman RC, Sejvar JJ, et al. Infectious disease hospitalizations among older adults in the United States from 1990 through 2002. Arch Intern Med 2005;165(21):2514–20.

6. Christensen KL, Holman RC, Steiner CA, et al. Infectious disease hospitalizations in the United States. Clin Infect Dis 2009;49(7):1025–35.

7. Levant S, Chari K, DeFrances CJ. Hospitalizations for patients aged 85 and over in the United States, 2000-2010. NCHS Data Brief, No. 182. Hyattsville (MD): National Center for Health Statistics; 2015.

8. Curns AT, Steiner CA, Sejvar JJ, et al. Hospital charges attributable to a primary diagnosis of infectious diseases in older adults in the United States, 1998 to 2004. J Am Geriatr Soc 2008;56(6):969–75.

9. Gohil SK, Datta R, Cao C, et al. Impact of hospital population case-mix, including poverty, on hospital all-cause and infection-related 30-day readmission rates. Clin Infect Dis 2015;61(8):1235–43.

10. National Center for Health Statistics. Health, United States, 2014: with special feature on adults aged 55-64. Hyattsville (MD): National Center for Health Statistics; 2015.

11. Appay V, Sauce D. Naive T cells: the crux of cellular immune aging? Exp Gerontol 2014;54:90–3.

12. Weiskopf D, Weinberger B, Grubeck-Loebenstein B. The aging of the immune system. Transpl Int 2009;22(11):1041–50.

13. Montgomery RR, Shaw AC. Paradoxical changes in innate immunity in aging: recent progress and new directions. J Leukoc Biol 2015;98(6):937–43.

14. Shaw AC, Goldstein DR, Montgomery RR. Age-dependent dysregulation of innate immunity. Nat Rev Immunol 2013;13(12):875–87.

15. Norman DC. Fever in the elderly. Clin Infect Dis 2000;31(1):148–51.

16. Roghmann MC, Warner J, Mackowiak PA. The relationship between age and fever magnitude. Am J Med Sci 2001;322(2):68–70.

17. Waalen J, Buxbaum JN. Is older colder or colder older? The association of age with body temperature in 18,630 individuals. J Gerontol A Biol Sci Med Sci 2011; 66(5):487–92.

18. High KP, Bradley SF, Gravenstein S, et al. Clinical practice guideline for the evaluation of fever and infection in older adult residents of long-term care facilities: 2008 update by the Infectious Diseases Society of America. Clin Infect Dis 2009; 48(2):149–71.

19. Singler K, Bertsch T, Heppner HJ, et al. Diagnostic accuracy of three different methods of temperature measurement in acutely ill geriatric patients. Age Ageing 2013;42(6):740–6.

20. Marco CA, Schoenfeld CN, Hansen KN, et al. Fever in geriatric emergency patients: clinical features associated with serious illness. Ann Emerg Med 1995; 26(1):18–24.

21. Tiruvoipati R, Ong K, Gangopadhyay H, et al. Hypothermia predicts mortality in critically ill elderly patients with sepsis. BMC Geriatr 2010;10:70.

22. Martin GS, Mannino DM, Moss M. The effect of age on the development and outcome of adult sepsis. Crit Care Med 2006;34(1):15–21.

23. Mayr FB, Yende S, Linde-Zwirble WT, et al. Infection rate and acute organ dysfunction risk as explanations for racial differences in severe sepsis. JAMA 2010;303(24):2495–503.

24. Opal SM, Girard TD, Ely EW. The immunopathogenesis of sepsis in elderly patients. Clin Infect Dis 2005;41(Suppl 7):S504–12.

25. Krabbe KS, Bruunsgaard H, Qvist J, et al. Hypotension during endotoxemia in aged humans. Eur J Anaesthesiol 2001;18(9):572–5.

26. Inoue S, Suzuki-Utsunomiya K, Okada Y, et al. Reduction of immunocompetent T cells followed by prolonged lymphopenia in severe sepsis in the elderly. Crit Care Med 2013;41(3):810–9.

27. Inoue S, Suzuki K, Komori Y, et al. Persistent inflammation and T cell exhaustion in severe sepsis in the elderly. Crit Care 2014;18(3):R130.

28. Kumar A, Ellis P, Arabi Y, et al. Initiation of inappropriate antimicrobial therapy results in a fivefold reduction of survival in human septic shock. Chest 2009; 136(5):1237–48.

29. Gaieski DF, Edwards JM, Kallan MJ, et al. Benchmarking the incidence and mortality of severe sepsis in the United States. Crit Care Med 2013;41(5):1167–74.

30. Walkey AJ, Wiener RS, Lindenauer PK. Utilization patterns and outcomes associated with central venous catheter in septic shock: a population-based study. Crit Care Med 2013;41(6):1450–7.

31. Angus DC, Linde-Zwirble WT, Lidicker J, et al. Epidemiology of severe sepsis in the United States: analysis of incidence, outcome, and associated costs of care. Crit Care Med 2001;29(7):1303–10.

32. Ginde AA, Moss M, Shapiro NI, et al. Impact of older age and nursing home residence on clinical outcomes of US emergency department visits for severe sepsis. J Crit Care 2013;28(5):606–11.

33. Wester AL, Dunlop O, Melby KK, et al. Age-related differences in symptoms, diagnosis and prognosis of bacteremia. BMC Infect Dis 2013;13:346.

34. Lee CC, Chen SY, Chang IJ, et al. Comparison of clinical manifestations and outcome of community-acquired bloodstream infections among the oldest old, elderly, and adult patients. Medicine (Baltimore) 2007;86(3):138–44.

35. Green JE, Ariathianto Y, Wong SM, et al. Clinical and inflammatory response to bloodstream infections in octogenarians. BMC Geriatr 2014;14:55.

36. Girard TD, Opal SM, Ely EW. Insights into severe sepsis in older patients: from epidemiology to evidence-based management. Clin Infect Dis 2005;40(5): 719–27.

37. El Solh AA, Akinnusi ME, Alsawalha LN, et al. Outcome of septic shock in older adults after implementation of the sepsis "bundle". J Am Geriatr Soc 2008;56(2): 272–8.

38. Dellinger RP, Levy MM, Rhodes A, et al. Surviving Sepsis Campaign: international guidelines for management of severe sepsis and septic shock: 2012. Crit Care Med 2013;41(2):580–637.

39. Liang SY, Kumar A. Empiric antimicrobial therapy in severe sepsis and septic shock: optimizing pathogen clearance. Curr Infect Dis Rep 2015;17(7):493.

40. Paul M, Shani V, Muchtar E, et al. Systematic review and meta-analysis of the efficacy of appropriate empiric antibiotic therapy for sepsis. Antimicrob Agents Chemother 2010;54(11):4851–63.

41. Kumar A, Roberts D, Wood KE, et al. Duration of hypotension before initiation of effective antimicrobial therapy is the critical determinant of survival in human septic shock. Crit Care Med 2006;34(6):1589–96.

42. Ferrer R, Artigas A, Suarez D, et al. Effectiveness of treatments for severe sepsis: a prospective, multicenter, observational study. Am J Respir Crit Care Med 2009;180(9):861–6.

43. Gaieski DF, Mikkelsen ME, Band RA, et al. Impact of time to antibiotics on survival in patients with severe sepsis or septic shock in whom early goal-directed therapy was initiated in the emergency department. Crit Care Med 2010;38(4): 1045–53.

44. Ferrer R, Martin-Loeches I, Phillips G, et al. Empiric antibiotic treatment reduces mortality in severe sepsis and septic shock from the first hour: results from a guideline-based performance improvement program. Crit Care Med 2014; 42(8):1749–55.
45. Weant KA, Baker SN. Emergency medicine pharmacists and sepsis management. J Pharm Pract 2013;26(4):401–5.
46. Rivers E, Nguyen B, Havstad S, et al. Early goal-directed therapy in the treatment of severe sepsis and septic shock. N Engl J Med 2001;345(19):1368–77.
47. Investigators A, Group ACT, Peake SL, et al. Goal-directed resuscitation for patients with early septic shock. N Engl J Med 2014;371(16):1496–506.
48. Pro CI, Yealy DM, Kellum JA, et al. A randomized trial of protocol-based care for early septic shock. N Engl J Med 2014;370(18):1683–93.
49. Mouncey PR, Osborn TM, Power GS, et al. Trial of early, goal-directed resuscitation for septic shock. N Engl J Med 2015;372(14):1301–11.
50. Rajapakse S, Rajapakse A. Age bias in clinical trials in sepsis: how relevant are guidelines to older people? J Crit Care 2009;24(4):609–13.
51. Potasman I, Grupper M. Leukemoid reaction: spectrum and prognosis of 173 adult patients. Clin Infect Dis 2013;57(11):e177–81.
52. Macdonald SP, Arendts G, Fatovich DM, et al. Comparison of PIRO, SOFA, and MEDS scores for predicting mortality in emergency department patients with severe sepsis and septic shock. Acad Emerg Med 2014;21(11):1257–63.
53. Lee WJ, Woo SH, Kim DH, et al. Are prognostic scores and biomarkers such as procalcitonin the appropriate prognostic precursors for elderly patients with sepsis in the emergency department? Aging Clin Exp Res 2015. [Epub ahead of print].
54. Cheng H, Fan WZ, Wang SC, et al. N-terminal pro-brain natriuretic peptide and cardiac troponin I for the prognostic utility in elderly patients with severe sepsis or septic shock in intensive care unit: a retrospective study. J Crit Care 2015; 30(3):654.e6-14.
55. Wang H, Li Z, Yin M, et al. Combination of acute physiology and chronic health evaluation II score, early lactate area, and N-terminal prohormone of brain natriuretic peptide levels as a predictor of mortality in geriatric patients with septic shock. J Crit Care 2015;30(2):304–9.
56. Iwashyna TJ, Cooke CR, Wunsch H, et al. Population burden of long-term survivorship after severe sepsis in older Americans. J Am Geriatr Soc 2012;60(6): 1070–7.
57. Iwashyna TJ, Ely EW, Smith DM, et al. Long-term cognitive impairment and functional disability among survivors of severe sepsis. JAMA 2010;304(16):1787–94.
58. Iwashyna TJ, Netzer G, Langa KM, et al. Spurious inferences about long-term outcomes: the case of severe sepsis and geriatric conditions. Am J Respir Crit Care Med 2012;185(8):835–41.
59. Prescott HC, Langa KM, Liu V, et al. Increased 1-year healthcare use in survivors of severe sepsis. Am J Respir Crit Care Med 2014;190(1):62–9.
60. Osler W. The principles and practice of medicine. 15th edition. New York: Appleton-Century Company, Inc.; 1994.
61. Jackson ML, Neuzil KM, Thompson WW, et al. The burden of community-acquired pneumonia in seniors: results of a population-based study. Clin Infect Dis 2004;39(11):1642–50.
62. Jackson ML, Nelson JC, Jackson LA. Risk factors for community-acquired pneumonia in immunocompetent seniors. J Am Geriatr Soc 2009;57(5):882–8.

63. Riquelme R, Torres A, el-Ebiary M, et al. Community-acquired pneumonia in the elderly. Clinical and nutritional aspects. Am J Respir Crit Care Med 1997;156(6): 1908–14.
64. Metlay JP, Schulz R, Li YH, et al. Influence of age on symptoms at presentation in patients with community-acquired pneumonia. Arch Intern Med 1997;157(13): 1453–9.
65. Fernandez-Sabe N, Carratala J, Roson B, et al. Community-acquired pneumonia in very elderly patients: causative organisms, clinical characteristics, and outcomes. Medicine (Baltimore) 2003;82(3):159–69.
66. Ewig S, Klapdor B, Pletz MW, et al. Nursing-home-acquired pneumonia in Germany: an 8-year prospective multicentre study. Thorax 2012;67(2):132–8.
67. Polverino E, Dambrava P, Cilloniz C, et al. Nursing home-acquired pneumonia: a 10 year single-centre experience. Thorax 2010;65(4):354–9.
68. Gutierrez F, Masia M, Mirete C, et al. The influence of age and gender on the population-based incidence of community-acquired pneumonia caused by different microbial pathogens. J Infect 2006;53(3):166–74.
69. Jain S, Self WH, Wunderink RG, et al. Community-acquired pneumonia requiring hospitalization among U.S. adults. N Engl J Med 2015;373(5):415–27.
70. El-Solh AA, Aquilina AT, Dhillon RS, et al. Impact of invasive strategy on management of antimicrobial treatment failure in institutionalized older people with severe pneumonia. Am J Respir Crit Care Med 2002;166(8):1038–43.
71. Miyashita N, Kawai Y, Tanaka T, et al. Detection failure rate of chest radiography for the identification of nursing and healthcare-associated pneumonia. J Infect Chemother 2015;21(7):492–6.
72. Mandell LA, Wunderink RG, Anzueto A, et al. Infectious Diseases Society of America/American Thoracic Society consensus guidelines on the management of community-acquired pneumonia in adults. Clin Infect Dis 2007;44(Suppl 2): S27–72.
73. Fine MJ, Auble TE, Yealy DM, et al. A prediction rule to identify low-risk patients with community-acquired pneumonia. N Engl J Med 1997;336(4):243–50.
74. Ewig S, Kleinfeld T, Bauer T, et al. Comparative validation of prognostic rules for community-acquired pneumonia in an elderly population. Eur Respir J 1999; 14(2):370–5.
75. Yealy DM, Auble TE, Stone RA, et al. Effect of increasing the intensity of implementing pneumonia guidelines: a randomized, controlled trial. Ann Intern Med 2005;143(12):881–94.
76. Renaud B, Coma E, Labarere J, et al. Routine use of the Pneumonia Severity Index for guiding the site-of-treatment decision of patients with pneumonia in the emergency department: a multicenter, prospective, observational, controlled cohort study. Clin Infect Dis 2007;44(1):41–9.
77. Lim WS, van der Eerden MM, Laing R, et al. Defining community acquired pneumonia severity on presentation to hospital: an international derivation and validation study. Thorax 2003;58(5):377–82.
78. Man SY, Lee N, Ip M, et al. Prospective comparison of three predictive rules for assessing severity of community-acquired pneumonia in Hong Kong. Thorax 2007;62(4):348–53.
79. Chalmers JD, Singanayagam A, Akram AR, et al. Severity assessment tools for predicting mortality in hospitalised patients with community-acquired pneumonia. Systematic review and meta-analysis. Thorax 2010;65(10):878–83.
80. Aujesky D, McCausland JB, Whittle J, et al. Reasons why emergency department providers do not rely on the pneumonia severity index to determine the

initial site of treatment for patients with pneumonia. Clin Infect Dis 2009;49(10): e100–108.

81. Chalmers JD, Rother C, Salih W, et al. Healthcare-associated pneumonia does not accurately identify potentially resistant pathogens: a systematic review and meta-analysis. Clin Infect Dis 2014;58(3):330–9.

82. Houck PM, Bratzler DW, Nsa W, et al. Timing of antibiotic administration and outcomes for Medicare patients hospitalized with community-acquired pneumonia. Arch Intern Med 2004;164(6):637–44.

83. Ochoa-Gondar O, Vila-Corcoles A, de Diego C, et al. The burden of community-acquired pneumonia in the elderly: the Spanish EVAN-65 study. BMC Public Health 2008;8:222.

84. Calle A, Marquez MA, Arellano M, et al. Geriatric assessment and prognostic factors of mortality in very elderly patients with community-acquired pneumonia. Arch Bronconeumol 2014;50(10):429–34.

85. Neupane B, Walter SD, Krueger P, et al. Predictors of in-hospital mortality and re-hospitalization in older adults with community-acquired pneumonia: a prospective cohort study. BMC Geriatr 2010;10:22.

86. Wyrwich KW, Yu H, Sato R, et al. Observational longitudinal study of symptom burden and time for recovery from community-acquired pneumonia reported by older adults surveyed nationwide using the CAP Burden of Illness Questionnaire. Patient Relat Outcome Meas 2015;6:215–23.

87. Caterino JM, Weed SG, Espinola JA, et al. National trends in emergency department antibiotic prescribing for elders with urinary tract infection, 1996-2005. Acad Emerg Med 2009;16(6):500–7.

88. Marques LP, Flores JT, Barros Junior Ode O, et al. Epidemiological and clinical aspects of urinary tract infection in community-dwelling elderly women. Braz J Infect Dis 2012;16(5):436–41.

89. Eriksson I, Gustafson Y, Fagerstrom L, et al. Prevalence and factors associated with urinary tract infections (UTIs) in very old women. Arch Gerontol Geriatr 2010;50(2):132–5.

90. Griebling TL. Urologic diseases in America project: trends in resource use for urinary tract infections in men. J Urol 2005;173(4):1288–94.

91. Laupland KB, Ross T, Pitout JD, et al. Community-onset urinary tract infections: a population-based assessment. Infection 2007;35(3):150–3.

92. Caljouw MA, den Elzen WP, Cools HJ, et al. Predictive factors of urinary tract infections among the oldest old in the general population. A population-based prospective follow-up study. BMC Med 2011;9:57.

93. Caterino JM, Ting SA, Sisbarro SG, et al. Age, nursing home residence, and presentation of urinary tract infection in U.S. emergency departments, 2001-2008. Acad Emerg Med 2012;19(10):1173–80.

94. Juthani-Mehta M, Quagliarello V, Perrelli E, et al. Clinical features to identify urinary tract infection in nursing home residents: a cohort study. J Am Geriatr Soc 2009;57(6):963–70.

95. Barkham TM, Martin FC, Eykyn SJ. Delay in the diagnosis of bacteraemic urinary tract infection in elderly patients. Age Ageing 1996;25(2):130–2.

96. Arinzon Z, Shabat S, Peisakh A, et al. Clinical presentation of urinary tract infection (UTI) differs with aging in women. Arch Gerontol Geriatr 2012;55(1):145–7.

97. Ha YE, Kang CI, Joo EJ, et al. Clinical implications of healthcare-associated infection in patients with community-onset acute pyelonephritis. Scand J Infect Dis 2011;43(8):587–95.

98. De Vecchi E, Sitia S, Romano CL, et al. Aetiology and antibiotic resistance patterns of urinary tract infections in the elderly: a 6-month study. J Med Microbiol 2013;62(Pt 6):859–63.
99. Fagan M, Lindbaek M, Grude N, et al. Antibiotic resistance patterns of bacteria causing urinary tract infections in the elderly living in nursing homes versus the elderly living at home: an observational study. BMC Geriatr 2015; 15:98.
100. Juthani-Mehta M, Tinetti M, Perrelli E, et al. Role of dipstick testing in the evaluation of urinary tract infection in nursing home residents. Infect Control Hosp Epidemiol 2007;28(7):889–91.
101. Gordon LB, Waxman MJ, Ragsdale L, et al. Overtreatment of presumed urinary tract infection in older women presenting to the emergency department. J Am Geriatr Soc 2013;61(5):788–92.
102. Wilson ML, Gaido L. Laboratory diagnosis of urinary tract infections in adult patients. Clin Infect Dis 2004;38(8):1150–8.
103. Mody L, Juthani-Mehta M. Urinary tract infections in older women: a clinical review. JAMA 2014;311(8):844–54.
104. Gupta K, Hooton TM, Naber KG, et al. International clinical practice guidelines for the treatment of acute uncomplicated cystitis and pyelonephritis in women: a 2010 update by the Infectious Diseases Society of America and the European Society for Microbiology and Infectious Diseases. Clin Infect Dis 2011;52(5): e103–120.
105. Lutters M, Vogt-Ferrier NB. Antibiotic duration for treating uncomplicated, symptomatic lower urinary tract infections in elderly women. Cochrane Database Syst Rev 2008;(3):CD001535.
106. Marwick C, Santiago VH, McCowan C, et al. Community acquired infections in older patients admitted to hospital from care homes versus the community: cohort study of microbiology and outcomes. BMC Geriatr 2013;13:12.
107. D'Agata E, Loeb MB, Mitchell SL. Challenges in assessing nursing home residents with advanced dementia for suspected urinary tract infections. J Am Geriatr Soc 2013;61(1):62–6.
108. Ginde AA, Rhee SH, Katz ED. Predictors of outcome in geriatric patients with urinary tract infections. J Emerg Med 2004;27(2):101–8.
109. Tal S, Guller V, Levi S, et al. Profile and prognosis of febrile elderly patients with bacteremic urinary tract infection. J Infect 2005;50(4):296–305.
110. Thigpen MC, Whitney CG, Messonnier NE, et al. Bacterial meningitis in the United States, 1998-2007. N Engl J Med 2011;364(21):2016–25.
111. Lai WA, Chen SF, Tsai NW, et al. Clinical characteristics and prognosis of acute bacterial meningitis in elderly patients over 65: a hospital-based study. BMC Geriatr 2011;11:91.
112. Domingo P, Pomar V, de Benito N, et al. The spectrum of acute bacterial meningitis in elderly patients. BMC Infect Dis 2013;13:108.
113. Cabellos C, Verdaguer R, Olmo M, et al. Community-acquired bacterial meningitis in elderly patients: experience over 30 years. Medicine (Baltimore) 2009; 88(2):115–9.
114. Erdem H, Kilic S, Coskun O, et al. Community-acquired acute bacterial meningitis in the elderly in Turkey. Clin Microbiol Infect 2010;16(8):1223–9.
115. Weisfelt M, van de Beek D, Spanjaard L, et al. Community-acquired bacterial meningitis in older people. J Am Geriatr Soc 2006;54(10):1500–7.

16. Magazzini S, Nazerian P, Vanni S, et al. Clinical picture of meningitis in the adult patient and its relationship with age. Intern Emerg Med 2012;7(4):359–64.

17. Wang AY, Machicado JD, Khoury NT, et al. Community-acquired meningitis in older adults: clinical features, etiology, and prognostic factors. J Am Geriatr Soc 2014;62(11):2064–70.

18. Tunkel AR, Hartman BJ, Kaplan SL, et al. Practice guidelines for the management of bacterial meningitis. Clin Infect Dis 2004;39(9):1267–84.

19. Brouwer MC, McIntyre P, Prasad K, et al. Corticosteroids for acute bacterial meningitis. Cochrane Database Syst Rev 2015;(9):CD004405.

20. Tunkel AR, Glaser CA, Bloch KC, et al. The management of encephalitis: clinical practice guidelines by the Infectious Diseases Society of America. Clin Infect Dis 2008;47(3):303–27.

121. Hjalmarsson A, Blomqvist P, Skoldenberg B. Herpes simplex encephalitis in Sweden, 1990-2001: incidence, morbidity, and mortality. Clin Infect Dis 2007; 45(7):875–80.

122. Poissy J, Wolff M, Dewilde A, et al. Factors associated with delay to acyclovir administration in 184 patients with herpes simplex virus encephalitis. Clin Microbiol Infect 2009;15(6):560–4.

123. Sili U, Kaya A, Mert A, HSV Encephalitis Study Group. Herpes simplex virus encephalitis: clinical manifestations, diagnosis and outcome in 106 adult patients. J Clin Virol 2014;60(2):112–8.

124. Hebant B, Miret N, Bouwyn JP, et al. Absence of pleocytosis in cerebrospinal fluid does not exclude herpes simplex virus encephalitis in elderly adults. J Am Geriatr Soc 2015;63(6):1278–9.

125. Schoonman GG, Rath JJ, Wirtz PW, et al. Herpes simplex virus encephalitis without cerebrospinal fluid pleocytosis is not unusual. J Am Geriatr Soc 2012; 60(2):377–8.

126. Weil AA, Glaser CA, Amad Z, et al. Patients with suspected herpes simplex encephalitis: rethinking an initial negative polymerase chain reaction result. Clin Infect Dis 2002;34(8):1154–7.

127. Erdem H, Cag Y, Ozturk-Engin D, et al. Results of a multinational study suggest the need for rapid diagnosis and early antiviral treatment at the onset of herpetic meningoencephalitis. Antimicrob Agents Chemother 2015;59(6):3084–9.

128. Raschilas F, Wolff M, Delatour F, et al. Outcome of and prognostic factors for herpes simplex encephalitis in adult patients: results of a multicenter study. Clin Infect Dis 2002;35(3):254–60.

129. Whitley RJ, Alford CA, Hirsch MS, et al. Vidarabine versus acyclovir therapy in herpes simplex encephalitis. N Engl J Med 1986;314(3):144–9.

130. McNamara DR, Tleyjeh IM, Berbari EF, et al. Incidence of lower-extremity cellulitis: a population-based study in Olmsted county, Minnesota. Mayo Clin Proc 2007;82(7):817–21.

131. Tsan L, Davis C, Langberg R, et al. Prevalence of nursing home-associated infections in the Department of Veterans Affairs nursing home care units. Am J Infect Control 2008;36(3):173–9.

132. Stevens DL, Bisno AL, Chambers HF, et al. Practice guidelines for the diagnosis and management of skin and soft tissue infections: 2014 update by the Infectious Diseases Society of America. Clin Infect Dis 2014;59(2): 147–59.

133. Reddy M, Gill SS, Wu W, et al. Does this patient have an infection of a chronic wound? JAMA 2012;307(6):605–11.

134. Khor HM, Tan J, Saedon NI, et al. Determinants of mortality among older adults with pressure ulcers. Arch Gerontol Geriatr 2014;59(3):536–41.
135. Bulger EM, May A, Bernard A, et al. Impact and progression of organ dysfunction in patients with necrotizing soft tissue infections: a multicenter study. Surg Infect (Larchmt) 2015;16(6):694–701.

# Evaluation and Management of Chest Pain in the Elderly

Rohit Gupta, MD*, Robert Munoz, MD

## KEYWORDS

- Geriatric • Elderly • Chest pain • Acute coronary syndrome • Aortic dissection
- Pulmonary embolism • Pneumothorax • Esophageal perforation

## KEY POINTS

- Causes of chest pain in the elderly are common and life threatening. Acute coronary syndromes are the leading cause of death worldwide. Aortic dissection is rare but life threatening.
- This article discusses presentation, diagnosis, and treatment of acute coronary syndromes, aortic dissection, pulmonary embolism, pneumothorax, and esophageal perforation in the elderly.
- The elderly frequently present atypically and suffer greater morbidity and mortality owing to being frail and comorbid, but benefit from aggressive treatment.

Chest pain is the second most common chief complaint accounting for more than 6 million visits annually to emergency departments (EDs) in the United States.[1] The elderly make up a significant percentage of our population comprising 14.1% of the US population in 2013.[1] This percentage is expected to increase as the United States ages and longevity increases. Fifteen percent of all ED visits are made by those over 65 years of age.[2] An extensive differential diagnosis from benign illnesses to life-threatening disorders must be considered in patients with chest pain. Many disease entities tend to present in an atypical fashion in the elderly.

The evaluation and management of chest pain must be initiated rapidly. Within 10 minutes of arrival, in addition to vital signs, the elderly patient with chest pain should receive an electrocardiogram, the single most important test in identifying life threats.[3] If unstable, stabilization should be initiated using basic life support and advanced cardiac life support. In stable patients, the physician should complete a thorough history and physical examination. Based on the results of the initial evaluation,

Disclosure Statement: The authors have nothing to disclose.
Department of Emergency Medicine, Advocate Christ Medical Center, 4440 West 95th Street, Oak Lawn, IL 60453, USA
* Corresponding author.
E-mail address: rogu_md@yahoo.com

Emerg Med Clin N Am 34 (2016) 523–542
http://dx.doi.org/10.1016/j.emc.2016.04.006
0733-8627/16/$ – see front matter © 2016 Elsevier Inc. All rights reserved.

emed.theclinics.com

appropriate testing and treatment should be started. While these tests are being performed, additional history and chart review can be performed to narrow and reorder the differential diagnosis.

The elderly typically have multiple comorbidities and less physiologic reserve—the elderly are often frail—increasing morbidity and mortality for many conditions. Consequently, a more extensive diagnostic workup is usually required in the elderly patient with a complaint of chest pain and often the final cause of chest pain will not be established in the ED, but will require additional evaluation. The careful ED physician should maintain a high index of suspicion for acute, life-threatening emergencies.

The differential diagnosis for chest pain in the elderly is broad. **Table 1** lists a complete differential organized by acuity and organ system. Several diagnoses are far more likely in the elderly than in younger patients. Cardiac etiologies are not the most common cause but account for the greatest mortality. The remainder of this article focuses on the presentation, diagnosis, and management of 5 causes of chest pain: acute coronary syndrome (ACS), aortic dissection, pulmonary embolism (PE), pneumothorax, and esophageal rupture.

## ACUTE CORONARY SYNDROME

Ischemic heart disease is the leading killer in the world claiming 7,000,000 lives annually and accounting for 12.7% of all deaths.[4] Its incidence and lethality increases dramatically with age. The elderly over age 75, account for 33% of all episodes of ACS and 60% of deaths.[5] Age is a powerful predictor of adverse events from ACS with the risk of death increasing by 70% with each decade increase of age.[6] Being both common and deadly, the emergency provider must consider ACS early and evaluate carefully in geriatric patients with chest pain. The diagnosis and management of ACS in the elderly is similar to that in younger patients, focusing on accurate, early diagnosis and aggressive management.

### Definition

ACS applies to a spectrum of diseases resulting from abrupt reduction in blood flow to the myocardium that cause symptoms attributable to myocardial ischemia, dysfunction, and infarction. ACS refers to diseases that are high risk, that mandate aggressive therapy, but that cannot always be distinguished at initial presentation. The term encompasses (1) unstable angina (UA), acute ischemia without infarction; (2) non–ST-elevation myocardial infarction, a similar pathophysiology in which ischemia progresses to infarction, and (3) ST-elevation myocardial infarction (STEMI),

| Table 1 Causes of chest pain | | |
|---|---|---|
| **Organ System** | **High Acuity** | **Lower Acuity** |
| Cardiovascular | Acute coronary syndrome Aortic dissection Aortic aneurysm | Angina Pericarditis Myocarditis |
| Pulmonary | Tension pneumothorax Pneumonia | — |
| GastroIntestinal | Esophageal perforation Esophagitis | GERD/gastro-peptic Biliary disease |
| Chest wall | — | Costochondritis Rib fractures/trauma Herpes zoster |

he acute closure of a coronary vessel causing transmural infarction and that is amenable to emergent reperfusion. In their 2014 guideline update, the American Heart Association (AHA) and American College of Cardiology (ACC) combined UA and non–STEMI, using the term non–ST-elevation ACS (NSTE-ACS), thus recognizing that UA and non–STEMI exist on a continuum with indistinguishable initial presentations and identical management.[3]

## Presentation

Chest pain is the most frequent chief complaint of elderly patients with ACS. Features of the pain that suggest ACS include radiation to both arms, pain similar to episodes of prior ischemia, and a changing pattern of pain over the prior 24 hours.[7] Response of the pain to nitroglycerin is not helpful in ruling in or out ACS. A pleuritic description reduces the risk. The frequency of chest pain at presentation decreases substantially in the elderly. In the National Registry of Myocardial Infarction, chest pain as chief complain decreases from 77% of patients younger than 65 years, to 50% between 65 and 75, to only 40% in patients greater than 85 years of age.[6] In the Global Registry of Acute Coronary Events (GRACE) the frequency of atypical presentation defined as not having chest pain at presentation increases from 5.3% in patients less than 65 years, to 12.3% between 65 and 75, to 14.3% in patients greater than 85 years of age.[8]

Importantly, ACS in the elderly often presents with other complaints. In the GRACE dataset, primary complaints in the elderly without chest pain include dyspnea (49%), diaphoresis (26%), nausea and vomiting (24%), and syncope (19%).[8] Other common complaints include weakness and delirium. In the elderly, atypical presentations of ACS are common. The physician must maintain a high index of suspicion.

The diagnosis of myocardial infarction (MI) is also complicated by the presence of comorbid conditions. ACS can develop in the elderly who have hemodynamic stress from another acute illness such as exacerbation of congestive heart failure (CHF), sepsis, pneumonia, exacerbation of chronic obstructive pulmonary disease (COPD), or a fall. The clinical presentation of the acute illness may predominate.

Traditional risk factors for coronary artery disease include smoking, hypertension, hyperlipidemia, and diabetes mellitus. Age is an important independent risk factor. Although traditional risk factors adequately assess for lifetime risk of coronary artery disease, they are less useful at predicting an ACS. The most predictive risk factors are a history of abnormal prior stress test and peripheral artery disease.[7]

The physical examination findings for ACS are nonspecific. Hypotension may signal the presence of cardiogenic shock, an ominous sign. Signs of acute CHF, including crackles, greater jugular venous distention, and peripheral edema may indicate severe ischemic compromise and increase risk of mortality. Reproducible pain on palpation does decrease the likelihood of ACS, but does not exclude it.[7]

## Diagnostic Testing

### Electrocardiograph

The single most important test to diagnose an ACS is the electrocardiograph (ECG). It should be obtained and interpreted in every elderly patient with chest pain within 10 minutes of presentation.[3] It should also be obtained early in elderly patients with a variety of other complaints, as detailed above. The diagnosis of STEMI is made based on the ECG. The diagnosis of NSTE-ACS may be suggested. A normal ECG reduces the risk of an ACS but does not rule it out.

Interpretation of the ECG in the elderly can be challenging because the elderly tend to have abnormalities at baseline. Prior MI, left ventricular hypertrophy, bundle branch blocks, nonspecific ST-T changes, and atrial fibrillation complicate ECG analysis. An old ECG should be obtained for comparison to determine whether abnormalities are new. The proportion of NSTE-ACS patients in the National Registry of Myocardial Infarction presenting with nondiagnostic ECGs increases from 23% in patients less than 65 years to 43% in patients greater than 85 years.[6]

The diagnosis of STEMI is equally complicated in the elderly. In the National Registry of Myocardial Infarction, ST segment elevation was present on the ECG of 96.3% of STEMI patients younger than age 65 but only 69.9% of those greater than age 85.[9] An left bundle branch block, obscuring ECG analysis, was present in 5% of younger patients but 33.8% of those greater than 85 years of age.[9]

### Cardiac enzymes

Biochemical markers provide useful diagnostic and prognostic information in the elderly. A low threshold should be maintained to check biomarkers given the variability of presentation. Released after myocardial cell necrosis, enzyme elevation distinguishes MI from UA and a pattern of rising biomarkers over hours marks the acuity.

Troponin I and T are contractile proteins found only in cardiac myocytes. Being exquisitely sensitive and reasonably specific for acute MI, troponins have become the gold standard for the diagnosis of MI. Troponins appear within 6 hours of infarction and remain elevated for 4 to 8 days. Sensitivity is only 50% when measured within 4 hours of symptom onset, but increases to greater than 95% after 8 hours.[10]

Troponin assays are excellent diagnostic tools, but elevated levels must be interpreted in the clinical setting and do not diagnose ACS independently. Ischemic elevation not owing to ACS may result from demand ischemia from tachyarrhythmias, hypoxia, hypoperfusion, and sepsis. Nonischemic elevation may be owing to CHF, hypertension, stroke, PE, or renal failure.[11]

Providing prognostic information in addition to diagnostic, troponin elevation in ACS is associated independently with worse outcomes, including death. A metaanalysis of almost 19,000 ACS patients, both STEMI and NSTE-ACS, found a 30 day odds ratio of 3.4 for death or MI with elevated troponin.[12]

### Risk Stratification

The immediate goal of every chest pain evaluation is to rapidly decide whether a patient is having an ACS. The decision is not an easy one. Missed or mistreated ACS is the leading cause of malpractice payout against emergency physicians. Consequently, most emergency physicians make the decision conservatively. After the initial evaluation patients should be placed into 1 of 4 working groups: definite ACS, probable ACS, probably not ACS, or definitely not ACS.

With a working diagnosis of definite or probable ACS, the EP must further risk stratify to optimally treat. Patients with an STEMI are in the highest risk group. The NSTE-ACS patients should be further risk stratified using validated scoring instruments such as the HEART score and the GRACE score.

The HEART score is a prospectively derived and widely validated scoring system that can be used to risk stratify undifferentiated chest pain patients predicting the 6-week risk of major adverse cardiovascular events.[13] The score is calculated by awarding points for features of History, ECG changes, Age, Risk factors, and initial Troponin and varies between 0 and 10 points. Scores from 0 to 3 are considered low risk and predict less than 2% risk of major adverse cardiovascular events and may be managed as outpatients. Elderly patients receive 2 points just for being older than 65 years. Most elderly patients have at least 1 risk factor and so very few elderly patients are classified as low risk.

The GRACE 2.0 score is another well-validated scoring system designed to predict in-hospital, 1-year, and 3-year mortality in patients with ACS.[14] Containing 8 variably weighted inputs, including age, heart rate, systolic blood pressure, CHF severity, creatinine, ECG changes, cardiac arrest, and cardiac enzyme elevation, the GRACE score is best calculated using an online calculator (eg, the one at http://gracescore.org). The GRACE score does not help to determine whether an undifferentiated ED patient has an ACS; rather, in patients with definite or probable ACS, it predicts risk and guides therapy. The ACC/AHA guidelines recommend GRACE score cutoffs when selecting therapy.

Risk stratification is a dynamic process. Accurate risk stratification guides the speed, type, and invasiveness of therapy matching higher risk, higher resource intensity therapy with higher risk patients. Patients in the probably not ACS and definitely not ACS category should be evaluated for alternate causes of chest pain.

## Management

Detailed guidelines have been published jointly by the ACC/AHA for the treatment of STEMI[15] and NSTE-ACS.[3] The guidelines are up to date, evidence based, and widely available. There is a paucity of data to guide treatment of ACS in the elderly. **Table 2** summarize the classification of recommendations in the guidelines.

## Overview of Therapy

Geriatric patients with ACS should be treated as aggressively as younger patients using the entire spectrum of guideline determined medical therapy including antiischemic, antiplatelet, and anticoagulation therapy. Elderly patients with STEMI should be immediately reperfused using percutaneous coronary intervention (PCI) or fibrinolysis. For NSTE-ACS, aggressive medical therapy followed by either an early invasive strategy or a more moderate ischemia-guided strategy is recommended.[3] Treatment in the elderly, who are often frail, should be individualized and take into account the patient's goals, comorbidities, functional and cognitive status, and life expectancy.

## Antiischemic Therapy

Antiischemic therapy aims to increase oxygen supply and decrease myocardial demand by decreasing workload. Oxygen should be administered for signs of hypoxemia including an $O_2$ saturation of less than 90%, respiratory distress, or cyanosis. Although recommended in the past for all patients, the benefit of oxygen for normoxic patients in ACS is being questioned.[16]

Nitrates reduce ischemia by reducing myocardial oxygen demand. Nitrates act by dilating coronary arteries, increasing blood flow; by dilating capacitance vessels, decreasing preload; and by dilating arterial circulation, decreasing afterload. Although

| Table 2 | |
| --- | --- |
| **Classification of recommendations by the American Heart Association/American College of Cardiology** | |
| Class I | There is evidence of general agreement that the treatment is useful and effective |
| Class II | There is conflicting evidence of divergence of opinion |
| IIa | The weight of evidence favors utility–efficacy |
| IIb | Utility–efficacy is less well-established |
| Class III | There is evidence of general agreement that the treatment is neither useful nor effective and may be harmful |

no studies have demonstrated direct survival benefit in the elderly, nitrates reduce anginal symptoms and their use is supported by extensive clinical experience. ACS patients with continuing ischemic pain and without contraindications should receive sublingual and intravenous nitroglycerin (class I).[3] Nitrates also treat exacerbations of common comorbid conditions including heart failure and hypertension. Nitrates should not be used in patients who have taken a phosphodiesterase inhibitor, such as sildenafil, or in patients with hypotension.

In addition to potent analgesic and anxiolytic properties, morphine may reduce cardiac workload by reducing heart rate and systolic blood pressure. Evidence supporting the use of morphine is limited. Clinical experience supports the use of morphine for analgesia in ACS (class IIB).[3]

Beta-blockers reduce ischemia and cardiac oxygen demand by reducing heart rate, contractility, and blood pressure. Beta-blockers prevent recurrent ischemia and life-threatening ventricular arrhythmias. Unfortunately, as demonstrated in the ClOpidogrel and Metoprolol in Myocardial Infarction (COMMIT) trial, early intravenous beta-blockade increases the risk of cardiogenic shock.[17] Recommendations on the use of beta-blockers have moderated. Intravenous use of beta-blockers may cause harm in patients with risk factors for shock (class III) including age greater than 70 years, heart rate greater than 110 bpm, systolic blood pressure greater than 120 mm Hg, and late presentation.[3] With age being an independent risk factor, the use of intravenous beta-blockers in the ED in the elderly is no longer routinely recommended.

### Antiplatelet Therapy

The data supporting the use of aspirin (ASA) is irrefutable. The benefits of ASA therapy extend across all age groups and its use is strongly recommended (class I for NSTE-ACS and STEMI).[3,15] Clopidogrel should be used in place of ASA in intolerant patients.

Thienopyridine class antiplatelet agents ($P2Y_{12}$ receptor inhibitors) interrupt platelet aggregation and formation and progression of thrombosis. The guidelines support the use of a $P2Y_{12}$ receptor inhibitor, either clopidogrel or ticagrelor, in addition to ASA as early as possible or at the time of PCI in STEMI and NSTE-ACS patients (class I).[3,15] For patients with UA, the Clopidogrel in Unstable angina to prevent Recurrent Events (CURE) trial established an absolute risk reduction of 2% and a relative risk reduction of 13.1% in patients greater than 65 years with the addition of clopidogrel.[18] Ticagrelor is favored over clopidogrel in NSTE-ACS (class IIa).[3] By binding reversibly, ticagrelor allows faster recovery of platelet function when discontinued and may cause fewer bleeding complications if a patient is referred for coronary artery bypass surgery. The use of prasugrel, another $P2Y_{12}$ receptor inhibitor, may cause harm (class III for STEMI), excess bleeding, in patients with a history of prior stroke or transient ischemic attack and did not show benefit in patients greater than 75 years of age.[19]

Additional antiplatelet therapy with glycoprotein IIb/IIIa inhibitors works by blocking the glycoprotein IIb/IIIa receptor, the final common and obligate pathway in platelet aggregation. In the most recent guidelines, there are no class I recommendations for their use in STEMI or NSTE-ACS.[3,15] The decision to use glycoprotein IIb/IIIa inhibitors should be made in conjunction with cardiology only when an early invasive strategy is selected and may be better initiated in the catheterization laboratory.[20] If used in the elderly, dosing must be managed carefully; excess dosing is common.

### Anticoagulation Therapy

Anticoagulation therapy in addition to antiplatelet therapy is recommended for patients without contraindications regardless of age for both STEMI and NSTE-ACS class I).[3,15] Anticoagulation therapy has traditionally used unfractionated heparin to inactivate thrombin and factor Xa indirectly by activating antithrombin. The use of heparin in STEMI and NSTE-ACS is well-supported.[3,15]

Low-molecular-weight heparin (LMWH), consisting of only the short chain polysaccharides of heparin, was approved in the late nineties and works indirectly by primarily inactivating factor Xa. The use of LMWH in the treatment of NSTE-ACS was established by the Efficacy and Safety of Subcutaneous Enoxaparin in Non-Q wave Coronary Events (ESSENCE) trial, which suggested that enoxaparin is superior to heparin,[21] especially in the elderly. The use of LMWH in STEMI treated with fibrinolysis is recommended though dosage should be adjusted in patients greater than age 75 years. LMWH is not recommended in STEMI patients treated with PCI.

Bivalirudin, an intravenous direct thrombin inhibitor, is now available and commonly used during PCI. In STEMI patients undergoing PCI, bivalirudin decreases 30-day cardiac mortality (1.8% vs 2.9%) and all-cause mortality (2.1% vs 3.1%) versus heparin and a GPIIb/IIIa inhibitor.[22] The benefit is attributable to a decreased rate of major bleeding.[22] For NSTE-ACS, the ACUITY trial demonstrated a benefit versus heparin and a GPIIb/IIIa inhibitor also owing to less major bleeding.[23] A recent study comparing bivalirudin with heparin or LMWH in ACS did not show benefit.[24] Upstream use in the ED and use in the elderly of direct thrombin inhibitors is not well-studied.

The risk of bleeding owing to anticoagulation in ACS is increased in the elderly. Consequently, anticoagulation should be reserved for higher risk patients who are in the definite ACS group. All elderly patients who are given anticoagulation are exposed to the risks of bleeding; however, only those with a true ACS benefit. Because only about 10% of the nearly 8,000,000 patients who are evaluated for chest pain are found to have an ACS,[7] a liberal anticoagulation policy may cause harm.

## Reperfusion Therapy

### ST-elevation myocardial infarction

For STEMI, the ED must select and initiate delivery of the reperfusion strategy. Reperfusion is the priority and time is muscle. All patients regardless of age with an STEMI should receive reperfusion therapy with symptom onset within 12 hours (class I) and up to 24 hours with symptom or ECG evidence of continuing ischemia (class IIa).[15] PCI with a door to balloon time of less than 90 minutes is preferred (class I).[15] Transfer for PCI should be arranged if the initial medical contact to balloon time can be kept at less than 120 minutes (class I).[15] If PCI is unavailable, fibrinolytic therapy should be administered within 30 minutes of hospital arrival (class I).[15]

Compared with thrombolytics, PCI is more effective at opening the target vessel, lowers the risk of recurrent ischemia and reocclusion, and is safer with less intracerebral bleeding. In the elderly, PCI reduces both short and long term mortality.[5] A meta-analysis of 10 trials showed that PCI reduces mortality by 50% in the elderly greater than age 70 years when compared with thrombolysis.[25]

Thrombolysis, although less beneficial than PCI, is superior to medical management. A reanalysis of a large dataset that included elderly patients receiving fibrinolysis according to modern guidelines showed a mortality benefit in the elderly greater than age 75 years that extended to patients greater than age 85 years.[26]

### Non–ST-elevation acute coronary syndrome

In patients with NSTE-ACS the same urgency to initiate reperfusion is not present. Most importantly reperfusion with fibrinolysis is contraindicated (class III).[3] The

ACC/AHA guidelines recognize 2 treatment pathways for NSTE-ACS. The early invasive strategy triages all patients to an invasive diagnostic evaluation with coronary angiography. The ischemia guided pathway calls for maximal medical management and invasive evaluation for those patients who fail medical therapy. The initial ED management is identical for both pathways and focuses on alleviating symptoms and minimizing infarction by providing optimal antiischemic, antiplatelet, and anticoagulation therapy.

Management decisions including the strategy used and the timing to intervention must be made in conjunction with cardiology. For the early invasive strategy, the ED specialist must be aware of indications for immediate reperfusion within 2 hours with PCI in NSTE-ACS patients. The indications are refractory angina despite treatment, signs, and symptoms of heart failure, hemodynamic instability, and sustained ventricular arrhythmia.[3]

Because they are sicker, elderly patients likely derive greater benefit from an early invasive strategy than their younger counterparts. In patients with NSTE-ACS greater than age 65 years, an early invasive strategy compared with an ischemia-guided strategy significantly reduces the rate of death or MI at 30 days (5.7% vs 9.8%) and 6 months (8.8% vs 13.6%). The benefit is even greater in patients greater than age 75 years (10.8% vs 21.6%), but the risk of major bleeding also increases (16.6% vs 6.5%).[27] Despite strong evidence of benefit, age is the best predictor of not receiving early invasive management.[3]

### Prognosis

The prognosis for the elderly with ACS is significantly worse than for younger patients. According to registry data, the 30-day mortality increases from 2% for patients with NSTE-ACS who are younger than 65, to 5% for patients between the ages of 65 and 74, to 8% from 75 to 84, to 15% for patients greater than age 85 years.[6] For STEMI, the 30-day mortality rate increased 10-fold from 3% for patients less than 65% to 30% for those greater than age 85 years.[9]

## AORTIC DISSECTION

An aortic dissection is a rare but life-threatening condition that can occur in the elderly. It is reported to occur at an incidence of 2.9 per 100,000 person-years.[28] It is a devastating illness that must be diagnosed early and managed aggressively to improve survival.

### Definition and Classification

An aortic dissection is defined as a tear in the intimal layer of the aortic wall with subsequent propagation of blood between the intimal and medial layers. The Stanford classification system, a common system used to differentiate aortic dissection, classifies dissections into type A or type B. A type A dissection is one that involves the ascending aorta, whereas type B dissections are localized to the descending aorta.[29]

### Epidemiology

Aortic dissections are most common in the elderly with a peak incidence in the seventh decade of life.[30] Unlike in younger patients, where collagen vascular diseases are major risk factors, the most important risk factor in the elderly is chronic hypertension. In the International Registry of Acute Aortic Dissection (IRAD), hypertension was present in more than 70% of patients with aortic dissection.[30] Other risk factors, common in the elderly, include atherosclerosis, bicuspid aortic valve, known aortic aneurysm, and previous aortic valve replacement.

## History and Physical Examination

The most common presenting symptom, present in 90% of patients with aortic dissection, is severe pain.[30] In the majority of cases, the pain is abrupt in onset and located in the chest. Back pain and abdominal pain are also reported at a lesser frequency. Unlike typically taught, "tearing" or "ripping" pain is not the most common descriptor of the pain. Sharp pain was cited more frequently.

The location of the dissection also seems to influence the sensation of pain. Type A dissections seem more likely to present with anterior chest pain, whereas type B dissections more frequently present with back or abdominal pain. Age plays a role in the perception of pain, with the elderly experiencing pain differently. Migratory pain, syncope, and focal neurologic deficits are also possible presenting symptoms but are less common.[31]

Physical examination findings can be highly variable depending on the location and extent of the dissection. Hypertension is a common vital sign abnormality; however, one-quarter of type A dissections may present initially with hypotension. Pulse deficits, defined as unequal or delayed pulses, were found to be present in 15% of patients.[30] Type A dissections are associated with an aortic insufficiency murmur 40% to 50% of the time.[29] They can also be associated with acute onset heart failure and cardiac tamponade.[30] Less commonly, neurologic deficits caused by a stroke from extension of the dissection into the carotid artery or by spinal cord ischemia can occur.[30]

## Initial Diagnostic Tests

Diagnosing aortic dissection requires a high index of suspicion. The relatively rare nature of this disease and the large differential diagnosis associated with chest pain makes this diagnosis challenging. The 2010 AHA guidelines delineated a risk-stratifying tool for patients suspected of aortic dissection (**Table 3**).[32] If concern for an aortic dissection is present, further diagnostic modalities are usually required for evaluation. The diagnostic modalities used are determined by the physician's pretest probability for acute aortic dissection.

### Electrocardiograph

Although usually abnormal in patients with aortic dissection, no ECG findings are pathognomonic. Common findings include nonspecific ST-segment or T-wave changes, left ventricular hypertrophy, or the presence of Q waves.[30] The ECG is most important to assess for ACS. ECGs may have most utility in ruling out more common diagnosis such as STEMI.

**Table 3**
**Risk assessment in aortic dissection**

| Predisposing Risk Factors | High-Risk Pain Features | High Risk Exam Features |
|---|---|---|
| Marfan syndrome<br>Connective tissue disease<br>Family history aortic disease<br>Known aortic valve disease<br>Recent aortic manipulation<br>Known thoracic aortic aneurysm | Chest back or abdominal pain described as: Abrupt in onset/severe in intensity and Ripping/tearing/sharp or stabbing quality | Evidence of perfusion deficit<br>Pulse deficit<br>Systolic BP differential<br>Focal stroke deficit<br>Murmur of aortic insufficiency (new and with pain)<br>Shock state or hypotension |

### D-Dimer

Speculation has gone into using a D-dimer level in the evaluation for aortic dissection. An elevated D-dimer is thought to indicate intravascular blood coagulation and fibrinolysis. Recent studies have been performed to evaluate whether a negative D-dimer can reliably rule out the presence of an aortic dissection. A recent systematic review and metaanalysis suggested that a negative D-dimer might be sufficient to rule out an aortic dissection in low risk patients.[33] D-Dimer testing is not sufficient in moderate to high-risk patients, however. Further studies to validate the safety of this strategy are still needed.

### Chest radiograph

Abnormalities on the chest radiograph are present in the majority of dissections. The most common abnormality is a widened mediastinum. Other radiographic abnormalities include an abnormal aortic contour, an abnormal cardiac contour, pleural effusions, or displaced calcification of the aorta.[30] Abnormalities on the chest radiography, unfortunately, are neither sensitive nor specific enough to diagnose an aortic dissection.

### Helical computed tomography

A computed tomography (CT) scan is the most commonly used imaging modality when evaluating for a dissection.[30] New multirow detector CT scans are very accurate at detecting aortic dissections. Recent data suggest a sensitivity of 99% and a specificity of 100%.[34] There are multiple advantages toward obtaining a CT scan: It is readily available in most EDs, it is relatively quick, it is noninvasive, it is not user dependent, and it can evaluate potentially for alternative diagnoses. Disadvantages include the need for a potentially unstable patient to leave the ED and exposing the patient to a contrast and radiation load.

### MRI

MRI is another, noninvasive, accurate imaging modality that may be used. It has a reported sensitivity of 100% for type A dissections and 96.5% for type B dissections. Specificity was reported as 98.6% for type A and 100% for type B dissection.[35] MRI may be beneficial in elderly patients who have contraindications to contrast-enhanced CT scan. However, certain limitations do exist. MRI is not readily available in all EDs. An MRI also takes longer than a CT scan to perform and potentially unstable patients would have to be out of the ED for a longer period of time.

### Echocardiography

Transesophageal echocardiography is an imaging modality that can be performed directly in the ED. It is fast and extremely accurate. A sensitivity of 98% and a specificity of 95% for the diagnosis of dissection have been reported.[36] When available, a transesophageal echocardiography may be the ideal imaging modality. Limited availability, however, is its major limitation. Transesophageal echocardiography requires the presence of experienced operators. The need for sedation in patients who may be hemodynamically unstable is another limitation.

In contrast, the use of transthoracic echocardiography exclusively is inadequate for diagnosis. It has a reported sensitivity of 59% and specificity of 83%.[36]

### Aortography

Aortography, the traditional gold standard, has largely been supplanted by other imaging modalities. In the IRAD database, aortography was only performed in 4% of patients.[30] It had a sensitivity of 88% and a specificity of 94%.[37] Major limitations include being time consuming, invasive, labor intensive, and expensive.

## Management

Early and aggressive management in aortic dissection is imperative for survival. A cardiothoracic surgeon should be notified as soon as the diagnosis is made, regardless of the location of dissection. Aggressive blood pressure and heart rate management is crucial. Elevated blood pressure and increased heart rate are thought to increase aortic wall stress, leading to further propagation and expansion of the dissection. The ACC/AHA guidelines published in 2010 recommend a heart rate goal of 60 bpm or less and a systolic blood pressure goal of 100 to 120 mm Hg.[32]

Intravenous beta-blockers are typically recommended as first-line agents to achieve these goals. Labetalol has the advantage of having α activity, in addition to β activity, thereby offering effective heart rate and blood pressure control with one agent. Esmolol is fast acting and has a very short half-life, making it more attractive for patients with potential contraindications.

A second antihypertensive agent is commonly required for optimal blood pressure control. A vasodilator, such as nitroprusside, is commonly recommended as a second-line agent. It is imperative to use to rate control agent before starting a vasodilator. Initial therapy with a vasodilator may cause a reflex tachycardia, leading to increased wall stress and further propagation of the dissection. Pain control with an opioid analgesic is also indicated. Uncontrolled pain leads to sympathetic activation resulting in blood pressure and heart rate elevation.

Definitive treatment of an aortic dissection depends on multiple factors, most important, the type of the dissection. Type A dissections are considered a surgical emergency. Operative treatment should not be restricted to younger patients; elderly patients seem to benefit.[31] In contrast, type B dissections are typically managed nonoperatively. Indications for surgical repair include persistent pain, aortic expansion, progression of the dissection, ischemia of end organs owing to arterial blockage from the dissection, and uncontrolled hypertension.

Patients with aortic dissection should be transferred to the intensive care unit for further monitoring and management.

## PULMONARY EMBOLISM

A PE must always be considered in the evaluation of an elderly patient with undifferentiated chest pain. The incidence of PE increases significantly as a person ages.[38] PEs are also associated with higher mortality in the elderly with age greater than 70 years being an independent risk factor for death.[39] Other risk factors frequently present in the elderly that are associated with PE include CHF, COPD, malignancy, and immobilization from previous stroke, surgery, or frailty.

## Presentation

As with many disease entities in geriatrics, presentation of PE can be variable. Classically, the most common symptom is dyspnea either at rest or with exertion. In 1 large prospective study, dyspnea was present in 76% of all patients with PE. Patients greater than 70 of age, however, reported it only 66% of the time.[40] Likewise, pleuritic chest pain was reported in 46% of patients younger than 70 compared with 35% in those older than 70. Two-pillow orthopnea was also more common in the younger cohort. Physical examination findings are nonspecific in PE. Tachypnea is present in 46% to 73% of cases.[40,41] Less commonly, patients may be tachycardic and may wheeze, cough, or have hemoptysis.

### Risk Stratification

The decision to pursue further evaluation for a PE should be determined by a patient's pretest probability based on the history and physical examination. A risk stratification tool, such as the Wells score, a well-validated instrument to assist in assigning the pretest probability, should be used.[42] As expected, with age the prevalence of a high pretest probability increases and that of a low pretest probability decreases. The performance of these risk stratification tools in the elderly however, seems to be similar to that in the younger population and their use in the elderly is recommended.[43] The clinical gestalt of an experienced ED physician successfully assigns pretest risk, as successfully as a validated tool.

### Diagnosis

Most diagnostic algorithms recommend the use of a D-dimer for low- to moderate-risk patients. A level of less than 500 ng/mL in most assays used is considered negative and makes a PE highly unlikely. The specificity of D-dimer in the elderly, however, is greatly decreased, resulting in many false-positive results. One study showed that the specificity for venous thromboembolism decreased from 70% in those younger than 40 years to 25% in those older than 60 years to less than 5% in those greater than 80 years of age.[44]

To make the test more useful in the elderly, an age-adjusted threshold may be used in patients over the age of 50. A prospective study, defining the age-adjusted cutoff as age × 10, demonstrated a failure rate of only 0.3% in patients whose D-dimer was greater than the usual cutoff but less than the age-adjusted threshold. Further, the study demonstrated a 5-fold increase in the proportion of patients over age 75 ruled out for PE.[45] Although an age adjusted D-dimer shows promise, there is need for further validation before it can be widely used.

Low-risk patients with a positive D-dimer or higher risk patients must be evaluated further for PE. CT pulmonary angiography is a common imaging modality used to diagnose PE. Its diagnostic accuracy does not seem to be affected by a patient's age.[46] Elderly patients, however, have an increased rate of renal insufficiency, which may preclude the use of CT pulmonary angiography. If a CT scan is negative for PE the diagnosis is considered ruled out.

A ventilation/perfusion (V/Q) scan is another modality that is commonly used. It is an alternative in patients who cannot undergo CT pulmonary angiography. Patients with a normal V/Q scan are ruled out. Low-, intermediate-, and high-risk V/Q scan results are interpreted according to the patient's pretest probability. Concordant results are considered diagnosed. Discordant results are nondiagnostic. Unfortunately, in the elderly higher rates of nondiagnostic V/Q scans are present.[47]

Other imaging modalities may be used if the initial studies are nondiagnostic. Options include traditional pulmonary angiography, MR pulmonary angiography, or lower extremity compression ultrasound examination. Many algorithms make a presumptive diagnosis of PE if a patient with intermediate to high probability for PE has a positive ultrasound examination.

### Treatment

Hemodynamically unstable patients with a presumptive or definitive diagnosis of PE should be treated with emergent thrombectomy or thrombolysis. Age greater than 75 years, however, is considered a relative contraindication to thrombolytics based on the increased rate of major bleeding in this population.[48] One study found that patients greater than 70 years of age had a 4-fold increase in the rate of major bleeding compared with those less than 50 years of age. It also found that the risk of major bleeding increases by 4% every year.[49] Thus, the use of thrombolytic therapy in the elderly patient with an acute PE should be considered carefully before administration. Other absolute and relative contraindications to thrombolysis are listed in **Box 1**.[50]

Hemodynamically stable patients with a PE should be treated with anticoagulation. In addition to age, other risk factors for bleeding that may preclude treatment include cancer, renal insufficiency, hepatic insufficiency, diabetes, prior cardiovascular accident, and frequent falls. When anticoagulation is appropriate, the College of Chest Physicians recommends the initiation of LMWH or fondaparinux over unfractionated heparin.[48] For patients who are high risk, treatment with anticoagulation should be started when the diagnosis is considered. Treatment should not be delayed until the diagnosis is confirmed.

Pulmonary embolus is a life-threatening condition. Elderly patients with PE who ate unstable hemodynamically, have massive PE, signs of heart strain, or significant comorbidity should be admitted to the intensive care unit.

## PNEUMOTHORAX

Pneumothorax, a cause of chest pain that can be life threatening, must be considered in geriatric patients. A pneumothorax is defined as the presence of air in the pleural space, a potential space between the visceral and parietal pleura that normally lie in

---

**Box 1**
**Absolute and relative contraindications to thrombolysis**

*Absolute*

- Prior intracranial hemorrhage
- Known structural intracranial cerebrovascular disease (ie, arteriovenous malformation)
- Malignant intracranial neoplasm
- Ischemic stroke within 3 months
- Suspected aortic dissection
- Active bleeding or bleeding diathesis
- Recent surgery encroaching on spinal canal or brain
- Recent significant closed head or facial trauma with radiological evidence of fracture or brain damage.

*Relative*

- On anticoagulation medication
- Noncompressible vascular punctures
- Traumatic or prolonged cardiopulmonary resuscitation (>10 minutes)
- Internal bleeding within 2 to 4 weeks
- History of uncontrolled hypertension
- Systolic blood pressure of greater than 180 mm Hg or diastolic blood pressure greater than 110 mm Hg
- Dementia
- Ischemic stroke greater than 3 months ago
- Major surgery in last 3 weeks.

close apposition. A pneumothorax may be spontaneous, iatrogenic or traumatic. A spontaneous pneumothorax (SP) occurs in the absence of an external precipitating cause. A primary SP occurs in individuals without lung disease. The incidence of a primary SP is 5 to 15 cases per 100,000 population.[51] A secondary SP complicates diseased lungs, most often in patients with COPD, asthma, or malignancy. The incidence of secondary SP is 2 to 6 cases per 100,000 population.[51] The frequency of secondary SP increases in the elderly because of increased comorbidity. A tension pneumothorax refers to any pneumothorax where the intrathoracic pressure builds up enough to exceed atmospheric pressure, compress the lung, and impair cardiac function. It is a true emergency.

### History and Physical Examination

The symptoms of a primary SP typically begin suddenly while at rest. Chest pain and dyspnea are common, but may be subtle. The chest pain may be pleuritic. Sudden onset, pleuritic chest pain was present in less than 20% of elderly patients with SP, but in almost two-thirds of younger patients.[52] Cough is common. Subtle symptoms often improve and delayed presentations are common. The most common finding on physical examination is sinus tachycardia. A large pneumothorax may present with decreased or absent breath sounds and hyperresonance to percussion. A small SP may be impossible to detect on physical examination.

A secondary SP usually presents with significant symptoms suggesting decompensation of the underlying medical condition. The addition of the pneumothorax to already diminished pulmonary reserve causes a significant decline. Dyspnea is generally present and may be severe. Ipsilateral chest pain is common.[51] Symptoms rarely resolve on their own. In secondary SP, the physical examination demonstrates findings attributable to the underlying medical condition. Hypoxia and cyanosis may be present. A pneumothorax should be considered immediately in elderly patients with decompensated COPD or asthma. The diagnosis in secondary SP can be challenging because findings often overlap with findings of the underlying medical condition.

A patient with a tension pneumothorax usually presents in extremis with severe dyspnea and chest pain. Signs of asphyxia with cyanosis and hypoxia, and cardiogenic shock with hypotension may be present. Tension pneumothorax may culminate in cardiac arrest, especially a pulseless electrical activity arrest. The diagnosis of tension pneumothorax should be made on the basis of clinical findings alone.

### Diagnostic Testing

The diagnosis of pneumothorax is made typically with chest radiography. The typical appearance is that of a thin pleural line running parallel to but separated from the chest wall by an area free of all lung markings. In the elderly with comorbidity, interpretation of the chest radiograph can be complicated by lung scarring, bullous changes, and fibrosis.

Thoracic ultrasound imaging can rapidly and accurately diagnose pneumothorax at the bedside.[53] In a normal lung, closely approximated parietal and visceral pleura will slide against each other creating a shimmering appearance. Absence of sliding at the pleural line confirms the diagnosis of pneumothorax.

A CT scan of the chest is considered the gold standard for diagnosis.

### Treatment

The treatment of a tension pneumothorax is an emergency and should be initiated as soon as the diagnosis is reasonably certain. Treatment should not be delayed for radiographic confirmation. Needle decompression to relieve tension should be performed as a temporizing measure by placing a large angiocath in the midclavicular line of the second intercostal space. Definitive management with tube thoracostomy should be performed as soon as possible to definitively relieve tension and prevent recurrence.

Stable patients with an initial episode of primary SP may be managed with observation and placement on 100% oxygen therapy. Oxygen increases pleural air absorption by a factor of 3 or 4. Patients who fail conservative therapy, patients with recurrent pneumothoraces, and patients with secondary SP should be definitively managed with tube thoracostomy. Common complications of chest tube placement include incorrect placement, pleural infection, and prolonged pain. In the elderly, a persistent air leak is seen in 85% of patients receiving tube thoracostomy. Intraoperative pleurodesis during tube placement may be warranted to reduce the complication.[54] Generally, the elderly, being frail, should be admitted for further management.

## Prognosis

The prognosis for patients with SP is excellent with most resolving within 7 days of tube thoracostomy. Treatment failure is more common in the elderly with secondary SP and recurrent pneumothorax. Recurrences are common with recurrence rates of 33% for primary SP[55] and 39% to 47% for secondary SP.[52]

## ESOPHAGEAL PERFORATION

Esophageal perforation is a rare and life-threatening emergency. Rupture of the esophagus leads to leakage of esophageal contents into surrounding structures with devastating consequences. When evaluating an elderly patient with chest pain, one must maintain a high index of suspicion to diagnose an esophageal perforation owing to its rare occurrence and high morbidity and mortality. It has a reported age-standardized incidence of 3.1 in 1,000,000 per year.[56] Most patients who suffer from an esophageal perforation are in their 60s.[57] Mortality rates for esophageal perforations have been reported at 20%, highlighting the need for early recognition and treatment.[58]

## Presentation

Patients with an esophageal rupture can present with nonspecific signs and symptoms based on the location and depth of rupture. Chest pain is a common symptom, present in approximately 70% of patients.[56] The pain is usually abrupt in onset, is severe in nature, is worse with swallowing, and often radiates to the neck, back, and shoulders.[59] Patients may present with vomiting and hematemesis.

A recent procedural history should be obtained. Esophageal rupture is commonly iatrogenic. Responsible for 50% of cases, endoscopic and surgical procedures near the esophagus are frequently at fault.[60] Spontaneous rupture (Boerhaave's syndrome) from increased intraabdominal pressure often from vomiting is responsible for about 15% to 33% of cases.[56,57] Other less common causes include foreign body ingestions, trauma, and esophageal tumors.

Patients may seem to be septic with tachycardia, fever, and tachypnea. Crepitus, present in two-thirds of cases, indicates subcutaneous emphysema. Crepitus may be appreciated in the neck and chest regions.[61] A Hamman crunch, a rare finding on cardiac auscultation caused by subcutaneous air, may be present as a crunching sound over the anterior chest wall. If esophageal contents leak into the peritoneum, patients may present with peritonitis.

### Diagnosis

Chest radiographs may suggest the presence of an esophageal rupture with findings of a pleural effusion, subcutaneous emphysema, pneumomediastinum, or a hydropneumothorax.[61] CT of the chest is a very accurate and commonly used imaging modality to diagnose an esophageal rupture.

Definitive diagnosis may be made by a contrast esophagography. Water-soluble contrast agents, such as gastrografin, should be used over barium to prevent barium-mediated inflammation of the mediastinum.[56]

### Treatment

Early management and resuscitation is critical in patients with an esophageal rupture. A delay in treatment for greater than 24 hours has been shown in multiple studies to increase morbidity and mortality significantly.[62] Patients should be given intravenous fluids and signs of shock should be addressed. All patients should be made NPO. Early intravenous antibiotic administration with broad-spectrum antimicrobial coverage is crucial. Esophageal rupture is considered a surgical emergency and a surgical consultation should be obtained in all patients diagnosed with an esophageal rupture. A subset of patients may be managed nonoperatively.[63] The decision should be made in consultation with surgery. Most patients with an esophageal rupture should be further managed and monitored in an intensive care unit.

### SUMMARY

Geriatric patients are at increased risk for serious morbidity and mortality from life-threatening causes of chest pain. As the geriatric population grows, providing care to this high risk population will require increasing resources. This article covers 5 life-threatening causes of chest pain in the elderly: ACS, aortic dissection, PE, pneumothorax, and esophageal rupture. The atypical presentations, the frailty, and the significant comorbidities that characterize the elderly simply make the diagnosis and treatment of these already complicated conditions even more complicated. The emergency provider must be vigilant and maintain a low threshold to test. When a diagnosis is made, treatment must be aggressive. The elderly benefit from optimal care.

### REFERENCES

1. Administration on Aging, Administration for Community Living. A profile of older Americans: 2014. Washington, DC: U.S. Department of Health and Human Services; 2014.
2. Albert M, McCaig LF, Ashman JJ. Emergency department visits by persons aged 65 and over: United States, 2009–2010. NCHS data brief, no 130. Hyattsville (MD): National Center for Health Statistics; 2013.
3. Amsterdam EA, Wenger NK, Brindis RG, et al. 2014 ACC/AHA guideline for the management of patients with non–ST-elevation acute coronary syndromes: a report of the American College of Cardiology/American Heart Association Task Force on Practice Guidelines. Circulation 2014;130:e344–426.
4. Finegold JA, Asaria P, Francis DP. Mortality from ischaemic heart disease by country, region, and age: Statistics from World Health Organisation and United Nations. Int J Cardiol 2013;168(2):934–45.
5. Jokhadar M, Wenger NK. Review of the treatment of acute coronary syndrome in elderly patients. Clin Interv Aging 2009;4:435–44.

6. Alexander KP, Newby LK, Cannon CP, et al. Acute coronary care in the elderly, part I non-ST-segment-elevation acute coronary syndrome. Circulation 2007; 115:2549–69.

7. Fanaroff AC, Rymer JA, Goldstein SA, et al. Does this patient with chest pain have acute coronary syndrome? The rational clinical examination systematic review. JAMA 2015;314(18):1955–65.

8. Brieger D, Eagle KA, Goodman SG, et al. Acute coronary syndromes without chest pain, an underdiagnosed and undertreated high-risk group: insights from the Global Registry of Acute Coronary Events. Chest 2004;126:46146–9.

9. Alexander KP, Newby LK, Armstrong PW, et al. Acute coronary care in the elderly, part II ST-segment-elevation myocardial infarction. Circulation 2007;115:2570–89.

10. Antman EM, Grudzien C, Sacks DB. Evaluation of a rapid bedside assay for detection of serum cardiac troponin T. JAMA 1995;273(16):1279–82.

11. Newby L, Jesse RL, Babb JD, et al. ACCF 2012 expert consensus document on practical clinical considerations in the interpretation of troponin elevations: a report of the American College of Cardiology foundation task force on clinical expert consensus documents. J Am Coll Cardiol 2012;60(23):2427–63.

12. Ottani F, Galvani M, Nicolini FA, et al. Elevated cardiac troponin levels predict the risk of adverse outcome in patients with acute coronary syndromes. Am Heart J 2000;140(6):917.

13. Backus BE, Six AJ, Kelder JC, et al. A prospective validation of the HEART score for chest pain patients at the emergency department. Int J Cardiol 2013;168(3):2153–8.

14. Fox KA, Dabbous OH, Goldberg RJ, et al. Prediction of risk of death and myocardial infarction in the six months after presentation with acute coronary syndrome: prospective multinational observational study (GRACE). BMJ 2006;333(7578):1091.

15. O'Gara PT, Kushner FG, Ascheim DD, et al. 2013 ACCF/AHA guideline for the management of ST-elevation myocardial infarction: a report of the American College of Cardiology Foundation/American Heart Association Task Force on practice guidelines. Circulation 2013;127:e362–425.

16. Cabello JB, Burls A, Emparanza JI, et al. Oxygen therapy for acute myocardial infarction. Cochrane Database Syst Rev 2010;(8):CD007160.

17. Chen ZM, Pan HC, Chen YP, et al. Early intravenous then oral metoprolol in 45852 patients with acute myocardial infarction: randomized placebo controlled trial. Lancet 2005;366:1622–32.

18. Yusuf S, Zhao F, Mehta SR, et al. CURE Investigators. Effects of clopidogrel in addition to aspirin in patients with acute coronary syndromes without ST segment elevation. N Engl J Med 2001;345:494–502.

19. Wiviott SD, Braunwald E, McCabe CH, et al. Prasugrel versus clopidogrel for acute coronary syndromes without revascularization. N Engl J Med 2007;357:2001–15.

20. Stone GW, Bertrand ME, Moses JW, et al. Routine upstream initiation vs deferred selective use of glycoprotein IIb/IIIa inhibitors in acute coronary syndromes: the ACUITY timing trial. JAMA 2007;297(6):591–602.

21. Cohen M, Demers C, Gurfinkel EP, et al. A comparison of low-molecular-weight heparin with unfractionated heparin for unstable coronary artery disease. Efficacy and Safety of Subcutaneous Enoxaparin in Non-Q-Wave Coronary Events Study Group. N Engl J Med 1997;337:447–52.

22. Stone GW, Witzenbichler B, Guagliumi G, et al, HORIZONS-AMI Trial Investigators. Bivalirudin during primary PCI in acute myocardial infarction. N Engl J Med 2008;358(21):2218–30.

23. Stone GW, McLaurin BT, Cox DA, et al, for the ACUITY Investigators. Bivalirudin for patients with acute coronary syndromes. N Engl J Med 2006;355:2203–16.

24. Valgimigli M, Frigoli E, Leonardi S, et al. Bivalirudin or unfractionated heparin in acute coronary syndromes. N Engl J Med 2015;373:997–1009.

25. Zijlstra F, Patel A, Jones M, et al. Clinical characteristics and outcome of patients with early (<2 h), intermediate (2–4 h) and late (>4 h) presentation treated by primary coronary angioplasty or thrombolytic therapy for acute myocardial infarction. Eur Heart J 2002;23:550.

26. White HD. Thrombolytic therapy in the elderly. Lancet 2000;356:2028–30.

27. Bach RG, Cannon CP, Weintraub WS, et al. The effect of routine, early invasive management on outcome for elderly patients with non-ST-segment elevation acute coronary syndromes. Ann Intern Med 2004;141(3):186–95.

28. Meszaros I, Morocz J, Szlavi J, et al. Epidemiology and clinicopathology of aortic dissection. Chest 2000;117:1271–8.

29. Nienaber CA, Eagle KA. Aortic dissection: new frontiers in diagnosis and management: Part I: from etiology to diagnostic strategies. Circulation 2003;108: 628–35.

30. Hagan PG, Nienaber CA, Isselbacher EM, et al. The international registry of acute aortic dissection (IRAD): new insights into an old disease. JAMA 2000;283: 897–903.

31. Golledge J, Eagle KA. Acute aortic dissection. Lancet 2008;372:55–66.

32. Hiratzka LF, Bakris GL, Beckman JA, et al. 2010 ACCF/AHA/AATS/ACR/ASA/ SCA/SCAI/SIR/STS/SVM guidelines for the diagnosis and management of patients with Thoracic Aortic Disease: a report of the American College of Cardiology Foundation/American Heart Association Task Force on Practice Guidelines, American Association for Thoracic Surgery, American College of Radiology, American Stroke Association, Society of Cardiovascular Anesthesiologists, Society for Cardiovascular Angiography and Interventions, Society of Interventional Radiology, Society of Thoracic Surgeons, and Society for Vascular Medicine. Circulation 2010;121:e266–369.

33. Asha SE, Miers JW. A systematic review and meta-analysis of D-dimer as a rule-out test for suspected acute aortic dissection. Ann Emerg Med 2015;66:368–78.

34. Hayter RG, Rhea JT, Small A, et al. Suspected aortic dissection and other aortic disorders: multi-detector row CT in 373 cases in the emergency setting. Radiology 2006;238:841–52.

35. Hartnell G, Costello P. The diagnosis of thoracic aortic dissection by noninvasive imaging procedures. N Engl J Med 1993;328:1637–8.

36. Keren A, Kim CB, Hu BS, et al. Accuracy of biplane and multiplane transesophageal echocardiography in diagnosis of typical acute aortic dissection and intramural hematoma. J Am Coll Cardiol 1996;28:627–36.

37. Cigarroa JE, Isselbacher EM, DeSanctis RW, et al. Diagnostic imaging in the evaluation of suspected aortic dissection. Old standards and new directions. N Engl J Med 1993;328:35–43.

38. Silverstein MD, Heit JA, Mohr DN, et al. Trends in the incidence of deep vein thrombosis and pulmonary embolism: A 25-year population-based study. Arch Intern Med 1998;158:585–93.

39. Goldhaber S. Acute pulmonary embolism: clinical outcomes in the international cooperative pulmonary embolism registry (ICOPER). Lancet 1999;353:1386–9.

40. Stein PD, Beemath A, Matta F, et al. Clinical characteristics of patients with acute pulmonary embolism: data from PIOPED II. Am J Med 2007;120:871-9.

41. Masotti L, Ray P, Righini M, et al. Pulmonary embolism in the elderly: a review on clinical, instrumental and laboratory presentation. Vasc Health Risk Manag 2008; 4:629-36.

42. Wells PS, Anderson DR, Rodger M, et al. Excluding pulmonary embolism at the bedside without diagnostic imaging: management of patients with suspected pulmonary embolism presenting to the emergency department by using a simple clinical model and D-dimer. Ann Intern Med 2001;135:98-107.

43. Righini M, Le Gal G, Perrier A, et al. Effect of age on the assessment of clinical probability of pulmonary embolism by prediction rules. J Thromb Haemost 2004;2:1206-8.

44. Harper PL, Theakston E, Ahmed J, et al. D-dimer concentration increases with age reducing the clinical value of the D-dimer assay in the elderly. Intern Med J 2007;37:607-13.

45. Righini M, Van Es J, Den Exter PL, et al. Age-adjusted D-dimer cutoff levels to rule out pulmonary embolism: the ADJUST-PE study. JAMA 2014;311:1117-24.

46. Stein PD, Beemath A, Quinn DA, et al. Usefulness of multidetector spiral computed tomography according to age and gender for diagnosis of acute pulmonary embolism. Am J Cardiol 2007;99:1303-5.

47. Calvo-Romero JM, Lima-Rodriguez BM, Bureo-Dacal P, et al. Predictors of an intermediate ventilation/perfusion lung scan in patients with suspected pulmonary embolism. Eur J Emerg Med 2005;12:129-31.

48. Kearon C, Akl EA, Comerota AJ, Prandoni P, Bounameaux H, Goldhaber SZ, et al. Antithrombotic therapy for VTE disease: antithrombotic therapy and prevention of thrombosis, 9th ed: American College of Chest Physicians evidence-based clinical practice guidelines. Chest 2012;141:e419S-94S.

49. Mikkola KM, Patel SR, Parker JA, et al. Increasing age is a major risk factor for hemorrhagic complications after pulmonary embolism thrombolysis. Am Heart J 1997;134:69-72.

50. Jaff MR, McMurtry MS, Archer SL, et al, American Heart Association Council on Cardiopulmonary, Critical Care, Perioperative and Resuscitation, American Heart Association Council on Peripheral Vascular Disease, American Heart Association Council on Arteriosclerosis, Thrombosis and Vascular Biology. Management of massive and submassive pulmonary embolism, iliofemoral deep vein thrombosis, and chronic thromboembolic pulmonary hypertension: a scientific statement from the American Heart Association. Circulation 2011;123:1788-830.

51. Sahn SA, Heffner JE. Spontaneous pneumothorax. N Engl J Med 2000; 342(12):868.

52. Liston R, McLoughlin R. Acute pneumothorax: a comparison of elderly with younger patients. Age Ageing 1994;353:1386-9.

53. Moore CL, Copel JA. Point-of-care ultrasonography. N Engl J Med 2011;364: 749-57.

54. Zhang Y, Jiang G, Chen C, et al. Surgical management of secondary spontaneous pneumothorax in elderly patients with chronic obstructive pulmonary disease: retrospective study of 107 cases. Thorac Cardiovasc Surg 2009;57(6): 347-52.

55. Schramel FM, Postmus PE, Vanderschueren RG. Current aspects of spontaneous pneumothorax. Eur Respir J 1997;10:1372.

56. Søreide JA, Viste A. Esophageal perforation: diagnostic work-up and clinical decision-making in the first 24 hours. Scand J Trauma Resusc Emerg Med 2011;19:66–72.
57. Bhatia P, Fortin D, Inculet RI, et al. Current concepts in the management of esophageal perforations: a twenty-seven year Canadian experience. Ann Thorac Surg 2011;92:209–15.
58. Ryom P, Ravn JB, Penninga L, et al. Aetiology, treatment and mortality after oesophageal perforation in Denmark. Dan Med Bull 2011;58:A4267.
59. Tintinalli JE. Chapter 80: esophageal emergencies, gastroesophageal reflux disease and swallowed foreign bodies. In: Tintinalli JE, editor. Tintinalli's emergency medicine: a comprehensive study guide. 7th edition. New York: McGraw-Hill; 2011. p. 551.
60. Vidarsdottir H, Blondal S, Alfredsson H, et al. Oesophageal perforations in Iceland: a whole population study on incidence, aetiology and surgical outcome. Thorac Cardiovasc Surg 2010;58:476–80.
61. Eroğlu A, Can Kürkçüoğlu İ, Karaoğlanoğlu N, et al. Esophageal perforation: the importance of early diagnosis and primary repair. Dis Esophagus 2004;17:91–4.
62. Brinster CJ, Singhal S, Lee L, et al. Evolving options in the management of esophageal perforation. Ann Thorac Surg 2004;77:1475–83.
63. Abbas G, Schuchert MJ, Pettiford BL, et al. Contemporaneous management of esophageal perforation. Surgery 2009;146:749–55.

# Dyspnea in the Elderly

Andrew R. Barbera, MD[1], Michael P. Jones, MD*

## KEYWORDS

- Elderly • Geriatric • Dyspnea • Respiratory • Congestive heart failure
- Chronic obstructive pulmonary disease • Oxygenation • Ventilation

## KEY POINTS

- Acute and Chronic Dyspnea is a frequent presentation of Elderly Patients to the Emergency Department.
- Elderly patients have several anticipated alterations in cardiac and pulmonary physiology that contribute to illness when presenting with acute dyspnea.
- Understanding the important historical and physical findings in certain diseases assist with evaluation and management of typical diseases that cause dyspnea in the elderly.

## KEYWORD DEFINITIONS

### Dyspnea

Throughout the medical literature and clinical practice, many terms and definitions are encompassed by the broad term of *dyspnea*. These descriptions range from breathlessness, to painful breathing, to air hunger, to shortness of breath. There are many more terms used by patients to try to express the symptoms that they are experiencing. To more broadly define dyspnea to fully include each individual experience this article will use the definition proposed by the American Thoracic Society: "Dyspnea is a term used to characterize a subjective experience of breathing discomfort that consists of qualitatively distinct sensations that vary in intensity."[1] Under this broad definition, each individual's personal and subjective description of any form of discomfort related to the physiologic act of breathing will be included in the term *dyspnea*.

### Elderly

Traditionally in medicine and society as a whole the term *elderly* is used to describe any person older than 65, regardless of their health or frailty score.[2] We will use this definition; however, special emphasis is given to those with elevated frailty scores or with multiple comorbid medical conditions that are prevalent in advanced age.

Disclosure statement: The authors have nothing to disclose.
Department of Emergency Medicine, Jacobi/Montefiore Medical Centers, Albert Einstein College of Medicine, 1400 Pelham Parkway South, Suite 1B-25, Bronx, NY 10461, USA
[1] Present address: 13814 Oxmoor Pl, Germantown, MD 20874.
* Corresponding author. 666 West End Avenue, #15W, New York, NY 10025.
*E-mail address:* Michael.Jones@nbhn.net

Emerg Med Clin N Am 34 (2016) 543–558
http://dx.doi.org/10.1016/j.emc.2016.04.007
0733-8627/16/$ – see front matter © 2016 Elsevier Inc. All rights reserved.
emed.theclinics.com

## INTRODUCTION

Over the last several decades, the aging population has continued to expand and grow. According to the US Census Bureau, by 2050 the elderly population is estimated to reach a staggering 20.9% of the US population with a total 83.739 million people.[3,4] With this boom of the geriatric population comes an increase in a new variety of geriatric-specific symptoms and conditions, along with an increase in encounters between the geriatric patients and acute care physicians. Among the top 3 complaints of these patients is dyspnea,[5] and with the projected increase of the geriatric population over the next 35 years, it can be expected that this number will continue to grow exponentially. With a substantial increase in this patient population, it is increasingly important to understand the unique characteristics of evaluating and treating elderly patients and specifically to understand the unique pathology and physiology of dyspnea in this patient population.

## RELEVANT PHYSIOLOGY IN THE GERIATRIC POPULATION

The growth of the aging population poses an ever-increasing need to adapt care and acute interventions while addressing the elderly patient in the acute care setting. To do this, one must first understand the differences in the physiology of the elderly patient versus the average adult patient, specifically, the physiology of the respiratory and cardiovascular system and this effect on the perception of dyspnea.

### Cardiovascular Physiology

Among the changes that occur to the cardiovascular system, several can have a direct or indirect effect on the symptoms of dyspnea.

As individuals age, the connective tissue that constitutes our cardiovascular system tends to stiffen and become less compliant.[6,7] This, in turn, leads to decreased compliance and overall stiffening of veins, arteries, and myocardium. There are consequences of this change on our cardiovascular system as a whole. Arterial stiffening causes increase in systolic hypertension and impaired impedance matching between the heart and the aorta and can lead to myocardial hypertrophy. Venous stiffening causes a decreased ability to maintain stable cardiac preload, which leads to increased volume and distribution dependence.

Myocardium stiffening can lead to diastolic heart failure. Additionally, within the myocardium, there is a stiffening and fibrosis of the cardiac skeleton, which can cause valvular, disease particularly with calcification at the base of the aortic valve.

Further effects of aging on the cardiovascular system include the decrease in the response to β-receptor stimulation. This decrease contributes to a reduced heart rate and contractile response to hypotension, exercise, and exogenous catecholamine administration.[7] Additionally, atrial pacemaker cells are reduced in function, which results in a decreased intrinsic heart rate.

These consequences of aging contribute to increased systolic blood pressures, decreased left ventricular end-diastolic volumes, decreased stroke volumes, and decreased cardiac outputs. Subsequently, the heart becomes dependent on volume status, which dampens the ability to physiologically respond to any changes within the cardiovascular system.[7]

### Respiratory Physiology

With age, the lungs undergo significant structural and physiologic changes, which include a decrease in elastic recoil and lung volumes, enlargement of air spaces, decrease in alveolar surface area, decreased compliance of chest wall, and reduction of respiratory muscle mass. These changes lead to the gradual increase of functional residual capacity, functional residual volume, and subsequently a decrease in lung vital capacity, leading to an overall decrease in physiologic reserve. The aging process also has a detrimental effect on the gas exchange properties at an alveolar level, leading to a decrease in arterial oxygenation, lower tidal volume, and reliance on higher respiratory rates.

The elderly airway receptors also undergo functional changes and become less likely to respond to medications (such as inhaled β-agonists or corticosteroids); these are commonly used in younger individuals to treat common pulmonary disorders but are less effective in the elderly population. Typically, elderly patients have a decreased sensation of dyspnea and are unable to mount rapid and appropriate responses to conditions of hypoxia or hypercapnia, increasing their susceptibility to ventilatory collapse during high demand periods (eg, heart failure, pneumonia). This process can contribute to worse outcomes than their younger counterparts.[8]

Additional changes include decrease in muscular pharyngeal support and decreased cough and swallowing reflexes. Often, these changes lead to increased risk of upper airway obstruction and aspiration, respectively.[6,9]

## APPROACH TO AN ELDERLY PATIENT WITH DYSPNEA

The evaluation and treatment of the elderly patient can be broken into 2 broad classifications that require different approaches and management in the acute care setting. These categories are the stable and the unstable patients.

## EVALUATION OF THE STABLE PATIENT

In the stable elderly patient with dyspnea, evaluation begins with the traditional approach. Before taking a history, it is often important to note the vital signs, age, and chief complaint and evaluate airway and work of breathing before proceeding to a focused history and physical examination.

### History

A general focused history of the patient is warranted and should include the following information: history of the onset, duration, and progression of symptoms. This history provides key information to the natural history of the illness and potential severity. Noting exacerbating or precipitating factors can yield diagnostic information and lead the physician toward the proper treatment modality.

Information specific to the elderly patient population that may assist with diagnostic evaluation includes the following:

- Lifetime exposures, including previous occupational environments with dust, asbestos, or noxious chemicals, may suggest underlying interstitial lung disease.[10]
- Worsening exercise tolerance or exertional dyspnea can indicate patient deconditioning or an overall cardiopulmonary disease process.[10]
- History of orthopnea (specifically note the number of pillows used at night) or increased peripheral edema can be a sign of decompensating heart failure.[10]
- Smoking history is of particular importance, as this can lead to chronic obstructive pulmonary disease, chronic bronchitis, trigger for asthma, and risk factor for coronary artery disease.
- Miscellaneous information, such as recent hospitalization or travel and a detailed medical history can assist the provider in evaluating risk factors for potential

infectious etiologies and progression or exacerbation of underlying disease, respectively.
- Information about medication changes or noncompliance may also reveal risk factors for any iatrogenic causes or exacerbation of undertreated disease.

### Physical Examination

The physical examination should focus primarily on the cardiopulmonary systems. Vital signs are of particular importance and, if abnormal, can immediately alert you to the severity of the disease (and alert the provider to the potentially unstable nature of the patient). However, as discussed above, vital signs may lag behind the progression of the disease process and should be repeated often and trended over time (with respect to both the current visit and previous visits, if the data are available). Work of breathing must also be noted along with factors that comprise it. This evaluation should include airway patency, respiratory rate, the patient's ability to speak in full sentences, any voice changes (perceived by the clinician, relatives of the patient, or the patient themselves), presence of audible respiratory noise, and the use of accessory respiratory muscles. For an experienced clinician, this evaluation takes only a moment and will guide the need for immediate or delayed intervention. The auscultation of heart and breath sounds is of great importance and provides pertinent clues as to the underlying physiology of the disease. Over-reliance on particularities of the physical examination (specifically characterizing lung sounds and the presence or absence of sounds) can potentially be avoided with the immediate availability of digital x-ray and point-of-care ultrasound scan.

Additional evaluation of the abdomen, extremities, and skin should be included in the physical examination of these patients. These can provide additional information pertinent to the cardiopulmonary system (**Table 1**).

### Adjuncts to Physical Examination

Many adjunct measures can help narrow the differential diagnosis and guide appropriate treatment during the evaluation of patients with dyspnea. These adjuncts are discussed here in order of importance and ease of obtaining. The importance of each test may change with particular disease etiologies. Additionally, availability will certainly vary based on the resources in a particular practice setting. Electrocardiogram (EKG) and chest radiograph are fast, readily available adjuncts that provide

**Table 1**
**Physical examination of stable elderly patient with dyspnea**

| Physical Examination | What to Evaluate |
| --- | --- |
| Vital signs | Heart rate, blood pressure, respiratory rate, oxygen saturation, glucose level, (end-tidal $CO_2$, if available) |
| General work of breathing | Respiratory rate, muscle use, overall patient comfort |
| Airway patency | Voice changes, secretions, edema, foreign body |
| Lung | Breath sounds, wheezing, crackles, rhonchi, rales, generalized vs focal |
| Heart | S3, murmur, rub, gallop, decreased, click |
| Abdominal | Abdominal muscle use during respiration, distention, fluid wave, tympani, tenderness, acute increase in girth, mass, rigidity |
| Extremity | Bilateral or unilateral edema, pain, wounds, splinter emboli, clubbing of digits |
| Skin | Rashes, wounds, lesions, scars, blisters |

pertinent information; these should be done on most elderly patients with dyspnea. The EKG aids in the evaluation of an arrhythmia or myocardial infarction (ST elevation or non-ST elevation, ST-segment elevation myocardial infarction or non–ST-segment elevation myocardial infarction, respectively). The provider must pay close attention to the EKG result, as this can show subtle evidence of myocardial ischemia, signs of new or progressive cardiopulmonary diseases (such as congestive heart failure, pulmonary embolism, pericarditis, pulmonary hypertension, or valve disease) The chest radiograph will give information as to heart size, cardiac/aortic silhouette, pulmonary infiltrate, masses, effusion, pneumothorax, hemothorax, or bony abnormalities.

End-tidal $CO_2$ monitoring is becoming increasingly available and should be used if available. Moment-to-moment information on the ventilation status of the patient and the perfusion dynamics can be interpreted from the end-tidal $CO_2$ waveform, and changes in that measurement can also provide clues to impending changes in hemodynamic status.

Ultrasound scan (point of care) is also becoming more widely available and can provide immediate and potentially life-saving information. Of particular importance are the cardiac and lung examinations. The cardiac examination can provide information about the presence of a pericardial effusion and potential tamponade physiology, basic evaluation of cardiac output based on heart chamber squeeze, and evidence of cardiac hypertrophy. The lung examination can identify the presence of a pneumothorax or hemothorax based on the absence of pleural sliding and the presence of pulmonary edema based on the presence of b-lines. Additionally, the rapid ultrasound in shock and hypotension or RUSH examination is easy and fast to perform and gives additional information as to cardiopulmonary status (including the information noted above). It also gives further information about volume status and the potential presence of deep vein thrombosis in the lower extremities. Although this information may not be required on stable patients, it should be kept in mind if there is any change in status of the patient or in the elderly patient with undifferentiated dyspnea and shock.

Laboratory data can readily assist in the evaluation and treatment of the stable patient with dyspnea; however, unless point-of-care testing is available, it is of limited utility in the unstable or metastable patient. A basic metabolic panel provides information on electrolyte abnormalities, kidney function, anion gap, and glucose level. These results also provide information on the acid-base status of the patient, particularly if used in conjunction with an arterial or venous blood gas. A complete blood count provides information about anemia, shows possible volume contraction, and indicates infection through the white blood cell count. A troponin (serial or single, as appropriate) is a marker for myocardial damage and an indicator of systemic organ damage. A creatine phosphokinase (CPK) evaluates for muscle breakdown and rhabdomyolysis. A D-dimer can be used as a marker for potential deep vein thrombosis or pulmonary embolism in low-risk patients, bearing in mind that there are suggestions that D-dimer cutoff levels need to be adjusted as patients age older than 50 to maintain sensitivity.[11] Liver function test evaluates albumin and protein and can give information of vascular oncotic pressure, generalized nutritional status, and acute hepatocyte damage. An arterial or venous blood gas test provides useful information as to the acid/base status, evaluation of oxygenation, and ventilation of the patient.

Further imaging, such as computed tomography (CT) imaging or a bedside formal echocardiogram or lower extremity deep vein thrombosis examination can be used, if available and appropriate. The necessary information for emergency diagnosis and disposition can be readily obtained from these studies alone. This evaluation includes testing for malignancy, pulmonary embolism (in high risk patients), pneumonia, and cardiac abnormalities.

### Evaluation of the unstable patient

In the unstable patient, the evaluation (specifically, the history and physical examination) is done in conjunction with management and treatment of symptoms and underlying causes. The information noted above about the stable patient is of importance and should eventually be obtained once feasible. In the unstable elderly patient, it is recommended to use a similar approach to adult advanced cardiac life support (ACLS) protocols with first evaluation and stabilization of airway, breathing, and circulation before moving on to additional history and evaluation of the patient.

### Evaluation

The initial evaluation for any elderly patient with a complaint of dyspnea should begin while walking into the examination room and looking at and listening to the patient. Inability of the patient to talk and increased work of breathing (including tachypnea, using supraclavicular or abdominal muscles, retractions, audible wheezing, crackles, grunting, stridor, or gasping), are all signs of impending respiratory compromise and may require emergent airway or ventilatory management before continuing the overall assessment. Breath sounds can give the provider clues to the underlying cause of dyspnea and guide management of the patient. Concurrently or immediately after assessment of airway and breathing, members of the treatment team should establish vascular access. Whether peripheral venous, central venous, or intraosseous access is required depends on the specific needs and ability to obtain based on the patient's anatomy and pathology. Once airway and ventilation status are controlled in the unstable dyspneic patient, the provider can move forward to further evaluation.

### History

Although history may be difficult to obtain in the unstable or nonverbal elderly patient, it is important to obtain a focused history including onset, duration, attempted therapy, previous causes of dyspnea, cardiac and respiratory history, a list of medications/compliance, and potential allergies. Often this information is limited in the acute setting or unobtainable from the patient. If immediately available, history from family members, emergency medical services report, chart review, nursing home chart review, or medication list review can be important and help guide appropriate management of the patient.

### Physical Examination

As mentioned above, the physical examination in an unstable elderly patient should be done in a similar approach to the advanced cardiac life supportprotocol. First, is the evaluation of airway, looking for airway patency, obstruction, edema, voice changes, and the ability to manage secretions. Next is the evaluation of breathing, including breath sounds, respiratory rate, and extrarespiratory muscle use. Cardiovascular examination, particularly evaluation of heart sounds/murmurs, pulses, and extremity edema should follow. Patients should be fully undressed and the skin examined, followed by the rest of the physical examination. Vital signs are of paramount importance and should be immediately available to the provider during initial examination.

### Adjuncts

In addition to the adjuncts in stable dyspnea discussed above, particularly useful in the unstable patient is the use of point-of-care ultrasound scan (particularly the RUSH examination) and end-tidal $CO_2$ capnography.

## Treatment

### Oxygen

Oxygen should be given to all patients with hypoxia ($O_2$ saturation <90%), and these patients should be titrated using nasal cannula, venturi mask, or nonrebreather as appropriate for the patient's condition with a goal saturation of 94%.[12] Additional use of humidified air may make high-flow oxygen therapy more tolerable, particularly for the elderly patient. Patients with a diagnosis of chronic obstructive pulmonary disease (COPD), especially those older than 70 are at risk of hypercapnic respiratory failure, and oxygen therapy should be used with caution.[12] In these cases, it is recommended that the goal saturation be reduced to 88% to 92% with frequent blood gas monitoring to reduce precipitating hypercapnea.[12]

### Noninvasive positive pressure ventilation

Noninvasive positive pressure ventilation (NIPPV) is an important treatment modality that provides ventilation assistance without invasive endotracheal intubation (bi-pap is the most commonly used form of NIPPV). Bi-pap provides ventilation assistance by providing 2 separate levels of positive airway pressure: a higher level with inspiratory breath and a lower level with expiratory breath.[13]

Some patients may begin to feel anxious or claustrophobic with NIPPV. Some providers advocate using small doses of a benzodiazepine to allay this feeling; however, particular caution should be used, as the patient can become overly sedated (a decreased mental status is a contraindication to using NIPPV) or paradoxically increasingly agitated (**Box 1**).

### Intubation

Intubation should be used in cases that require a definitive airway to protect the airway from collapse (eg, in cases such as airway edema, mental status decline and inability to manage secretions) or from acute or pending respiratory failure (**Box 2**).

---

**Box 1**
**Contraindications and indications for NIPPV**

*Contraindications for NIPPV*

Patients without spontaneous respiratory drive

Inability to protect airway (decreased mental status, vomiting, epistaxis, increased secretions, facial trauma)

Pneumothorax

Recent oral intake

Hypotension (relative contraindication)

*Indications for NIPPV*

Acute respiratory distress

Pulmonary edema (congestive heart failure, acute pulmonary edema)

COPD/asthma (can use albuterol/Atrovent concurrently)

Pneumonia

Metabolic abnormalities

Sepsis

> **Box 2**
> **Indications for intubation**
>
> Acute or pending respiratory failure/arrest
>
> Failure of NIPPV
>
> Inability to maintain airway
>
> Imminent loss of airway (eg, anaphylaxis, hypersecretions, traumatic airway injury)
>
> Decreased mental status
>
> Aspiration risk
>
> Hypercapnia with increasing acidosis

## CAUSES OF ACUTE DYSPNEA IN ELDERLY PATIENTS

The list below is not a complete list; however, the most common causes of dyspnea in the elderly include the following.

### Pulmonary

#### Chronic obstructive pulmonary disease

COPD typically affects the elderly population, and over the last several decades, COPD was a leading cause of morbidity and mortality among elderly adults.[14] Although traditionally an elderly male disease, the prevalence in women is now almost equal to that of men. COPD is often unrecognized and untreated until the disease progresses to more severe symptoms.[14] It is important to maintain a high degree of suspicion for patients presenting with progressive dyspnea and risk factors for COPD.

Patients with COPD exacerbations almost exclusively have an extensive history of heavy tobacco smoking. The patients often describe their dyspnea with symptoms of coughing, wheezing, or shortness of breath. It is important, if the patient has a previous history of COPD, to ask about recent medication changes or noncompliance, as this may lead to an acute exacerbation of the condition. Physical examination is focused on lung examination auscultation for wheezing (which is usually diffuse). Decreased breath sounds from poor air movement and air trapping may also be heard. Patients will also have a prolonged expiratory phase. Chest radiographs may show hyperinflated lungs or focal consolidations if a lobar pneumonia is a concomitant (and potentially exacerbating) illness. Additionally, noting the presence of large alveolar blebs versus possible pneumothoraces is important.

Treatment of these patients begins with inhaled β-agonists (such as albuterol) along with inhaled anticholinergics (such as ipratropium bromide). Patients with worse symptoms often require systemic steroids (Solu-Medrol or prednisone can be administered based on whether the patient can tolerate oral medications or requires intravenous administration). Antibiotic therapy is found to have an important effect on clinical recovery and outcome and should be started at the beginning of treatment.[15] Patients requiring further treatment may benefit from a trial of NIPPV as long as there are no contraindications (**Table 2**).

### Asthma

Approximately 6.3% of patients older than 65 have asthma (approximately 2.719 million).[16] In a study done by Quadrelli and Roncoroni,[17] elderly patients with long-standing asthma were found to have an increased requirement for systemic steroid use and a worse forced expiratory volume in first second of expiration

**Table 2**
**Typical characteristics of patients presenting with COPD**

| History | Physical Examination | Adjuncts | Treatment |
|---------|---------------------|----------|-----------|
| Tobacco smoke | Wheezing | Peak flow decreased | Albuterol/Atrovent |
| Cough | Decreased breath sounds | Chest radiography hyperinflated | Solu-Medrol vs prednisone |
| Wheezing | Prolonged expiratory phase | EKG normal vs nonspecific, or evidence of cor pulmonale | Antibiotics |
| Medication Changes | — | — | NIPPV |
| Exposure to allergen | — | — | — |

(FEV$_1$) with a decreased best FEV1. It was also found that these patients had less over-all time between symptoms and symptom free time. Symptoms were generally more frequent and more severe than patients with asthma younger than 65.

Elderly patients with acute asthma exacerbations often have a previous diagnosis of reactive airway disease. These patients typically complain of symptoms of cough and wheezing. Patients may also have recent medication changes or noncompliance with medications leading to an acute exacerbation. Physical examination again is focused on the patient's work of breathing and lung examination. Wheezing is typically auscultated diffusely or bilaterally in the lower lobes, or there is minimal air movement heard. Patients often exhibit a prolonged expiratory phase along with accessory respiratory muscle use. Peak flow measurements are an important adjunct in the evaluation of patients with asthma. Noting an initial peak flow measurement and comparing that with the patient's baseline best peak flow measurement and changes over time with therapeutic interventions, can help appropriately guide disposition and further management. Chest radiograph is also an important diagnostic modality.

The treatment of these patients includes inhaled β-agonists and anticholinergics as well as systemic steroids. If an exacerbation is severe or not improving, intravenous magnesium can be given, although caution must be taken in dosing for patients with severe renal failure, as magnesium is cleared renally and accumulation can cause toxicity. Additionally, NIPPV may be trialed (**Table 3**).

*Parenchymal lung disease*
Elderly patients with parenchymal lung disease often have a previous history of pneumotoxic exposures. These exposures are often environmental and often related to

**Table 3**
**Typical characteristics of patients presenting with asthma**

| History | Physical Examination | Adjuncts | Treatment |
|---------|---------------------|----------|-----------|
| Reactive airway disease | Wheezing | Peak flow decreased | Albuterol/Atrovent |
| Cough | Decreased BS | Chest radiography | Solu-Medrol vs prednisone |
| Wheezing | Prolonged expiratory phase | EKG nonspecific | Magnesium |
| Medication change | Accessory respiratory muscle use | — | NIPPV |
| Exposure to allergen/trigger | — | — | — |

previous work exposures (asbestos, chemicals, and metal or wood dust). Additional exposures such as tobacco smoke, inhalant abuse, radiation, or pneumotoxic medications are additional risk factors. A patient's duration of exposure is often indicative of future severity of symptoms.[18] The physical examination often finds clubbing of the digits and bibasilar crackles, which are often described as *velcro crackles*. Along with the basic medical workup, chest radiograph and chest CT scan can find parenchymal lung disease and, in concordance with the patient's symptoms, can reveal the severity of the disease. Patients should be given supplemental oxygen to help maintain their oxygen saturation and help decrease symptoms.[19]

### Pneumonia

Elderly patients with pneumonia do not typically present with the same complaints and symptoms as their younger counterparts. In fact, they often present with significantly fewer respiratory symptoms and commonly with only cough or pleuritic chest pain, until they begin to decompensate.[20,21] History and risk factors suggestive of pneumonia including fever, chills, cough with or without nausea and vomiting, increased sputum production, fatigue, myalgias, aspiration risk factors, and delirium. Additionally, patients with history of falls, alcoholism, high frailty score, asthma, and immunosuppression are at higher risk of severe complications of pneumonia.[20,22] The physical examination often holds many suggestions that will guide in this diagnosis. The vital signs can have many abnormalities including fever, tachycardia, tachypnea, and decreased oxygen saturation. However, these signs may not be present or may be masked (either because of physiologic changes or pharmacologic interactions) in the elderly patient. When auscultating the lungs one should listen particularly for focal decreased breath sounds, crackles, or rales. Bronchial breathing and pleural friction rub may also be present. The patient may also have dullness to percussion over the affected lobe and tactile or vocal fremitus. Increased or decreased white blood cell count can be suggestive of infection; however, this is a nonspecific marker. Chemistry panel may show electrolyte abnormalities secondary to the infection, whereas lactate measurement and trending can help illustrate the severity of illness. Chest radiograph is often the diagnostic image of choice and can show a focal consolidation or generalized haziness. Antibiotic therapy is necessary for these patients with specific agent choice dependent on risk factors (eg, community-acquired vs health care–associated pneumonia, aspiration, immunosuppression, sepsis) Supplemental oxygen and other resuscitative measures should be used as clinically appropriate.[22]

### Pulmonary embolism

Elderly patients often present with atypical symptoms of pulmonary embolism that can lead to delays in diagnosis and treatment. This delay can potentially lead to increased disease severity at time of diagnosis. In a study done by Timmons and colleagues,[23] it was found that a significant percentage (24%) of elderly patients with pulmonary embolism present with collapse compared with only 3% of their younger counterparts. It was also discovered that elderly patients presented more often with cyanosis and hypoxia compared with the younger population. However, they had similar heart rate, respiratory rate, and mean arterial pressure compared with to the younger population. Also noted was that the complaint of pleuritic chest pain was less prevalent in the elderly with pulmonary embolism when compared with younger patients with pulmonary embolism. However, pleuritic chest pain and dyspnea remain the most frequent complaints in both populations.[24]

Physical examination can be most significant for tachycardia, tachypnea, or decreased oxygen saturation. Risk factors and symptoms for pulmonary embolisms are often extrapolated during the history. It is important to ask for the Pulmonary Embolism Rule-out Criteria risk factors (while these factors may increase the pretest probability of disease, the actual Pulmonary Embolism Rule-out Criteria rule does not apply to the geriatric population, as one of the factors is age >50 years old), additional history of chest pain, hemoptysis, cough, or decreased mobility. Electrocardiograms should be performed on most elderly patients with complaint of dyspnea. In the setting of a pulmonary embolism, EKG may show a S1Q3T3 pattern, sinus tachycardia, right bundle branch block, or other nonspecific ST-T abnormalities. Chest radiograph should be obtained, as cardiomegaly, pleural effusion, and wedge-shaped consolidation might be noted. Arterial blood gas may be used for evaluating hypoxemia and hypocapnia. A d-dimer is helpful in low-risk patients to further investigate, although it can be falsely elevated in elderly patients, particularly those with multiple comorbid illnesses. An extremity duplex positive for deep vein thrombosis can assist when pulmonary CT or ventilation/perfusion (VQ) scan are difficult to obtain. Troponin (single or serial trend) along with cardiac ultrasound scan to evaluate right heart strain may also be used to risk stratify severity of the pulmonary embolism. Patients with either definitive diagnosis of pulmonary embolism or high suspicion of this diagnosis should be treated with anticoagulation. This can initially be done with heparin bolus and drip or low-molecular-weight heparin depending on the patient's comorbidities as well as institutional preferences and patient stability. Elderly patients who are at an increased risk of falling or potentially life-threatening hemorrhages should have an appropriate risk and benefit evaluation to identify the best anticoagulation treatment course. Additionally, in-hospital and out-of-hospital assessments and interventions to reduce falls should occur. Long-term anticoagulation versus inferior vena cava filter are often indicated but will not be reviewed here[25] (**Fig. 1**).

## Pneumothorax

Pneumothorax can occur either spontaneously or owing to trauma. Patients with traumatic pneumothoraces usually have a known history of trauma, although in frail elderly patients this may include falls from a chair, bed, or standing. Patients with spontaneous pneumothorax often have a history of COPD, tobacco use, or inhalation drug abuse. Symptoms will often present with tachycardia, tachypnea, hypotension, or hypoxia. The physical examination often finds unilateral or focal decreased breath sounds and hyper-resonance with percussion over affected lobes. One may also find a deviated trachea in severe cases of tension pneumothorax. Examination of the skin and chest wall may find ecchymosis, abrasions, wounds, or other signs of traumatic injury. One may also see decreased chest wall recoil with exhalation. High suspicion by history and physical examination may warrant immediate tube thoracostomy if the patient is unstable. However, if the patient remains stable, chest x-ray is often diagnostic, and a bedside ultrasound scan can also be used to support the diagnosis. If a patient is found to have a spontaneous pneumothorax a nonemergent chest CT may be indicated to further evaluate for underlying lung parenchyma disease. Supplemental oxygen should also be used to help correct hypoxia. For a simple, nontraumatic pneumothorax, a small pig-tail catheter can be used or thoracostomy can even be deferred in favor of observation in certain cases.

## Allergic reaction

Elderly patients with allergic reactions often have a history of known allergies and may have a known exposure to this allergen. Vital signs often are significant for tachycardia, and as disease progresses there may be hypotension, tachypnea, and hypoxia. On physical examination there may be hives, wheezing, cough, or stridor. This

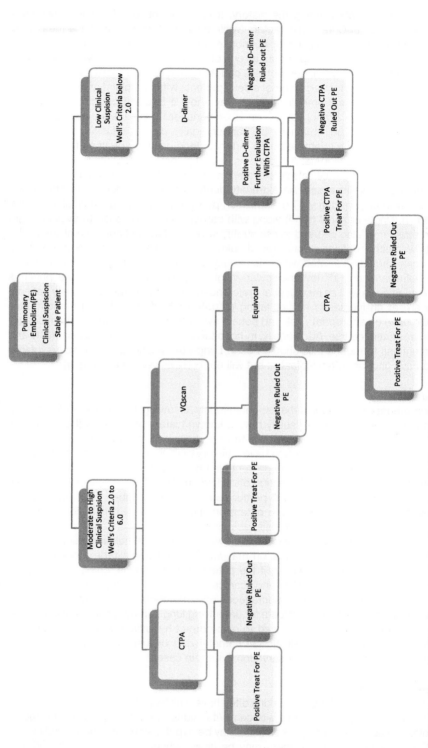

**Fig. 1.** Decision algorithm for suspected pulmonary embolism (PE). *CTPA*, computed tomography pulmonary angiogram.

diagnosis is often based solely on clinical appearance with adjuncts being used to rule out additional conditions. Respiratory distress in patients with allergic reactions is always indicated in increased severity of disease and should warrant the clinician preparing for a possible emergent airway (and, unfortunately, in this case, for one that may be difficult). Medications typically used include antihistamines (diphenhydramine), H2 receptor antagonists (famotidine, ranitidine), corticosteroids (Solu-Medrol or prednisone), and, in severe reactions, epinephrine. Although many clinicians may be cautious in giving epinephrine to elderly patients, when respiratory distress and potential anaphylaxis are of concern, the risks of a rapid adrenergic surge are far outweighed by the potential of avoiding complete airway occlusion, and epinephrine should be administered.

## Cardiovascular

### Heart failure (right, left, or biventricular)
Congestive heart failure is a progressive disease and is usually diagnosed in the aging or geriatric population. The patient's comorbidities are often clues to suggest heart failure such as previous coronary artery disease and untreated hypertension. The most common presentation is worsening dyspnea, orthopnea, weight gain, and decreased exercise tolerance. Patients may also complain of worsening peripheral edema of gravity-dependent body parts (bilateral lower extremities, buttocks, or the scrotum). If they have a previous history of heart failure, medication changes or noncompliance often precede an acute exacerbation. Auscultation of the lungs often reveals crackles or decreased breath sounds in the lower lobes. S3 heart sound and murmurs may be audible when listening to heart sounds. Patients often have jugular venous distention and as equally distributed edema in gravity-dependent body parts. Important adjuncts to evaluation of potential heart failure exacerbation include EKG, cardiac ultrasound scan, chest radiograph, electrolyte panel, blood urea nitrogen/creatinine, and pro- B-type Natriuretic Peptide (pro-BNP). Acute exacerbations are treated with diuresis (furosemide), nitrates, noninvasive positive pressure ventilation, and, in some cases, angiotensin-converting enzyme inhibitors.

### Myocardial infarction/coronary artery disease
Patients with acute myocardial infarction often have chest pain, whether acute or episodic in nature. Patients often express worsening dyspnea on exertion and decreased exercise tolerance. The patient may report nausea, vomiting, or diaphoresis during these episodes. It is also important to note medical history for risk factors including previous coronary artery disease, tobacco use, hypertension, diabetes, and hyperlipidemia. The physical examination is typically unrevealing but important to evaluate for other worrisome cardiopulmonary entities (signs of heart failure such as jugular venous distension, crackles, or edema). An EKG is the most important adjunct in this setting and should be viewed immediately in patients complaining of symptoms concerning for myocardial ischemia, particularly dyspnea. If any previous EKG is available, comparison should be made and any changes noted along with signs suggesting need for emergent cardiac catheterization. Serial EKGs should also be used, as a myocardial infarction is progressive and may not show any signs on the initial EKG. Serial cardiac enzymes, chest radiograph, and ultrasound scan are also important in evaluation and decision making for these patients, particularly in identifying the need for urgent or emergent cardiac catheterization. Patients with suspected or confirmed myocardial infarction should be treated immediately with aspirin and oxygen and other stabilizing therapies. Additionally, the emergency physician should ensure rapid involvement of a cardiologist for cardiac catheterization (for

| Box 3 |
|---|
| **Additional causes of dyspnea** |
| *Cardiovascular* |
| Pulmonary hypertension |
| Other valvular abnormalities |
| Septal defect |
| Pericarditis |
| Arrhythmia |
| *Miscellaneous* |
| Systemic infection |
| Metabolic disorders |
| Trauma |
| Deconditioning |
| Neuromuscular disorders |
| Anxiety |
| Hyperventilation |

diagnosis/characterization and reperfusion). One should also consider additional antiplatelet agents (clopidogrel) and anticoagulation (unfractionated vs low-molecular-weight heparin).[26]

### Valvular dysfunction (aortic stenosis)

There are many types of valvular dysfunction that can lead to complaints of dyspnea. They may all affect geriatric patients; however, aortic stenosis has the highest prevalence, with approximately 12.4% of the elderly population afflicted and nearly 3.4% with severe aortic stenosis, which may require surgical intervention.[27] Patients often have extensive medical histories and may have had aortic stenosis diagnosed previously. Comorbid conditions such as diabetes, hypertension, and hyperlipidemia along with tobacco use are often noted on history. In additional to complaints of dyspnea, the patient often expresses symptoms of worsening dyspnea and angina on exertion, orthopnea, syncope, and decreased exercise tolerance. Physical examination may find pulsus parvus et tardus, S3 or S4 heart sounds, or a crescendo-decrescendo systolic murmur along the left sternal border. Important adjuncts include chest radiography to evaluate for possible cardiomegaly or pulmonary effusions. An EKG may show evidence of left ventricular hypertrophy with early repolarization, bundle branch blocks, or dysrhythmias (typically atrial fibrillation). A cardiac ultrasound scan may show valvular thickening, left ventricular hypertrophy, trileaflet or bileaflet aortic valve, or aortic valve outflow obstruction. Treatment of valvular dysfunction is based on a patient's clinical picture and may include volume resuscitation, supportive management, use of dobutamine or other cardiac/vasopressor support medications, and urgent cardiology evaluation.[28]

See **Box 3** for additional causes of dyspnea.

### SUMMARY

The evaluation of elderly patients with acute dyspnea should follow a systematic approach. It is important to first identify potentially ill patients and stabilize them and then to consider the broad range of conditions that can contribute to dyspnea in the elderly. Because of the changes in the physiology of the geriatric population, the onset of symptoms may occur late, and the severity of symptoms may be blunted and not correlate with the severity of the condition. It is important to recognize quickly the unstable patients and resuscitate them appropriately and, if needed, quickly establish a definitive airway before continued evaluation and treatment of underlying causes. Through a careful history and physical examination and use of the proper adjuncts, one can begin to work through the differential diagnosis and initiate the appropriate treatment of these patients.

## REFERENCES

1. Dyspnea. Mechanisms, assessment, and management: a consensus statement. American Thoracic Society. Am J Respir Crit Care Med 1999;159(1):321–40.
2. Available at: http://geriatricresearch.medicine.dal.ca/pdf/Clinical%20Faily%20Scale.pdf. Accessed October 10, 2015.
3. West LA, Cole S, Goodkind D, et al. 65+ in the United States: 2010. US Department of commerce, economics and Statistics administration. US Census Bureau; 2014. Available at: https://www.census.gov/content/dam/Census/library/publications/2014/demo/p23-212.pdf.
4. Albert M, Mccaig LF, Ashman JJ. Emergency department visits by persons aged 65 and over: United States, 2009-2010. NCHS Data Brief 2013;(130):1–8.
5. Pines JM, Mullins PM, Cooper JK, et al. National trends in emergency department use, care patterns, and quality of care of older adults in the United States. J Am Geriatr Soc 2013;61(1):12–7.
6. Alvis BD, Hughes CG. Physiology considerations in geriatric patients. Anesthesiol Clin 2015;33(3):447–56.
7. Rooke GA. Cardiovascular aging and anesthetic implications. J Cardiothorac Vasc Anesth 2003;17(4):512–23.
8. Sharma G, Goodwin J. Effect of aging on respiratory system physiology and immunology [review]. Clin Interv Aging 2006;1(3):253–60.
9. Sprung J, Gajic O, Warner DO. Review article: age related alterations in respiratory function - anesthetic considerations. Can J Anaesth 2006;53:1244–57.
10. Morgan WC, Hodge HL. Diagnostic evaluation of dyspnea. Am Fam Physician 1998;57(4):711–6.
11. Righini M, Van Es J, Den Exter PL, et al. Age-adjusted D-Dimer cutoff levels to rule out pulmonary embolism: the ADJUST-PE study. JAMA 2014;311(11):1117–24.
12. O'driscoll BR, Howard LS, Davison AG. BTS guideline for emergency oxygen use in adult patients. Thorax 2008;63(Suppl 6):vi1–68.
13. Kirkland L. Noninvasive positive-pressure ventilation. ACP Hospitalist 2010.
14. Chronic obstructive pulmonary disease (COPD). WHO; 2015. Available at: http://www.who.int/respiratory/copd/en/.
15. Ram FS, Rodriguez-Roisin R, Granados-Navarrete A, et al. Antibiotics for exacerbations of chronic obstructive pulmonary disease. Cochrane Database Syst Rev 2006;(12):CD010257.
16. Centers for Disease Control and Prevention. Most recent asthma data. Centers for Disease Control and Prevention; 2015. Available at: http://www.cdc.gov/asthma/asthmadata.htm.
17. Quadrelli S, Roncoroni AJ. Is asthma in the elderly really different? Respiration 1998;65:347–53.

18. Meyer KC. Management of interstitial lung disease in elderly patients. Curr Opin Pulm Med 2012;18(5):483–92.

19. Papanikolaou IC, Drakopanagiotakis F, Polychronopoulos VS. Acute exacerbations of interstitial lung diseases. Curr Opin Pulm Med 2010;16(5):480–6.

20. Metlay JP, Schulz R, Li YH, et al. Influence of age on symptoms at presentation in patients with community-acquired pneumonia. Arch Intern Med 1997;157(13): 1453–9.

21. Berman AR. Pulmonary embolism in the elderly. Clin Geriatr Med 2001;17(1): 107–30.

22. Gubbins PO, Li C. The influence of influenza and pneumococcal vaccines on community-acquired pneumonia (CAP) outcomes among elderly patients. Curr Infect Dis Rep 2015;17(12):49.

23. Timmons S, Kingston M, Hussain M, et al. Pulmonary embolism: Differences in presentation between older and younger patients. Age Ageing 2003;32:601–5.

24. Kokturk N, Oguzulgen IK, Demir N, et al. Differences in clinical presentation of pulmonary embolism in older vs younger patients. Circ J 2005;69(8):981–6.

25. Masotti L, Ray P, Righini M, et al. Pulmonary embolism in the elderly: a review on clinical, instrumental and laboratory presentation. Vasc Health Risk Manag 2008; 4(3):629–36.

26. Carro A, Kaski JC. Myocardial infarction in the elderly. Aging Dis 2011;2(2): 116–37.

27. Osnabrugge RJ, Mylotte D, Head SJ, et al. Aortic stenosis in the elderly: disease prevalence and number of candidates for transcatheter aortic valve replacement: a meta-analysis and modeling study. J Am Coll Cardiol 2013;62(11):1002–12.

28. Maganti K, Rigolin VH, Sarano ME, et al. Valvular heart disease: diagnosis and management. Mayo Clin Proc 2010;85(5):483–500.

# Abdominal Pain in the Geriatric Patient

Phillip D. Magidson, MD, MPH[a,b], Joseph P. Martinez, MD[c,d],*

## KEYWORDS

- Geriatrics • Abdominal pain • Elderly • Emergency

## KEY POINTS

- Geriatric patients with abdominal disease or pathologic conditions present to the emergency department atypically.
- There is increased morbidity and mortality associated with geriatric patients who are seen in the emergency department with abdominal pain compared with younger patients.
- Further diagnostics and admission are frequently warranted in elderly patients who present with abdominal pain.

## INTRODUCTION AND EPIDEMIOLOGY

Between 2000 and 2010, the population older than 65 years grew at a rate of more than 15% compared with just 10% for the entire population.[1] As the geriatric population increases, so do emergency department (ED) visits by the elderly. According to the last National Hospital Ambulatory Care Survey in 2011, more than 20 million or nearly 15% of all ED visits were by patients older than 65 years.[2]

After chest pain and shortness of breath, abdominal pain is the third most common chief complaint in patients older than 65 years who present to the ED.[2] ED clinicians (EDCs) must have a robust understanding of diseases that present with abdominal pain. These diseases are more complex, in both presentation and treatment, in geriatric patients than in their younger counterparts.

---

Disclosures: None.
[a] Department of Emergency Medicine, University of Maryland Medical Center, 6th Floor, Suite 200, 110 South Paca Street, Baltimore, MD 21201, USA; [b] Department of Medicine, University of Maryland Medical Center, 6th Floor, Suite 200, 110 South Paca Street, Baltimore, MD 21201, USA; [c] Department of Emergency Medicine, University of Maryland School of Medicine, 6th Floor, Suite 200, 110 South Paca Street, Baltimore, MD 21201, USA; [d] Department of Medicine, University of Maryland School of Medicine, 6th Floor, Suite 200, 110 South Paca Street, Baltimore, MD 21201, USA
* Corresponding author. Departments of Emergency Medicine and Medicine, University of Maryland School of Medicine, 6th Floor, Suite 200, 110 South Paca Street, Baltimore, MD.
E-mail address: jmartinez@som.umaryland.edu

Emerg Med Clin N Am 34 (2016) 559–574
http://dx.doi.org/10.1016/j.emc.2016.04.008
0733-8627/16/$ – see front matter © 2016 Elsevier Inc. All rights reserved.
emed.theclinics.com

Geriatric patients seen in the ED for abdominal pain have higher rates of admission, up to 60%, as well as longer length of stays in the ED and inpatient units when admitted. Of geriatric patients admitted for abdominal pain, nearly 20% underwent an invasive procedure or surgery.[3] These patients generate more charges and cost the health care system more compared with younger patients.[4,5]

Geriatric patients not only require more aggressive workups and treatment, they tend to fare less well when compared with younger patients. For geriatric patients discharged from the hospital who presented with abdominal pain, nearly 1 in 10 will return within 2 weeks for similar complaints.[4] Of those geriatric patients presenting to the ED for abdominal pain who undergo surgical intervention, 17% will die, with mortality approaching 40% for patients older than 80 years.[4,6–8]

## PRESENTATION
### Physiology

Numerous physiologic changes occur with age. It is necessary for the EDC to have a clear understanding of these changes and how they complicate the workup of abdominal pain.

A fever may be helpful to the EDC when considering the differential diagnosis of abdominal pain in the elderly because its presence may suggest an underlying bacterial infection. Additionally, the presence of a fever is a component of some clinical decision tools (identification of systemic inflammatory response syndrome or Charcot triad) that may help guide further management. However, geriatric patients are less able to mount a fever. In fact, 20% to 30% of older patients with an active infection may have a blunted fever response.[9–11] This blunted response starts with a lower baseline body temperature but may also be secondary to decreased temperature regulation by the central nervous system, decreased response to both endogenous and exogenous pyrogens, as well as decreased conservation of heat.[11]

Geriatric patients' immune systems are less adept at fighting infections. Although the total number of T cells may not decrease significantly with age, their functionality, specifically their ability to respond to new antigens, does decrease.[12]

Both bowel and bladder functionality decreases with age. Elderly patients have a decrease in colonic motility and transit time, as well as pelvic floor dysfunction, leading to much higher rates of constipation in this age group.[13,14] Furthermore, the risk of acute urinary retention (AUR), particularly in men, increases with age. For men older than 70 years, the risk of AUR per year is nearly 35% for those who experience moderate or severe benign prostate hypertrophy symptoms. Those with only mild symptoms still have a 10% risk of AUR.[15]

Finally, pain perception is also less sensitive in geriatric patients, particularly in abdominal disease or pathologic conditions.[16,17] This can delay the presentation of serious disease.

### Polypharmacy

Of patients older than 65 years, nearly 40% report taking 5 or more drugs within the past month. This can serve to complicate both objective and subjective signs of disease.

For example, geriatric patients are more likely to be on beta blockers that may inhibit tachycardic response in the setting of infection or pain. Nearly a quarter of patients older than 65 years report taking beta blockers.[18] Use of opioid analgesia, which may mask serious pathologic conditions by blunting the pain response, is used by adults older than 60 years at nearly a 50% higher rate than in younger adults.[19]

More than 20% of patients older than 75 years are on some form of anticoagulation, which increases the risk of gastrointestinal (GI) bleeding and major bleeding in the setting of seemingly mild trauma.[18] Antibiotics may cause pain, diarrhea, or vomiting as well as *Clostridium difficile* infection. Anticholinergic medications can increase the risk of urinary retention, leading to lower abdominal pain and, potentially, urinary tract infections. There are many other examples of medications causing or masking disease. It is important for the EDC to obtain a complete medication history, including prescribed and nonprescribed medications.

## SPECIFIC CONDITIONS
### Peptic Ulcer Disease or Upper Gastrointestinal Bleeding

One-half of all ulcers in the elderly initially present with a complication such as perforation or hemorrhage. Upper GI bleeding (UGIB), defined as bleeding above the ligament of Treitz, is the most common cause of GI bleeding in geriatric patients. Two-thirds of all GI bleeding is UGIB, with more than 70% of all cases occurring in patients older than 60 years.[20,21] Although some studies have suggested that the mortality associated with nonvariceal UGIB has decreased in younger patients in the past 10 years, these decreases in mortality have not been appreciated in patients older than 80 years.[22]

Peptic ulcer disease (PUD) is the most frequent cause of painful UGIB in geriatric patients.[23] The most common risk factors associated with PUD and UGIB in geriatric patients include nonsteroidal anti-inflammatory drugs (NSAIDs) as well as *Helicobacter pylori* infection. The odds ratio for bleeding peptic ulcers in geriatric patients who used NSAIDs is 4.9 compared with those patients without NSAID use. For geriatric patients infected with *H pylori*, the odds ratio for bleeding peptic ulcers is 1.8 compared with patients without said infection. With both NSAID use and *H pylori infection*, this increases to 6.1.[24] Additionally, use of NSAIDs with oral anticoagulants increases the risk of hemorrhagic PUD in elderly patients 13-fold compared with patients not on either medication.[25]

Other causes of UGIB that should be considered include gastritis and Mallory-Weiss tear. Esophageal or gastric varices may produce significant UGIB, although pain is a less common presenting symptom and patients with this condition tend to be younger.[22]

Evaluation and management in the ED should focus on resuscitation and identification of any immediate surgical emergencies. Immediate interventions should include multiple, large-bore, peripheral intravenous (IV) access sites; crystalloid administration; or blood transfusion in hypotensive patients, as well as consideration of platelet transfusions or other anticoagulation reversal agents in patients on blood thinners. The utility of IV proton pump inhibitors (PPIs) is a matter of debate with respect to whether this intervention decreases rebleeding or improves mortality.[26] However, many EDCs begin PPI therapy as part of initial stabilization in patients with UGIB. Laboratory studies looking for anemia, thrombocytopenia, or other coagulopathies can further guide management. An upright chest radiograph to look for intraperitoneal air is a reasonable first step, although this finding may be absent in 40% of geriatric patients with a perforated viscus.[27] An electrocardiogram should also be obtained because up to 14% of acute myocardial infarction may occur in the setting of acute GI hemorrhage.[28]

### Biliary Disease

The prevalence of biliary disease increases in geriatric patients, in part due to physiologic changes in the biliary tract. Nearly one-third of patients older than 65 years will have some degree of gallstone burden.[29] Biliary disease is the primary cause for emergent abdominal surgery in the geriatric population.[30,31]

One challenge faced by the EDC lies in the fact many of the cardinal signs of serious biliary disease, such as Charcot triad, may not be present in the geriatric population. This triad is suggestive of cholangitis and includes fevers, right upper-quadrant pain, and jaundice. It is present in only 30% to 45% of all geriatric patients, even those with advanced cholangitis.[32–34] As mentioned previously, a leukocytosis may also be absent in these patients.

Ultrasound is generally the preferred first step in imaging of patients with suspected gallbladder disease due to its noninvasive nature, relative availability, expeditious manner in which it can be accomplished, and high sensitivity and specificity.[35] A 2006 study showed that the EDC can detect gallstones with bedside ultrasound with 94% and 96% sensitivity and specificity, respectively.[36] For patients with suspected complications of gallbladder disease or with an equivocal ultrasound but continued high clinical suspicion, a computed tomography (CT) scan should be obtained (**Fig. 1**).[37] **Table 1** outlines the pros and cons of various imaging modalities.

If acute cholangitis is suspected, immediate administration of broad spectrum antibiotics targeted to cover anaerobic and gram-negative organisms should be initiated. Prompt evaluation by a gastroenterologist, general surgeon, or interventional radiologist is also necessary for consideration of further invasive, source control measures. Geriatric patients, even when treated aggressively for cholangitis, have higher rates of mortality than younger patients.[33]

Uncomplicated cholelithiasis in geriatric patients can also pose difficulties for EDCs. Patients diagnosed with this condition in the ED, who are otherwise stable with relatively well controlled pain, may be discharged home with outpatient surgical follow-up. A recent study, however, showed that many of these patients that have been discharged do not obtain timely surgical follow-up. This leads to repeat ED visits, further emergent imaging, and urgent or emergent cholecystectomy in nearly 13% of these patients.[38] Geriatric patients who are discharged home with a diagnosis of uncomplicated cholelithiasis should always have a clear follow-up plan in place.

### Pancreatic Disease

Pancreatitis is a common disorder in geriatric patients, with one-third of all cases of acute pancreatitis occurring in elderly patients.[39] Gallstones cause 75% of cases of

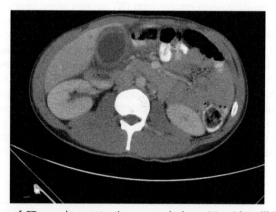

**Fig. 1.** Axial image of CT scan demonstrating acute cholecystitis with gallbladder wall thickening and pericholecystic fluid.

**Table 1**
**Imaging modalities for geriatric patients with abdominal pain**

| | Imaging in Abdominal Pain in the Elderly | | |
|---|---|---|---|
| Modality | Pros | Cons | Ideal for Evaluation of |
| Plain Radiographs | • Portable<br>• Widely available<br>• Quick to interpret<br>• Economical | • Lacks sensitivity and specificity compared with other modalities | • Bowel obstruction<br>• Foreign body identification<br>• Free intraperitoneal air (if of sufficient quantity) |
| CT Scan | • High sensitivity and specificity for numerous abdominal conditions<br>• Quickly accomplished | • May require nephrotoxic contrast<br>• May not be readily available | • Abdominal aortic aneurysm<br>• Appendicitis<br>• Diverticular disease<br>• Bowel obstruction |
| Ultrasound | • Portable<br>• No contrast required | • Operator-dependent<br>• Body habitus limitations | • Gallbladder disease<br>• Abdominal aortic aneurysm<br>• Bowel obstruction |
| MRI | • High-resolution images<br>• Avoidance of nephrotoxic contrast | • Not readily available<br>• Time consuming<br>• Expensive | • Diverticular disease<br>• Abdominal aortic aneurysm |
| Angiography | • Useful in both diagnosis and treatment | • Invasive<br>• Nephrotoxic contrast | • Mesenteric ischemia |

acute pancreatitis in patients older than 85 years.[40] Iatrogenic causes of pancreatitis from medication administration must also be considered in this population. Some of these medications are from classes commonly used by the elderly, including angiotensin-converting enzyme (ACE) inhibitors, diuretics, and statins.[41]

Pancreatitis in elderly patients may also present differently. Many elderly patients do not have the typical periumbilical pain with radiation to the back. As many as 10% may simply present with altered mental status or hypotension.[12,40] In some studies, typical abdominal pain is absent in 90% of cases of pancreatitis in subjects older than 65 years.[39]

The utility of routine imaging in cases of mild, uncomplicated pancreatitis has been called into question. In the older patient, CT scan imaging is likely prudent in most cases. Fatal acute pancreatitis has a 3-fold higher incidence of occurrence in patients older than 60 years compared with younger patients (**Fig. 2**).[42] Also, unlike in younger patients, pancreatic cancer is a more common cause of both acute and chronic pancreatitis in older patients with a median age of diagnosis of 72 years.[43]

Chronic pancreatitis is less common in geriatric patients. It is most commonly caused by chronic alcohol abuse and generally presents during the fourth or fifth decade of life rather than older than 65 years.

Treatment of pancreatitis is similar in all age groups, with avoidance of oral intake, pain control, and IV hydration. Of note, geriatric patients are more likely to suffer from congestive heart failure and require cautious resuscitation to avoid iatrogenic pulmonary edema.

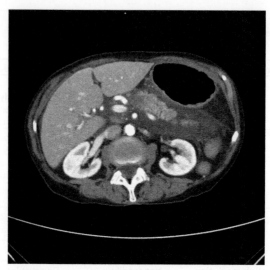

**Fig. 2.** Axial image of CT scan showing hypoattenuation in proximal portion of pancreas with a large amount of fluid surrounding the organ. Findings are consistent with acute necrotic pancreatitis.

## *Bowel Obstruction*

Symptoms of bowel obstruction in geriatric patients are similar to those in younger patients. These include abdominal pain and distention, nausea and vomiting, as well as constipation. Small bowel obstructions (SBOs) are significantly more common than large bowel obstructions (LBOs)[12] (**Table 2**).

Up to 75% of SBO are directly related to past abdominal surgery with subsequent adhesions.[44] Other causes of SBO include malignancies and Crohn disease. Narcotic medication use may lead to small bowel ileus development. Complication rates of SBO increase with age so it is imperative that the EDC identify these patients and provide appropriate care.[45]

Although the physical examination is relatively nonspecific, abdominal distention and abnormal bowel sounds are the 2 physical examination findings that are the greatest predictors of SBO.[46]

Upright abdominal plain radiographs are generally the first imaging choice in the ED, despite their sensitivity for SBO being only 50% to 60%.[47] Depending on available resources and the skill of the EDC, bedside ultrasound has been shown to have good sensitivity (91%) and specificity (84%) when used in the ED to diagnose SBO. Findings

**Table 2**
**Large versus small bowel obstruction**

|  | Large Bowel | Small Bowel |
|---|---|---|
| Incidence | Less common, 20% of total | Most common, 80% of total |
| Cause | Diverticular disease or malignancy, fecal impaction | Most commonly adhesions from prior surgery; also incarcerated hernia |
| Symptoms | Distention, abdominal pain, later symptoms of nausea, vomiting | Distention, abdominal pain, earlier onset of nausea, vomiting |

n ultrasound include dilated loops of bowel adjacent to normal loops of bowel as well
as either absent or significantly reduced bowel peristalsis.[48,49] Numerous studies have
shown CT scan has a sensitivity and specificity that approaches nearly 100%, making
it the ideal imaging study.[44]

LBO, although less common than SBO, is seen more frequently in geriatric patients
than in younger people. The primary causes of LBO are GI malignancy or diverticulitis,
both of which occur more frequently in older patients.[50] Of note, given the increased
volume of the large bowel, nausea and vomiting may either be absent or a late symptom of an LBO in contrast to SBO.[51]

Treatment of both SBO and LBO is similar. The EDC should focus on pain management, decompression with a nasogastric tube, supportive care with antibiotics, fluids
or pressers if indicated, and prompt surgical evaluation.

## Volvulus

After GI malignancy and diverticulitis, sigmoid volvulus is the third most common
cause of LBO and the most common type of volvulus. Geriatric patients are much
more likely to be diagnosed with volvulus compared with younger adults. This is in
large part because geriatric patients suffer from diseases more likely to slow gut
motility, such as Parkinson disease and diabetes, which predispose to volvulus formation. Additionally, more than 60% of these patients have comorbid neurologic and
psychiatric conditions.[52] The clinical presentation is similar to that of SBO and LBO
with the earliest and most common sign being abdominal pain. Because volvuli may
spontaneously reduce, 60% of geriatric patients who present with volvulus have a history of similar episodes.[53]

Diagnosis of sigmoid volvulus may be made by plain radiograph in up to 80% of
cases but it is less reliable in cecal volvulus (**Fig. 3**).[54] Contrast enema may be used
for diagnosis when plain radiographs are not definitive but the EDC must do this in
consultation with radiology and surgery.

Treatment includes supportive care, decompression, fluids, broad-spectrum antibiotics, and surgical evaluation. Most cases of sigmoid volvulus can be decompressed
emergently with either sigmoidoscopy or contrast enema. The recurrence rate is 50%
to 60%, so many patients will eventually need a definitive surgical procedure.

## Diverticulitis

Diverticular disease is a common problem in geriatric patients, especially in Western
cultures. The prevalence of the disease increases with age with 50% of patients older
than 60 years and up to 70% of patients older than 80 years having the disease.[55,56]
The pathophysiology is not well understood but diets low in fiber are epidemiologically
related to the underlying process of outpouching of colonic mucosa.[57]

Most patients with diverticular disease display no symptoms but up to 25% will
become symptomatic at some time.[57,58] Because 90% of diverticular disease in Western countries affects the sigmoid and descending colon, patients classically present
with left lower quadrant pain.[59]

In geriatric patients, many may report a known history of diverticular disease. An
elevated white blood cell count and/or fever may be present but their absence does
not exclude serious abdominal pathologic conditions, including diverticular disease.
Advanced disease process may present with diffuse abdominal tenderness or, in
the setting of diverticular perforation, guarding, rigidity, and frank peritonitis.

CT scan is the imaging modality of choice in the diagnosis of diverticulitis.[60] Despite
a preference of most EDCs to get imaging, there are clinical decision rules that may
suggest a diagnosis of diverticulitis and obviate imaging. Acute diverticulitis is likely

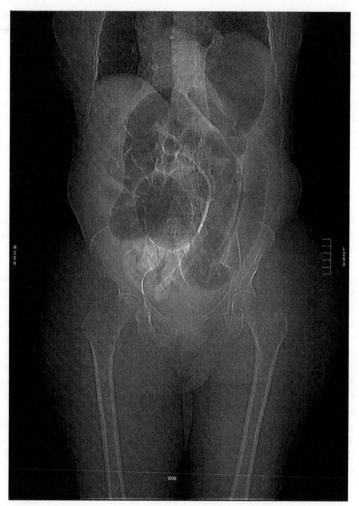

**Fig. 3.** Scout film from a CT scan demonstrating the classic bent inner tube bowel gas pattern of sigmoid volvulus.

in patients with isolated lower left quadrant tenderness, a C-reactive protein level greater than 50 mg/L, and the absence of vomiting.[61] Treatment may range from antibiotic therapy alone (a common regimen is ciprofloxacin plus metronidazole) to percutaneous drainage or open surgical procedures, depending on the severity and complexity of the case.

### Appendicitis

Only 5% to 10% of all cases of appendicitis are diagnosed in patients older than 65 years but these patients have mortality rates 5 to 8 times higher than younger patients.[62,63] Even among geriatric patients, complications remain highest among the oldest. In a study comparing younger geriatric patients (younger than 79 years) to older geriatric patients (80 years and older), delay to diagnosis was longer, and the rates of appendix perforation and postoperative mortality were higher in the older group.[64]

The classic triad of appendicitis is anorexia, fever, and right lower quadrant pain. In the elderly, however, this triad is present in just 20% of patients with appendicitis at presentation.[65] Up to 25% of elderly patients with appendicitis will have no right lower quadrant pain and less than 25% of geriatric patients with appendicitis presented with a fever higher than 37.7°C.[66–68]

Geriatric patients present later in the course of their illness, with 85% presenting after 24 hours of pain.[66] This delay in diagnosis leads to higher rates of perforation; 72% in geriatric patients as opposed to 20% to 30% in younger populations.[62,69]

CT scan remains the imaging modality of choice for the evaluation of appendicitis. Early surgical consultation should be obtained even in the absence of clear radiographic signs of acute appendicitis. The primary treatment of appendicitis has been prompt surgical intervention by way of an appendectomy. Although there has been a movement in recent years towards observation and medical management, there remains little to no data on the longitudinal morbidity and mortality of geriatric patients treated with this method.[69] Studies from the 1990s have clearly demonstrated improved outcomes with appendectomy over periods of observation.[70,71]

## Abdominal Aortic Aneurysm

Up to 10% of men older than 65 years will be diagnosed with an abdominal aortic aneurysm (AAA).[72] Because age is among the greatest risk factors associated with AAA, a broad differential for abdominal pain in the geriatric patient must include this diagnosis. However, the triad of back pain with associated abdominal pain, hypotension, and a pulsatile abdominal mass may only be present in 25% to 50% of patients with this condition, making the diagnosis challenging.[73,74] In fact, 30% of AAAs are missed on initial presentation with renal colic being the most common misdiagnosis.[12,73] The consequence of a missed AAA is significant. A ruptured AAA, the most common complication, portends mortality in up to 90% of patients.[74]

In addition to the triad of symptoms listed previously, patients with AAA or ruptured AAA may present with neurologic symptoms of the lower extremities due to compromised blood flow (numbness, cold extremities), groin or testicular pain, testicular ecchymosis (scrotal sign of Bryant), or Grey-Turner sign that is suggestive of retroperitoneal hematoma.[75–78]

Radiological evaluation for AAA may be accomplished with ultrasound or CT scan, ideally with IV contrast (**Fig. 4**). As bedside ultrasound becomes more readily available in the ED, its use as the initial imaging tool seems most prudent. Numerous studies have demonstrated EDC can quickly and accurately diagnose AAA with bedside ultrasound.[79] For stable patients in whom ultrasound may not be conclusive and IV contrast cannot be given, MRI may be used to evaluate abdominal vascular structures. Of course, this imaging modality is time-consuming and, in a patient with significant pain, may be limited by motion artifact.

For unstable patients with suspected ruptured AAA, a vascular surgeon should be consulted immediately along with simultaneous volume resuscitation. Operative intervention is the only treatment option for these patients. For hemodynamically stable patients, over-resuscitation should be avoided with some degree of permissive hypotension. Some research has suggested that too much fluid resuscitation may inhibit clot formation, contribute to coagulopathy, and ultimately worsen intra-abdominal bleeding.[80]

## Mesenteric Ischemia

Like AAA, acute mesenteric ischemia (AMI) presents diagnostic challenges to the EDC. Patients present with nonspecific symptoms that are often seen in other, less

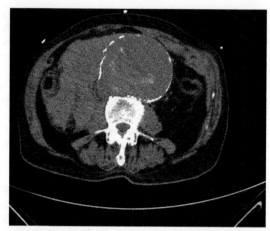

**Fig. 4.** Axial image of CT scan showing a large, heavily calcified AAA with free fluid consistent with rupture.

serious, disease processes. These symptoms may include generalized abdominal pain, vomiting and/or diarrhea, and a history of previous cardiac conditions such as atrial fibrillation. Overall, AMI is more common in the elderly, with 67% of events seen in patients older than 80 years.[81] In total, AMI represents 1% of all admissions for acute abdomen in patients older than 65 years.[82] Mortality associated with AMI is high, up to 80%. The earlier the disease is identified and infarction prevented the better the survival rate.[81]

Mesenteric ischemia can be classified within 4 specific categories, the most common of which is superior mesenteric artery (SMA) embolus. Acute SMA emboli accounts for up to 50% of all causes of AMI. The most common presentation is a very acute, unrelenting onset of abdominal pain. Many patients can state exactly when the pain started. Causes of embolic processes, such as atrial fibrillation or valvular disease, are often contributing factors.[81,83]

Nonocclusive mesenteric ischemia (NOMI) makes up about 20% of cases of AMI and is caused from hypoperfusion or shock states such as sepsis, cardiogenic shock (either from acute myocardial infarction (MI) or longstanding congestive heart failure), or hypovolemia secondary to dehydration. NOMI is more commonly found in the hospitalized patient, although these patients may present to the ED. Dialysis is a predisposing factor, especially in those patients who have an episode of intradialytic hypotension.[84]

SMA thrombus is often a process that evolves over time. This disease process is seen in patients with atherosclerotic vascular disease and accounts for 20% of all cases of AMI. Nearly 80% of patients will have a history of postprandial abdominal pain, or intestinal angina. Acute abdominal pain develops after a plaque breaks free and obstructs blood flow within the SMA.[83,85]

Thrombosis of the superior mesenteric vein is the least common cause of AMI, accounting for only 5% to 10% of cases. The cause is usually secondary to an underlying medical condition that causes a hypercoagulable state such as sepsis, malignancy, or liver disease. Mortality with venous thrombosis is significantly less than with SMA embolus, thrombosis, and NOMI.[86]

Abnormal laboratory values, such as an elevated white count, lactate, amylase, base excess, D dimer, and low pH, have been associated with AMI.[87] No single test s sensitive enough to make the diagnosis. The current standard for diagnosis is CT angiography. Although percutaneous thrombolytic treatment has been used for AMI, the primary treatment is surgery.[88] For most patients with AMI, and certainly those with signs of sepsis, early antibiotics are also key.

## Extra-Abdominal Causes

There are numerous causes of abdominal pain that may be secondary to pathologic conditions beyond the abdomen, so the astute EDC will keep a broad differential list.

One of the most serious causes is cardiac. Many elderly patients with MI present atypically, with abdominal pain or GI symptoms as the chief complaint. According to 1 study, 33% of older women diagnosed with MI presented with abdominal pain as the chief complaint.[89]

Some common infectious causes of abdominal pain include urinary tract infections, which occur at a much higher annual incidence in elderly patients, from 10% to 30% in patients living in nursing homes or long-term care facilities.[90] Herpes zoster, which is more common in the elderly, presents with trunk lesions 60% of the time and should be considered.[91]

Other causes can include lower lobe pneumonia, malignancy, metabolic abnormalities (diabetic ketoacidosis or adrenal insufficiency), and withdrawal from medications. **Table 3** lists common extra-abdominal causes of pain in the elderly that should be considered.

## General Management Strategies

The approach to elderly patients with abdominal pain requires an individualized approach. Although many patients are volume-depleted from poor oral intake combined with excessive losses due to vomiting or diarrhea, the higher incidence of congestive heart failure in this population requires careful attention to fluid balance rather than indiscriminant large boluses of crystalloid. Fluid hydration is a significant aspect of management, however, especially because many of these patients will require IV contrast for imaging studies. Small sequential boluses with frequent re-evaluation of the patient's cardiopulmonary status are appropriate.

Urinalysis is an important part of the work-up, yet many geriatric patients will have difficulty with providing a sample, much less a clean, uncontaminated sample. However, urinary catheters should not be used simply to obtain urine for testing if a patient is able to void on their own. If a catheter is used, it should not be left indwelling merely for convenience. The elderly are at higher risk than the general public for catheter-associated urinary tract infections.

Analgesia is an important component of the management of abdominal pain. Elderly patients are screened less often for pain and are often provided inadequate

| Table 3 | |
|---|---|
| **Extra-abdominal causes of abdominal pain in the elderly** | |
| Cardiac | Myocardial infarction, pericarditis, heart failure |
| Pulmonary | Lower lobe pneumonia, pneumothorax, pulmonary embolism |
| Metabolic | Diabetic ketoacidosis, adrenal insufficiency, hypercalcemia, uremia |
| Infectious | Herpes zoster, cellulitis, urinary tract infections |
| Genitourinary | Prostatitis, neurogenic bladder, uterine prolapse |
| Medication | Narcotic withdrawal, iron overdose, antibiotics |
| Hematologic | Acute leukemia, rectus sheath hematoma (anticoagulated patients) |

analgesia.[92] Several medications that are frequently used in the management of patients with abdominal pain (eg, metoclopramide and ketorolac) are determined by the Beers Criteria to be potentially inappropriate medications in the elderly.[93]

Patients who are ill-appearing are best served by early surgical consultation, in parallel with the ongoing evaluation. The same is true for those who are thought to be high-risk (by history, physical examination, and risk factor analysis) for life-threatening conditions such as ruptured AAA or mesenteric ischemia. Many patients will require prolonged evaluations and thorough work-ups that include serial examinations. As such, observation or admission may be required. For those that are discharged home, clear discharge instructions and a definitive follow-up plan are crucial.

## SUMMARY

The geriatric patient with abdominal pain presents a unique set of challenges, including atypical presentations, distinctive physiology, and life-threatening disease. A broad differential with rapid evaluation and aggressive use of laboratory and radiologic testing is necessary to effectively evaluate and treat this population.

## REFERENCES

1. US Census Bureau. Age and Sex Composition: 2011. Available at: http://www.census.gov/prod/cen2010/briefs/c2010br-03.pdf. Accessed November 1, 2015.
2. National Center for Health Statistics. Health, United States, 2014. Hyattsville (MD): U.S. Department of Health and Human Services; 2014. Available at: http://www.cdc.gov/nchs/data/hus/hus14.pdf#086.
3. Bugliosi TF, Meloy TD, Vukov LF. Acute abdominal pain in the elderly. Ann Emerg Med 1990;19(12):1383–6.
4. Lewis LM, Banet GA, Blanda M, et al. Etiology and clinical course of abdominal pain in senior patients: a prospective, multicenter study. J Gerontol A Biol Sci Med Sci 2005;60(8):1071–6.
5. Singal BM, Hedges JR, Rousseau EW, et al. Geriatric patient emergency visits part I: comparison of visits by geriatric and younger patients. Ann Emerg Med 1992;21(7):802–7.
6. Marco CA, Schoenfeld CN, Keyl PM, et al. Abdominal pain in geriatric emergency patients: variables associated with adverse outcomes. Acad Emerg Med 1998; 5(12):1163–8.
7. Fenyo G. Acute abdominal disease in the elderly. Am J Surg 1982;143(6):751–4.
8. van Geloven AA, Biesheuvel TH, Luitse JSK, et al. Hospital admissions of patients aged over 80 with acute abdominal complaints. Eur J Surg 2000;16(11):866–71.
9. Norman DC, Grahn D, Yoshikawa TT. Fever and aging. J Am Geriatr Soc 1995; 80(1):53–67.
10. Chung MH, Huang CC, Vong SC, et al. Geriatric fever score: a new decision rule for geriatric care. PLos One 2014;9(10):e110927.
11. Carpenter CR, Katz ED. Fever and immune function in the elderly. In: Meldon SW, Ma OJ, Woolard R, editors. Geriatric emergency medicine. New York: McGraw-Hill; 2004. p. 55–69.
12. Martinez JP, Mattu A. Abdominal pain in the elderly. Emerg Med Clin North Am 2006;24(2):371–88.
13. Roque MV, Bouras EP. Epidemiology and management of chronic constipation in elderly patients. Clin Interv Aging 2015;10:919–30.

14. Camilleri M, Lee JS, Viramontes B, et al. Insights into the pathophysiology and mechanisms of constipation, irritable bowel syndrome and diverticulosis in older people. J Am Geriatr Soc 2000;48(9):1142–50.
15. Roehrborn CG. The epidemiology of acute urinary retention in benign prostatic hyperplasia. Rev Urol 2001;3(4):187–92.
16. Cooper GS, Shales DM, Salata RA. Intraabdominal infection: differences in presentation and outcome between younger patients and the elderly. Clin Infect Dis 1994;19(1):146–8.
17. McCleane G. Pain perception in the elderly patient. Clin Geriatr Med 2008;24(2): 203–11.
18. National Center for Health Statistics. Health, United States, 2013: with special feature on prescription drugs. Available at: http://www.cdc.gov/nchs/data/hus/hus13.pdf#092. Accessed November 1, 2015.
19. Frenk SM, Porter KS, Paulozzi LJ. Prescription opioid analgesic use among adults: United States, 1999-2012. NCHS Data Brief 2015;189:1–8. Available at: http://www.cdc.gov/nchs/data/dataBriefs/db189.pdf.
20. Hoffman ME. Peptic ulcer disease and gastrointestinal bleeding. In: Meldon SW, Ma OJ, Woolard R, editors. Geriatric emergency medicine. New York: McGraw-Hill; 2004. p. 179–84.
21. Yachimski PS, Friedman LS. Gastrointestinal bleeding in the elderly. Nat Clin Pract Gastroenterol Hepatol 2008;5(2):80–93.
22. Ahmed A, Stanley AJ. Acute upper gastrointestinal bleeding in the elderly: aetiology, diagnosis and treatment. Drugs Aging 2012;29(12):993–1040.
23. Thomopoulos KC, Vagenas KA, Vagianos CE, et al. Changes in aetiology and clinical outcome of acute upper gastrointestinal bleeding during the last 15 years. Eur J Gastroenterol Hepatol 2004;16(2):177–82.
24. Huang JQ, Sridhar S, Hunt RH. Role of *Helicobacter pylori* infection and non-steroidal anti-inflammatory drugs in peptic ulcer disease: a meta-analysis. Lancet 2002;359(9300):14–22.
25. Shorr RK, Ray WA, Daugherty JR, et al. Concurrent use of nonsteroidal anti-inflammatory drugs and oral anticoagulants places elderly persons at high risk for hemorrhagic peptic ulcer disease. Arch Intern Med 1993;153(14):1665–70.
26. Laine L, Jensen DM. Management of patients with ulcer bleeding. Am J Gastroenterol 2012;107(3):345–60.
27. McNamara RM. Acute abdominal pain. In: Sanders AB, editor. Emergency care of the elder person. St Louis (MO): Beverly Cracom Publications; 1996. p. 219–43.
28. Bellotto F, Fagiuoli S, Pavei A, et al. Anemia and ischemia: myocardial injury in patients with gastrointestinal bleeding. Am J Med 2005;118(5):548–51.
29. Shah BB, Agrawal RM, Goldwasser B, et al. Biliary disease in the elderly. Pract Gastroenterol 2008;32(9):14–6, 19,20,22–24,26.
30. Ross SO, Forsmark CE. Pancreatic and biliary disorders in the elderly. Gastroenterol Clin North Am 2001;30(2):531–45.
31. Rosenthal RA, Anderson DK. Surgery in the elderly: observations on the pathophysiology and treatment of cholelithiasis. Exp Gerontol 1993;28(4–5):459–72.
32. Sharma BC, Kumar R, Agarwal N, et al. Endoscopic biliary drainage by nasobiliary drain or by stent placement in patients with acute cholangitis. Endoscopy 2005;37(5):439–43.
33. Agarwal N, Chander Sharma B, Sarin SK. Endoscopic management of acute cholangitis in elderly patients. World J Gastroenterol 2006;12(40):6551–5.

34. Morrow DJ, Thompson J, Wilson SE. Acute cholecystitis in the elderly. Arch Surg 1978;113:114–52.

35. Shea JA, Verlin JA, Escarce JJ, et al. Revised estimates of diagnostic test sensitivity and specificity in suspected biliary tract disease. Arch Intern Med 1994; 154(22):2573–81.

36. Miller AH, Pepe PE, Brockman R, et al. ED ultrasound in hepatobiliary disease. J Emerg Med 2006;30(1):69–74.

37. Bennett GL, Balthazar EJ. Ultrasound and CT evaluation of emergent gallbladder pathology. Radiol Clin North Am 2003;41(6):1203–16.

38. Williams TP, Dimou FM, Adhikari D, et al. Hospital readmissions after emergency room visits for cholelithiasis. J Surg Res 2015;197(2):318–23.

39. Shah BB, Farah KF, Goldwasser B, et al. Pancreatic disease in the elderly. Pract Gastroenterol 2008b;32(10):18–23, 27–30,32.

40. Gloor B, Zulfiqar Z, Waldemar U, et al. Pancreatic disease in the elderly. Best Pract Res Clin Gastroenterol 2002;16(1):159–70.

41. Kaurich T. Drug-induced acute pancreatitis. Proc (Bayl Univ Med Cent) 2008; 21(1):77–81.

42. Corfield AP, Cooper MJ, Williams RC. Acute pancreatitis: a lethal disease of increasing incidence. Gut 1985;26(7):724–9.

43. Petrowsky H, Clavien PA. Should we deny surgery for malignant hepato-pancreatico-biliary tumors to elderly patients? World J Surg 2005;29(9): 1093–100.

44. Taylor MR, Lalani N. Adult small bowel obstructions. Acad Emerg Med 2013; 20(6):528–44.

45. Fevang BT, Fevang J, Stangeland L, et al. Complications and death after surgical treatment of small bowel obstruction. Ann Surg 2000;231(4):529–37.

46. Eskelinen M, Ikonen J, Lipponen P. Contributions of history-taking, physical examination, and computer assistance to diagnosis of acute small-bowel obstruction. Scand J Gastroenterol 1994;29(8):715–21.

47. Brant WE, Helms CA. Fundamentals of diagnostic radiology. Philadelphia: Lippincott Williams & Wilkins; 2007.

48. Jang BT, Schindler D, Kaji A. Bedside ultrasonography for the detection of small bowel obstruction in the emergency department. Emerg Med J 2011;28(8): 676–8.

49. Schmutz GR, Benko A, Fournier L, et al. Small bowel obstruction: role and contribution of sonography. Eur Radiol 1997;7(7):1054–8.

50. Simmons WN, Putzer GJ. Bowel obstruction. In: Meldon SW, Ma OJ, Woolard R, editors. Geriatric emergency medicine. New York: McGraw-Hill; 2004. p. 198–201.

51. Richards WO, Willaims LF. Obstruction of the large and small intestine. Surg Clin North Am 1988;68(2):355–76.

52. Halabi WJ, Jafari MD, Kang CY, et al. Colonic volvulus in the United States: trends, outcomes, and predictors of mortality. Ann Surg 2014;259(2):293–301.

53. Frizelle FA, Wolff BG. Colonic volvulus. Adv Surg 1996;29:131–9.

54. Jones IT, Fazio VW. Colonic volvulus. Etiology and management. Dig Dis 1989; 7(4):203–9.

55. Ferzoco LB, Raptopoulos V, Silen W. Current concepts: acute diverticulitis. N Engl J Med 1998;338(21):1521–6.

56. Liu CK, Hsu HH, Cheng SM. Colonic diverticulitis in the elderly. Int J Gerontol 2009;3(1):9–15.

57. Hobson KG, Roberts PL. Etiology and pathophysiology of diverticular disease. Clin Colon Rectal Surg 2004;17(3):147–53.

58. Farrell RJ, Farrell JJ, Morrin MM. Gastrointestinal disorders in the elderly. Gastroenterol Clin North Am 2001;30(2):475–96.

59. Stollman NH, Raskin JB. Diverticular disease of the colon. J Clin Gastroenterol 1999;29(3):241–52.

60. Cho KC, Morehouse HT, Alterman DD, et al. Sigmoid diverticulitis: diagnostic role of CT–comparison with barium enema studies. Radiology 1990;176(1):111–5.

61. Laméris W, van Randen A, van Gulik TM, et al. A clinical decision rule to establish the diagnosis of acute diverticulitis at the emergency department. Dis Colon Rectum 2010;53(6):896–904.

62. Ghnnam WM. Elderly versus young patients with appendicitis 3 years experience. Alexandria J Med 2012;48(1):9–12.

63. Gupta H, Dupuy D. Abdominal emergencies: has anything changed? Surg Clin North Am 1997;77:1245–64.

64. Young YR, Chiu TF, Chen JC, et al. Acute appendicitis in the octogenarians and beyond: a comparison with younger geriatric patients. Am J Med Sci 2007; 334(4):255–9.

65. Horattas MC, Guyton DP, Wu D. A reappraisal of appendicitis in the elderly. Am J Surg 1990;160(3):291–3.

66. Sidman RD, Roche CN, Meldon SW. Acute appendicitis. In: Meldon SW, Ma OJ, Woolard R, editors. Geriatric emergency medicine. New York: McGraw-Hill; 2004. p. 220–6.

67. La Mura F, Di Patrizi MS, Farinella E, et al. Acute appendicitis in the geriatric patient. BMC Geriatr 2009;9(Suppl I):A70.

68. Elangovan S. Clinical and laboratory findings in acute appendicitis in the elderly. J Am Board Fam Parct 1996;9(2):75–8.

69. Omari AH, Khammash MR, Qasaimeh GR, et al. Acute appendicitis in the elderly: risk factors for perforation. World J Emerg Surg 2014;9(1):6.

70. Forde KA. The role of laparoscopy in the evaluation of the acute abdomen in critically ill patients. Surg Endosc 1992;6(5):219–21.

71. Koruda MJ. Appendicitis: laparoscopic strategy in diagnosis and treatment. N C Med J 1992;53(5):196–8.

72. Cosford PA, LEng GC. Screening for abdominal aortic aneurysm. Cochrane Database Syst Rev 2007;(2):CD002945.

73. Marston WA, Ahlquist R, Johnson G, et al. Misdiagnosis of ruptured abdominal aortic aneurysm. J Vasc Surg 1992;16(1):17–22.

74. Assar AN, Zarins CK. Ruptured abdominal aortic aneurysm: a surgical emergency with many clinical presentations. Postgrad Med J 2009;85(1003):268–73.

75. Kamano S, Yonezawa I, Arai Y, et al. Acute abdominal aortic aneurysm rupture presenting as transient paralysis of the lower legs: a case report. J Emerg Med 2005;29(1):53–5.

76. Borrero E, Queral LA. Symptomatic abdominal aortic aneurysm misdiagnosed as nephroureterolithiasis. Ann Vasc Surg 1988;2(2):145–9.

77. Lynch RM. Ruptured abdominal aortic aneurysm presenting as groin pain. Br J Gen Pract 2002;52(477):320–1.

78. Sufi PA. A rare case of leaking abdominal aneurysm presenting as isolated right testicular pain. CJEM 2007;9(2):124–6.

79. Costantino TG, Bruno EC, Handly N. Accuracy of emergency medicine ultrasound in the evaluation of abdominal aortic aneurysm. Ann Emerg Med 2007; 49(4):547.

80. Moll FL, Powell JT, Fraedrich G, et al. Management of abdominal aortic aneurysms clinical practice guidelines of the European Society for Vascular Surgery. Eur J Vasc Endovasc Surg 2011;41(Suppl 1):S1–58.
81. Oldenburg WA, Lau LL, Rodenberg TJ, et al. Acute mesenteric ischemia. Arch Intern Med 2004;164:1054–62.
82. Ruotolo RA, Evans SR. Mesenteric ischemia in the elderly. Clin Geriatr Med 1999; 15(3):527–57.
83. Vitin AA, Metzner JI. Anesthetic management of acute mesenteric ischemia in elderly patients. Anesthesiol Clin 2009;27(3):551–67.
84. Diamond S, Emmett M, Henrich WL. Bowel infarction as a cause of death in dialysis patients. JAMA 1986;256:2545.
85. Manko JA, Levy PD. Mesenteric ischemia. In: Meldon SW, Ma OJ, Woolard R, editors. Geriatric emergency medicine. New York: McGraw-Hill; 2004. p. 227–36.
86. Clavien PA, Durig M, Harder F. Venous mesenteric infarction: a particular entity. Br J Surg 1988;75(3):252–5.
87. Brandt LJ, Boley SJ. AGA technical review on intestinal ischemia. Gastroenterology 2000;118(5):954–68.
88. Stoker J, van Randen A, Lameris W, et al. Imaging patients with acute abdominal pain. Radiology 2009;253(1):31–46.
89. Lusiani L, Perrone A, Pesavento R, et al. Prevalence, clinical features, and acute course of atypical myocardial infarction. Angiology 1994;45(1):49–55.
90. Cove-Smith A, Almond M. Management of urinary tract infections in the elderly. Trends in Urology, Gynaecology & Sexual Health 2007;12(4):31–4.
91. Yawn BP, Saddier P, Wollan PC, et al. A population-based study of the incidence and complication rates of herpes zoster before zoster vaccine introduction. Mayo Clin Proc 2007;82(11):1341–9.
92. Hwang U, Platts-Mills TF. Acute pain management in older adults in the emergency department. Clin Geriatr Med 2013;29(1):151–64.
93. American Geriatrics Society updated Beers Criteria for potentially inappropriate medication use in older adults. J Am Geriatr Soc 2012;60(4):616–31.

# Neurologic Emergencies in the Elderly

Lauren M. Nentwich, MD*, Benjamin Grimmnitz, MD

## KEYWORDS

- Neurologic diseases • Geriatric patients • Neurologic emergencies

## KEY POINTS

- Neurologic diseases are a major cause of death and disability in elderly patients.
- Due to the physiologic changes and increased comorbidities that occur as people age, neurologic diseases are more common in geriatric patients and a frequent cause of emergency department (ED) presentation.
- The care of geriatric patients with neurological emergencies in challenging and complicated. ED physicians can improve outcomes and quality of life in these patients through aggressive and directed care in conjunction with specialists consultation.

## INTRODUCTION

Neurologic diseases are a major cause of death and disability in elderly patients. Due to the physiologic changes and increased comorbidities that occur as people age, neurologic diseases are more common in geriatric patients and a major cause of death and disability in this population. This article discusses the elderly patient presenting to the emergency department with acute ischemic stroke (AIS), transient ischemic attack (TIA), intracerebral hemorrhage (ICH), subarachnoid hemorrhage (SAH), chronic subdural hematoma (CSDH), traumatic brain injury, seizures, and central nervous system (CNS) infections. This article reviews the subtle presentations, difficult workups, and complicated treatment decisions as they pertain to our older patients.

## ACUTE ISCHEMIC STROKE

Stroke is the fourth leading cause of death and the leading cause of long-term disability in the United States, and approximately 795,000 Americans suffer a new or recurrent stroke annually.[1] AIS makes up approximately 87% of all strokes, and occurs when a thrombotic or embolic event causes sudden loss of blood supply to an area of the brain with resulting focal neurologic deficits.[1,2] AIS tends to be a

Disclosures: None.
Department of Emergency Medicine, Boston Medical Center, Dowling 1 South, 1 Boston Medical Center Place, Boston, MA 02143, USA
* Corresponding author.
E-mail address: lauren.nentwich@bmc.org

Emerg Med Clin N Am 34 (2016) 575–599
http://dx.doi.org/10.1016/j.emc.2016.04.009     emed.theclinics.com
0733-8627/16/$ – see front matter © 2016 Elsevier Inc. All rights reserved.

disease of the elderly, with average first stroke occurring at age 75 for women and 71 for men,[1] and 30% of all strokes occurring in patients older than 80 years.[3] Additionally, it is estimated that the incidence of stroke will more than double between 2010 and 2050, with most of the increase occurring in patients with age older than 75 years.[4] AIS in geriatric patients is also associated with much worse outcomes than in younger patients[1] (**Box 1**). Given the high incidences of AIS with associated increases in morbidity and mortality in geriatric patients, it is important that these patients are rapidly diagnosed and treated so as to offer them the greatest likelihood of a good outcome.

The diagnosis of AIS is made using a combination of patient history, physical examination, and imaging studies. Patients suffering an AIS may present with a variety of focal neurologic deficits, and elderly patients are more complicated as they may present with known focal neurologic symptoms or less specific atypical signs and symptoms[2,5] (**Box 2**). In addition to presenting with atypical symptoms, geriatric patients are significantly less likely to know signs and symptoms of stroke,[6] and more likely to delay going to the hospital.[5] A high degree of suspicion should always be maintained in evaluating elderly patients with focal neurologic symptoms and possible AIS.

Elderly patients presenting with suspected AIS should be triaged at the highest priority and undergo immediate evaluation by an emergency physician followed by urgent stroke team consultation. Initial evaluation should begin with a primary survey and immediate stabilization of the airway, breathing, circulation (ABCs) as needed with concurrent point-of-care blood glucose testing. A precise but expedited history should be obtained from the patient or accompanying family or caregivers, with special attention given to the time of symptom onset and/or the time that the patient was last seen at his or her neurologic baseline, as well as any potential contraindications to intravenous (IV) recombinant tissue plasminogen activator (rt-PA)[7] (**Box 3**). A rapid and thorough physical examination must be completed and the focused neurologic examination is enhanced by the use of a formal stroke score or scale, such as the National Institutes of Health Stroke Scale (NIHSS)[8] (access at: https://www.ninds.nih.gov/doctors/NIH_Stroke_Scale.pdf). Laboratory testing should include coagulation studies, platelets, and renal function. Given the increased risk of cardiac arrhythmias, especially atrial fibrillation, and cardiac ischemia in the elderly, a 12-lead electrocardiogram, cardiac monitoring, and cardiac enzymes should be performed in all elderly patients with suspected AIS.[7] This initial workup should not delay urgent brain imaging, especially in patients with onset of symptoms within the past 3 to 6 hours.

Patients presenting with possible AIS should undergo urgent brain imaging by computed tomography (CT) or MRI is necessary to exclude the presence of hemorrhage as the cause of the patient's focal neurologic symptoms and may help to guide

---

**Box 1**
**Worsened outcomes in patients suffering an ischemic stroke**

- Increased risk-adjusted mortality
- Increased disability
- Longer hospitalizations
- Less evidence-based care
- Less likely to be discharged to their initial residence

*Data from* Mozaffarian D, Benjamin EJ, Go AS, et al. Heart disease and stroke statistics—2015 update: a report from the American Heart Association. Circulation 2015;131(4):e29–322.

---

**Box 2**
**Signs/symptoms of acute ischemic stroke (AIS) in geriatric patients**

- Motor weakness
- Sensory loss
- Aphasia
- Dysarthria
- Neglect
- Vertigo/dizziness
- Visual field deficits
- Falls[a]
- Reduced mobility[a]
- Altered mental status[a]
- Urinary incontinence[a]

[a] Atypical signs/symptoms of AIS that may be seen in geriatric patients.
*Data from* Pare JR, Kahn JH. Basic neuroanatomy and stroke syndromes. Emerg Med Clin North Am 2012;30(3):601–15; and Muangpaisan W, Hinkle JL, Westwood M, et al. Stroke in the very old: clinical presentations and outcomes. Age Ageing 2008;37(4):473–5.

---

treatment (**Fig. 1**). Noncontrast brain CT is rapid with high accuracy in excluding hemorrhage and may be preferred in geriatric patients with cardiac pacemakers or other ferromagnetic metallic implanted substances that are contraindications for MRI. However, MRI is more specific and accurate for the diagnosis of AIS in patients in whom the diagnosis is less certain.[9]

In 1996, the Food and Drug Administration (FDA) approved the use of IV rt-PA for patients suffering an AIS.[10] The treatment of elderly patients with IV rt-PA is more complicated than for younger patients. Although geriatric patients are at increased risk for stroke-related death and disability, they may also be at increased risk for hemorrhagic complications after treatment with IV rt-PA.[11] The 1995 National Institutes of Neurological Disorders and Stroke (NINDS) IV rt-PA trial for treatment of patients with AIS within 3 hours of symptom onset enrolled 44 patients older than 80 years; these elderly patients were 2.87 times more likely than younger patients to experience symptomatic intracranial hemorrhage within 36 hours of treatment.[12] Due to these findings, when the European Cooperative Acute Stroke Study III (ECASS III) expanded the treatment window for IV rt-PA to 3.0 to 4.5 hours of symptom onset, the investigators excluded geriatric patients older than 80 years due to concern for increased risk of hemorrhagic complications.[13] However, multiple studies have shown a benefit of treatment with IV rt-PA in elderly patients older than 80 years within 3 hours of symptom onset.[11,14–16] Treating elderly patients with IV rt-PA within 3 hours of symptom onset is accepted treatment, but the treatment window should not be expanded to 4.5 hours in patients older than 80 years.[17]

Five positive trials published in 2015 have brought significant changes to the management of certain patients suffering an AIS. These 5 trials found a benefit to using stent retrievers for mechanical thrombectomy of proximal large-vessel occlusions and increased treatment options for selected patients presenting with AIS as well has helped to broaden the time window for possible therapeutic intervention.[18–22]

The first positive endovascular trial in the treatment of AIS, Multicenter Randomized Clinical Trial of Endovascular Treatment for Acute Ischemic Stroke (MR CLEAN), was

---

**Box 3**
**Contraindications to intravenous recombinant tissue plasminogen activator administration for AIS within 3 hours of symptom onset**

*Absolute exclusion criteria:*

- Significant head trauma or prior stroke in previous 3 months
- Symptoms suggestive of subarachnoid hemorrhage
- Arterial puncture at noncompressible site in previous 7 days
- History of previous intracranial hemorrhage
- Intracranial neoplasm, arteriovenous malformation, or aneurysm
- Recent intracranial or intraspinal surgery
- Elevated blood pressure (systolic >185 mm Hg or diastolic >110 mm Hg)
- Active internal bleeding
- Acute bleeding diathesis
- Platelet count less than 100,000/mm$^3$
- Heparin use within 48 hours, resulting in abnormally elevated activated partial thromboplastin time
- Current use of anticoagulant with international normalized ratio >1.7 or prothrombin time >15 seconds
- Current use of direct thrombin inhibitors or direct factor Xa inhibitors
- Blood glucose concentration <50 mg/dL or >400 mg/dL that cannot be corrected
- Computed tomography demonstrates multilobar infarction (hypodensity greater than one-third cerebral hemisphere)

*Relative exclusion criteria:*

- Minor or rapidly improving stroke symptoms
- Pregnancy
- Seizure at onset with postictal residual neurologic impairments
- Major surgery or serious trauma within previous 14 days
- Gastrointestinal or urinary tract hemorrhage within previous 21 days
- Myocardial infarction within previous 3 months

*Data from* Jauch EC, Saver JL, Adams HP, et al. Guidelines for the early management of patients with acute ischemic stroke: a guideline for healthcare professionals from the American Heart Association/American Stroke Association. Stroke 2013;44(3):870–947.

---

published in early 2015 and evaluated the role of endovascular treatment plus standard medical therapy up to 6 hours from symptom onset for patients with proximal large vessel intracranial arterial occlusion. Modified Rankin scores (mRS) at 90 days showed a significant increase in the rate of functional independence (mRS = 0–2) in the intervention arm (32.6% vs 19.1%). All patients enrolled in the MR CLEAN study had imaging of their cerebral vessels before enrollment. There was no age cutoff for this trial and the mean age of enrollment was just older than 65. A predefined subgroup analysis examining cohorts of patients older than and younger than 80 found consistent treatment effect in both groups.[18]

The other 4 interventional trials were all stopped early due to the positive MR CLEAN trial. Despite differences in methodology and smaller sample sizes, the combined

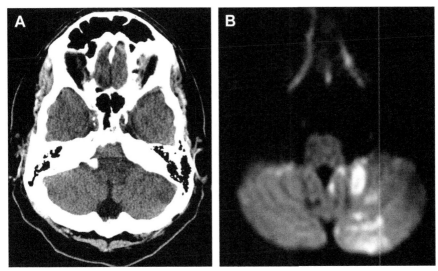

**Fig. 1.** Stroke on CT and MRI. (*A*) Noncontrast brain CT shows hypodensity in the left cerebellum consistent with recent stroke. (*B*) Diffusion-weighted MRI shows acute left cerebellum stroke.

results of these 5 studies show that mechanical thrombectomy of large-vessel occlusive AIS results in improved neurologic outcomes compared with rt-PA alone.[18–22] Four of the 5 trials ran prespecified subgroup analysis dividing patients at age 70 or 80 years, and all 4 found no change in the treatment effect between subgroups.[18,19,21,22] A prespecified meta-analysis looking at patient-level data from 4 of the trials in which Solitaire (Covidien, Irvine, CA) was the only or the predominant device used showed no reduced treatment effect in the elderly and a clinically and significant 20% absolute reduction in mortality for treated patients with age 80 or older.[23] A meta-analysis from the pooled patient-level data of all 5 trials showed the endovascular thrombectomy is favored over control in patients aged 80 years or older with a common odds ratio of 3.68 (95% confidence interval 1.95–6.92).[24–27] These 5 landmark trials and the following meta-analyses show that endovascular therapy should be strongly considered in elderly patients presenting with acute large-vessel occlusive ischemic stroke.

There have been a number of studies examining early hemicraniectomy in patients suffering a malignant middle cerebral artery (MCA) infarction with excessive brain edema, elevated intracranial pressure (ICP), and concern for herniation.[24–27] Initial trials performed on patients younger than 60 showed lower risks of death and disability, although there were increased numbers of severely disabled.[24,28,29] The DESTINY II trial focused on early hemicraniectomy (within 48 hours) in older patients suffering a malignant MCA infarct with edema and enrolled patients older than 60. In this trial, early hemicraniectomy in elderly patients significantly increased the probability of their survival, but most survivors had substantial disability with no patients attaining an mRS of 0 to 2.[29,30] On the basis of this study, it seems problematic to state an absolute cutoff of 60 years. However, due to the high morbidity in elderly patients, each patient should be evaluated individually with full discussion with patients' family members regarding the potential attitudes of the patient toward a life-saving procedure with potentially associated severe disabilities.[29]

## TRANSIENT ISCHEMIC ATTACK

A TIA is defined as a "transient episode of neurologic dysfunction caused by focal brain, spinal cord, or retinal ischemia, without acute infarction."[31] As with AIS, the incidence of TIA markedly increases with age, from 1 to 3 cases per 100,000 in those younger than 35 years to up to 600 to 1500 cases per 100,000 in those patients older than 85 years.[31,32] The importance of diagnosing TIA in the elderly is due to the significantly elevated risk of AIS after TIA,[33] and the pooled early risk of stroke after TIA has been reported as 3.1% to 3.5% at 2 days, 5.2% at 7 days, 8.0% at 30 days, and 9.2% at 90 days.[34,35] It is important that all elderly patients presenting with transient neurologic symptoms be worked up for TIA so as to optimize their current health and implement necessary treatments to prevent future stroke in these high-risk patients.

In elderly patients presenting with potential TIA, rapid triage and evaluation, initial history, physical examination, and diagnostic testing should mirror the evaluation of AIS. The diagnosis of TIA is clinical, and the history should focus on the nature and duration of focal neurologic deficits, whereas the physical examination should include a complete neurologic examination to determine if full neurologic function has been restored. All patients should undergo an evaluation and workup by a persons with clinical stroke expertise (**Box 4**). Neuroimaging, preferably by MRI, should be within 24 hours of symptom onset and include imaging of the cervicocephalic vessels.[31,36–38] Patients suffering a TIA should be evaluated via inpatient hospitalization, an observation unit, or a dedicated outpatient 24-hour TIA clinic to ensure that all necessary tests and monitoring is completed.[36,38] Given the high morbidity and mortality of elderly patients who suffer a TIA, it is prudent to consider hospitalization or admission to an observational unit to facilitate the rapid workup for secondary prevention as well as close monitoring for recurrent symptoms.

The treatment of patients suffering a TIA focuses on the prevention of future AIS by looking for definitive secondary causes amenable to intervention. Reviewing all potential interventions and treatments for patients suffering a TIA is outside the scope of this

---

**Box 4**
**Workup of patients suffering a transient ischemic attack (TIA)**

- Routine Laboratory Testing
  - Including platelet and coagulopathy studies

- Electrocardiogram
  - Screen for cardiac arrhythmias, particularly atrial fibrillation

- Brain Imaging
  - MRI preferred: diffusion-weighted imaging lesions are a risk marker for early stroke recurrence
  - Vascular imaging of the cervicocephalic vessels: therapeutic intervention for certain stenosis

- Echocardiography
  - Reserved for patients without a clear cause of TIA after workup or patients with high suspicion of cardiac etiology

- Cardiac Monitoring
  - In appropriate patients, to monitor for paroxysmal atrial fibrillation and other cardiac arrhythmias

- Risk Factor Screening
  - Screen for diabetes mellitus (HbA1c)
  - Screen for hypercholesterolemia and hyperlipidemia

*Data from* Refs.[31,36–38]

article, but there are a few specific interventions that have shown to be beneficial or specific to elderly patients.[39] All patients with TIA who are medically fit to undergo surgery receive benefit from carotid endarterectomy (CEA) for ipsilateral severe (70%–99%) carotid stenosis. Medically fit patients older than 75 years with recent TIA also receive benefit from undergoing CEA in cases of ipsilateral moderate (50%–69%) stenosis, and should be evaluated for the possibility of this procedure.[40] Additionally, atrial fibrillation is a common cause of embolic TIA and is the leading cardiac arrhythmia found in older patients. Elderly patients with TIA with known atrial fibrillation or who are found to have atrial fibrillation on cardiac monitoring should be considered for anticoagulation to prevent recurrent stroke. Due to other comorbidities, many older patients may not be able to take oral anticoagulation and these patients should be treated with aspirin.[39]

## NONTRAUMATIC INTRACEREBRAL HEMORRHAGE

ICH is defined as spontaneous, nontraumatic bleeding into the brain parenchyma.[41] It accounts for 10% to 15% of all first-ever strokes and remains a significant cause of morbidity and mortality, with 30-day mortality rates of 35% to 52% and only 20% of patients functionally independent at 6 months.[42] ICH is classified as primary or secondary, dependent on whether or not there is an underlying congenital lesion as the cause.

ICH is an important disease of the elderly with an incidence that increases with age and doubles each decade after 35 years of age.[43] Risk factors for ICH include older age, as well as a number of other factors that are often seen in elderly patients, such as cerebral amyloid angiopathy, hypertension, previous stroke, and oral anticoagulation use.[44]

The clinical presentation of ICH depends on its location, size, and rapidity of development.[45] Similar to AIS, ICH causes sudden onset of focal neurologic deficits with certain initial findings more likely to be associated with ICH[46,47] (**Box 5**). However, many patients suffering an ICH lack these distinctive clinical findings and ICH can only definitively be made through the use of brain imaging.[47]

---

**Box 5**
**Clinical findings more likely to be associated with intracranial hemorrhage over AIS**

- Symptom progression over minutes to hours
- Loss of consciousness
- Coma
- Neck stiffness
- Seizure at onset of neurologic symptoms
- Systolic blood pressure >220 mm Hg
- Diastolic blood pressure >110 mm Hg
- Vomiting
- Severe headache

*Data from* Unchey S, McGee S. Does this patient have a hemorrhagic stroke? Clinical findings distinguishing hemorrhagic stroke from ischemic stroke. JAMA 2010;303(22):2280–6; and Hemphill JC, Greenberg SM, Anderson CS, et al. Guidelines for the management of spontaneous intracerebral hemorrhage: a guideline for healthcare professionals from the American Heart Association/American Stroke Association. Stroke 2015;46(7):2032–60.

Initial evaluation of patients with known or suspected ICH should mirror that outlined for AIS with triage as highest priority and immediate emergency physician evaluation with stabilization followed by urgent neurology and neurosurgical consultation. Given the high prevalence of hypertension as well as oral anticoagulation therapy in the elderly, special attention should be paid to blood pressure (BP) and coagulation studies as part of the initial workup. Elderly patients presenting with concern for ICH should undergo rapid brain imaging by noncontrast CT or gradient-echo (GRE) and T2* susceptibility-weighted MRI. Once ICH is diagnosed, additional neuroimaging, such as CT angiography/venography or MR angiography/venography, may be performed in select patients to evaluate for secondary causes of ICH that are amenable to intervention, such as aneurysms, arteriovenous malformations, fistulas, or cerebral venous thrombosis.[47]

Acutely elevated BP is common in patients with ICH, especially in elderly patients, and may lead to adverse outcomes via hematoma expansion or perihematomal edema formation. Early studies showed that early intensive lowering of BP in patients suffering an ICH is clinically feasible and safe.[48,49] INTERACT2, a phase 3 trial investigating the efficacy of aggressive BP lowering in patients suffering an ICH with systolic BP (SBP) between 150 and 220 within 6 hours of onset, did not show a significant reduction in the rate of death or severe disability but did continue to show that it was safe with surviving patients showing a modestly better functional recovery.[47,50] Based on these studies, current American Heart Association (AHA) class I recommendations on BP management in patients with ICH state that if SBP is 150 to 220 mm Hg without contraindications to acute BP treatment, lowering the SBP to less than 140 mm Hg is safe and may be effective in improving functional outcomes.[47]

Special consideration must be given to the patient on anticoagulation who suffers an ICH. Medication-related coagulopathy, via vitamin K antagonists (VKAs), low molecular weight heparin (LMWH), or the new oral anticoagulants (OACs), is more common in the geriatric population and increases the risk of ICH, and patients taking OACs constitute 12% to 20% of patients with ICH. LMWH is a direct factor Xa inhibitor given via subcutaneous injection, whereas the remainder of the anticoagulants are given orally. The oldest oral anticoagulant is warfarin, a VKA. The new OACs include direct factor IIa inhibitors (dabigatran) and direct factor Xa inhibitors (rivaroxaban, apixaban, and edoxaban). These new OACs appear to be associated with a lower risk of ICH than VKAs. However, in patients on anticoagulation suffering an ICH, the offending agent should be discontinued immediately and medical management should be targeted for early correction of their coagulopathy and to prevent continued bleeding. A brief overview of the pharmacokinetics and target reversal of anticoagulants in listed in **Table 1**. Anticoagulant activity typically dissipates after 4 to 5 half-lives, and patients should be monitored closely during this time.[51,52] For patients who are taking the antiplatelet agents, the usefulness of platelet transfusion in patients with ICH is uncertain and currently being evaluated in randomized clinical trials.[11]

All elderly patients diagnosed with ICH should undergo urgent neurology and neurosurgical consultation, or be transferred to a hospital with full neurology, neuroradiology, and neurosurgical capabilities. Studies have shown that one of the most important prognostic variables in determining outcome after ICH is the level of medical support provided, and patients who are initially predicted to have a poor outcome can achieve reasonable recovery if they are treated aggressively.[55] Limiting care in response to early Do Not Resuscitate (DNR) orders, withdrawal of care, or deferral of life-sustaining interventions is independently associated with both short-term and long-term mortality after ICH, independent of other predictors of death.[56] Per the AHA guidelines, aggressive care early after ICH onset with postponement of new

**Table 1**
**Pharmacokinetics and reversal of anticoagulants**

| Anticoagulant | Mechanism | Excretion | Half-Life, h | Reversal |
|---|---|---|---|---|
| Warfarin | Vitamin K antagonist | Hepatic (100%) | 36–42 | IV Vitamin K + PCCs (or FFP) |
| LMWH (enoxaparin) | Factor Xa inhibitor | Renal (100%) | 4.5–7 | Protamine Andexanet α[d] |
| Dabigatran | Direct Factor IIa inhibitor | Renal (85%) | 12–17 | Idarucizumab[a] May consider • Dialysis[b] • PCCs[c] |
| Rivaroxaban | Direct Factor Xa inhibitor | Renal (66%) Hepatic (33%) | 9–13 | Andexanet α[d] May consider: • Plasma exchange • PCCs[c] |
| Apixaban | Direct Factor Xa inhibitor | Renal (25%) Hepatic (75%) | 8–15 | Andexanet α[d] May consider: • Plasma exchange • PCCs[c] |
| Edoxaban | Direct Factor Xa inhibitor | Renal | 8–10 | Andexanet α[d] May consider: • Plasma exchange • PCCs[c] |

*Abbreviations:* FFP, fresh frozen plasma; IV, intravenous; LMWH, low molecular weight heparin; PCCs, prothrombin complex concentrates.
[a] Idarucizumab: Granted accelerated approval for emergency reversal by the Food and Drug Administration (FDA) in October 2015 after clinical trials showed complete reversal of the anticoagulant effect of dabigatran within minutes.[53]
[b] Dialysis may be considered in critical situation when reversal agent no available; 50% of dabigatran removed after 4 hours of dialysis.
[c] PCCs may be partially effective in reversal of the target-specific oral anticoagulants but have not been evaluated in large-scale clinical trials and have the potential risk of thrombosis.
[d] A recent trial showed that andexanet α was safe and reversed the activity of apixaban and rivaroxaban in healthy study participations within minutes.[54] A current trial is ongoing, with planned end date of November 2022, evaluating the utility of andexanet α in patients with acute major bleeding (clinicaltrials.gov) and andexanet α does not have yet have FDA approval.
*Data from* Yates S, Sarode R. Reversal of anticoagulant effects in patients with intracerebral hemorrhage. Curr Neurol Neurosci Rep 2015;15(1):504; and Abo-Salem E, Becker RC. Reversal of novel oral anticoagulants. Curr Opin Pharmacol 2016;27:86–91.

Do Not Attempt Resuscitation (DNAR) orders until at least the second full day of hospitalization is probably recommended, and DNAR status should not limit appropriate medical and surgical interventions unless otherwise explicitly indicated. This current recommendation does not apply to elderly patients with established DNAR orders.[47]

## ANEURYSMAL SUBARACHNOID HEMORRHAGE

Aneurysmal subarachnoid hemorrhage (aSAH) is characterized by extravasation of blood into the cerebrospinal fluid (CSF) from a ruptured intracranial aneurysm. It accounts for approximately 2% to 5% of all new strokes and has high morbidity and mortality with an average case fatality rate of 51% and approximately one-third of survivors requiring lifelong care. aSAH is an important disease in the elderly, as incidence increases with age.[57] Not only is there a higher prevalence of intracranial aneurysms in patients older than 60, but age-related risk factors, such as increased atherosclerosis and hypertension, likely compound the risk of formation and rupture in elderly patients.[58] Elderly patients suffering an aSAH have worsened outcomes, as advanced age is one of the major negative prognostic factors.[57]

Patients suffering an aSAH may present typically with a sudden onset severe headache that may be associated with nausea, vomiting, and/or brief loss of consciousness. The physical examination may show retinal hemorrhages, restlessness, diminished level of consciousness, nuchal rigidity, photophobia, and focal neurologic signs.[59] Disorders of consciousness are more frequently seen in geriatric patients than in the general population.[58]

Like AIS and ICH, initial evaluation of patients with suspected aSAH should start with the highest level triage with immediate physician evaluation and stabilization. Patients who present with the "typical" acute-onset severe headache with signs and symptoms of increased ICP offer little diagnostic dilemma, but patients presenting without these typical signs and symptoms are often misdiagnosed.[59] Misdiagnosis of aSAH is most commonly due to failure to obtain a noncontrast head CT. Noncontrast head CT is paramount in making the diagnosis of aSAH and should be performed in all patients with suspected aSAH[57] (Fig. 2). The sensitivity of CT decreases over time from onset of symptoms as CSF flow and spontaneous red-cell lysis can result in rapid clearing of subarachnoid blood.[59] As such, lumbar puncture (LP) should be performed in any patient with suspected aSAH and negative CT results.[57] If SAH is diagnosed by CT or LP, a CT angiography should be considered to investigate for an aneurysm and further characterize it to guide decisions regarding the type of aneurysm repair: surgical clipping versus endovascular approaches.[60]

Once the diagnosis is made, the acute management of aSAH in the emergency department (ED) focuses on management of hypertension, reversal of coagulopathy for patients on OACs (reviewed in detail in the ICH section and Table 1), and timely

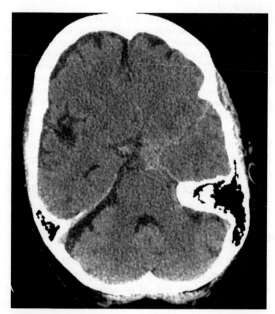

Fig. 2. aSAH seen on head CT. Diffuse subarachnoid hemorrhage involving the left cerebral hemisphere.

consultation for definitive management. Risk of rebleeding is maximal in the first 2 to 2 hours and is associated with poor outcome and high mortality,[60] with rebleeding rates in elderly patients higher and earlier than in younger patients.[58] Acute hypertension should be controlled from the time of diagnosis of aSAH until aneurysm obliteration using a titratable antihypertensive to balance the risk of stroke, hypertension-related rebleeding, and maintenance of cerebral perfusion pressure; parameters for BP control have not been clearly defined, but AHA guidelines recommend a goal SBP lower than 160 mm Hg.[60]

Early obliteration of the aneurysm is required to prevent rebleeding. Although the data are conflicting, some suggest that patients older than 70 years are ideal candidates for coiling rather than clipping.[60] If elderly patients are carefully selected, endovascular coiling or microsurgical clipping can lead to a positive outcome.[58] All patients with aSAH should be admitted to an intensive care unit. Neurologic complications are common after aSAH and include symptomatic vasospasm, hydrocephalus, rebleeding, and seizures.[57] Due to their advanced age and resulting comorbidities, elderly patients suffering an aSAH are at increased risk for both neurologic and general complications and should be monitored closely.[58]

## CHRONIC SUBDURAL HEMATOMA

CSDH is an abnormal collection of blood and liquefied blood degradation located in the subdural space between the dura matter and the arachnoid that may result in brain tissue compression and subsequent neurologic sequelae.[61–63] It is predominantly a disease of the elderly and advancing age is a major risk factor for CSDH. The incidence of CSDH is rising due to the combination of an aging population and the increasing use of anticoagulant and antiplatelet medications.[61] In the elderly, CSDH is usually caused by minor trauma, but a history of direct head trauma is absent in approximately 30% to 50% of patients, and age-related changes in the elderly brain (such as decreased elasticity and fragility of cerebral vessel as well as increased stress placed on venous structures due to cerebral atrophy) are a likely contributing cause.[62]

Due to its varied presentations, CSDH has been described as "the great neurologic imitator."[64] Presenting symptoms are listed in **Box 6**, and onset and progression can vary from days to weeks to even months.[61,62,65]

In most cases, the diagnosis of CSDH is usually not suspected on initial presentation and a high index of suspicion should be maintained in elderly patients presenting with change in mental status, worsening preexistent neurologic or psychological illness, new focal neurologic deficits, new headache, gait disturbance, or frequent falls.[62] The mainstay for diagnosis of CSDH is head CT, where a CSDH is seen as a hypodense crescentic collection along the convexity[61] (**Fig. 3**).

The treatment of CSDH begins with correction of coagulopathy for patients on OACs (reviewed in detail in the ICH section and **Table 1**) to reduce the risks of bleeding during operative intervention and minimize recurrence. Patients with symptoms that are attributed to a CT-confirmed CSDH should be treated surgically. The operative treatment of CSDH is evacuation of the hematoma via percutaneous twist-drill bedside drainage, operative theater burr holes, or craniotomy. Patients with mild symptoms and relatively small CSDH may not require surgery and can be medically managed with close observation. A recent meta-analysis of more than 34,000 patients showed that percutaneous bedside twist-drill drainage is a relatively safe and effective first-line management option for CSDH. This management option may be especially beneficial in the treatment of elderly patients, as it is less invasive and eliminates the associated risks related to general anesthesia.[61,63] All elderly patients diagnosed

---

**Box 6**
**Presenting symptoms of chronic subdural hematoma**

- Altered mental state
  - Confusion
  - Cognitive decline
  - Drowsiness
  - Coma
  - Delirium
  - Psychiatric symptoms (eg, paranoia, depression)
- Focal neurologic deficits[a]
  - Speech Impairment
  - Limb weakness/hemiparesis
  - Hemisensory deficit
- Gait disturbance
- Falls
- Headache
- Seizures

[a] Usually focal neurologic symptoms start insidiously and progress gradually. May also present as transient neurologic deficits.
*Data from* Refs.[61,62,65]

---

with a CSDH should undergo consultation by a neurosurgeon to determine proper management based on clinical status and comorbidities.

CSDH in the elderly is a sentinel event and often a marker of other chronic diseases, similar to hip fracture. Elderly patients who suffer a CSDH continue to have excessive mortality up to 1 year following hospital discharge, with observed overall mortality rates of 32% in one study.[66] Given the deceptively poor prognosis for elderly patients

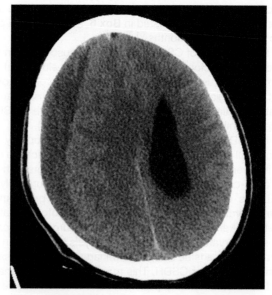

**Fig. 3.** CSDH seen on head CT.

suffering from CSDH, it is essential that these patients are treated urgently to optimize their care and outcomes.

## TRAUMATIC BRAIN INJURY

Traumatic brain injury (TBI) is a significant problem in elderly patients, causing more than 80,000 ED visits per year.[67] The leading causes of TBI in elderly patients are falls, accounting for 81% of all elderly patients' hospital visits for TBI, followed by blunt head strikes and motor vehicle crashes. Elderly patients suffering a TBI have the highest rates of hospitalization and death,[68] and older age has long been recognized as one of the more important factors predicting worsened outcomes from TBI.[69]

TBI is defined as an alteration in brain function, or other evidence of brain pathology, caused by an external force.[70] The pathophysiology of TBI can be either focal, occurring at the site of impact with resultant focal neurologic deficits in those areas, or diffuse, caused by diffuse shearing of axons in the cerebral white matter, gray-white junction, corpus callosum, and/or brainstem with resulting nonlateralizing neurologic deficits. TBI is often classified by severity, usually based on the Glasgow Coma Score (GCS)[71] (**Table 2**), In patients with moderate to severe TBI, the disease state also may be further delineated by abnormalities found on head CT, if present[71,72] (**Box 7**).

The workup of patients presenting with TBI differs based on the mechanism, severity, and patient's age. All patients presenting with moderate to severe TBI should undergo immediate head CT. For patients presenting with mild TBI, 3 common decision rules have been derived and are used to identify which patients should undergo head CT. All 3 studies excluded patients older than 60 or 65 years due to a higher rate of intracranial abnormalities in this patient population.[73–75] Brain imaging by head CT should be obtained in all elderly patients presenting with TBI, regardless of the severity of injury or the clinical presentation.

The ED management of geriatric patients who have suffered a severe TBI is similar to younger patients, with many of the recommendations provided by guidelines developed and maintained by the Brain Trauma Foundation (www.braintrauma.org)[76–78] (**Table 3**). Trauma surgery and neurosurgery consultation should be considered early, as these services are often involved in the care of patients with severe TBI. A lower threshold for trauma surgery consultation should be used in the evaluation of elderly patients suffering a TBI due to concomitant comorbidities, age-related biological differences, and worsened outcomes in older patients. Neurosurgery should be consulted for cases with evidence of elevated ICP or abnormalities on brain imaging for evaluation on the necessity of ICP monitoring and/or surgical intervention.[79] Disposition of elderly patients suffering a TBI is dependent on the comorbidities, injuries, and clinical status.

Like ICH, special attention must be paid to the patient on anticoagulation who suffers a moderate to severe TBI with associated intracranial hemorrhage.

| Table 2 Classification of traumatic brain injury by severity | |
|---|---|
| **Severity** | **Glasgow Coma Scale** |
| Mild | 13–15 |
| Moderate | 9–12 |
| Severe | 3–8 |

*Data from* Decuypere M, Klimo P. Spectrum of traumatic brain injury from mild to severe. Surg Clin North Am 2012;92(4):939–57. ix.

---

**Box 7**
**Abnormalities found on brain imaging**

- Skull fractures

- Diastasis of the skull

- Intracranial hemorrhage
  - Epidural hematoma
  - Subdural hematoma
  - Intracerebral hematoma
  - Intraventricular hemorrhage
  - Brain contusion
  - Traumatic subarachnoid hemorrhage

- Cerebral edema

- Pneumocephalus

- Traumatic infarction

- Diffuse axonal injury

*Data from* Decuypere M, Klimo P. Spectrum of traumatic brain injury from mild to severe. Surg Clin North Am 2012;92(4):939–57. ix; and Holmes JF, Hendey GW, Oman JA, et al. Epidemiology of blunt head injury victims undergoing ED cranial computed tomographic scanning. Am J Emerg Med 2006;24(2):167–73.

---

Medication-related coagulopathy is common in the geriatric population and increases the risk of post-TBI hemorrhage. In cases of TBI hemorrhage complicated by medication-related coagulopathy, the offending drug should be discontinued and medical management should be targeted to normalize hemostasis and avert hematoma expansion (as reviewed in detail in ICH section and **Table 1**).[51,52]

## SEIZURES

Compared with any other age group, elderly patients have the highest incidence of new-onset seizures, epilepsy, and status epilepticus with an incidence that increases with advancing age.[80–82] In fact, epilepsy represents the third most common neurologic condition in elderly patients after dementia and stroke.[83] Although relatively common in geriatric patients, diagnosing and treating seizures in the elderly is complex due to age, comorbid conditions, and adverse medication effects. New seizures in the elderly have increased mortality and morbidity, and many of the etiologic factors leading to a new seizure in elderly patients cause an enduring predisposition to seizures.[81] Similar to younger individuals presenting with a seizure, a clinical distinction must be made between a provoked seizure (due to an acute systemic or brain insult) and an unprovoked seizure.[81,84] A cause for acute seizure can usually be found in the geriatric patients, and approximately 75% of elderly patients suffering a new-onset seizure have a known provoking etiology[81,82,85,86] (**Box 8**).

Seizures are classified into 2 groups, generalized or partial (focal), depending on where they originate in the brain. Most new seizures in elderly patients are partial with or without secondary generalization.[87] Complex partial seizures in the elderly may manifest as simple motor or sensory symptoms, memory lapses, episodes of confusion, periods of inattention, apparent syncope, or a blank stare with transient disturbance of consciousness.[81,88] They are often misdiagnosed as altered mental status, confusion, or syncope, and epilepsy is not the initial suspected diagnosis in almost half of all elderly patients who are ultimately diagnosed.[81,85]

**Table 3**
**Emergency department management of elderly patients with severe TBI**

| Clinical Target | Management |
|---|---|
| GCS | Measure initially<br>Monitor continuously for clinical change |
| Airway and breathing | Evaluate and stabilize<br>Correct hypoxemia (SpO2 <90%)<br>Intubate for:<br>• GCS <9<br>• Inability to maintain an adequate airway<br>• Hypoxemia not corrected by supplemental oxygen<br>For intubated patients:<br>• Maintain normal breathing rates (unless signs of cerebral herniation)<br>• Maintain ETCO2 35–40 mm Hg |
| Physical Exam | Monitor vital signs<br>• Rapidly correct hypotension (SBP <90 mm Hg)<br>• Avoid hyperthermia<br>Assess for secondary trauma<br>Pupillary examination for asymmetry and reactivity to light<br>Frequent reassessment for signs of cerebral herniation, including:<br>• Dilated and unreactive pupils<br>• Asymmetric pupils<br>• Motor examination with extensor posturing or no response<br>• Progressive neurologic deterioration |
| IV and laboratory testing | Complete blood count<br>Metabolic panel (renal and hepatic function)<br>Type and screen<br>Toxicology screens<br>INR/PTT<br>• Elevated INR should be rapidly corrected in patients with intracranial hemorrhage |
| Consultation | Trauma surgery<br>Neurosurgery<br>* Consider transfer to designated trauma center if services unavailable |
| Prevent elevated ICP (target ICP <20 mm Hg) | Head of the bed elevation to 30°<br>Optimize cerebral venous drainage<br>• Keep neck in neutral position<br>• Loosen tight neck braces<br>Monitor central venous pressure<br>Sedation as needed to prevent agitation<br>Avoid excess hypervolemia<br>Consider ICP monitoring in high-risk patients<br>Consider mannitol, hypertonic saline, surgery for elevated ICP |

*Abbreviations:* ETCO2, end tidal $CO_2$ (carbon dioxide); GCS, Glasgow Coma Scale; ICP, intracranial pressure; INR, international normalized ratio; IV, intravenous; PTT, partial thromboplastin time; SBP, systolic blood pressure; TBI, traumatic brain injury.
*Data from* Refs.[76–78]

Workup of acute seizures in geriatric patients can be difficult and time-consuming. Many other medical disorders may mimic and coexist with seizure activity and the differential diagnosis for an elderly patient presenting with concern for new-onset seizure is broad[89] (**Box 9**). Initial evaluation should include vital signs, electrocardiogram, cardiac monitoring, laboratory testing (including thyroid-stimulating hormone), and brain imaging.[85,88,90] Electroencephalography (EEG) is an important diagnostic test in evaluating a patient with possible epilepsy, but the EEG findings do not always lead to a definitive diagnosis, especially in elderly patients. EEG is less specific and sensitive than neuroimaging in the evaluation of elderly people with seizure. With advancing age, 12% to 38% of patients develop EEG abnormalities in the absence of a seizure, and few elderly patients with seizures have abnormal interictal EEGs.[85]

Pharmacologic treatment for elderly patients with new epilepsy should be made in conjunction with neurologic consultation.[85,90] Physiologic aging accompanied by comorbidities and the concomitant polypharmacy alters the pharmacodynamics and pharmacokinetics of antiepileptic drugs (AEDs), and special care should be given in choosing the proper drug and dosing in elderly patients. Generally, AEDs are effective in lower doses in elderly patients, and most elderly patients remain seizure free with monotherapy. Lamotrigine, levetiracetam, and controlled-released carbamazepine should be considered as first-0line treatment in patients with late-onset epilepsy.[83]

Status epilepticus (SE) is a medical emergency, and up to 30% of acute seizures in the elderly present as SE with an increased mortality rate of up to 50%.[85,90,91] SE in elderly patients is usually caused by stroke, hypoxia, metabolic insult, or low AED concentrations. When an elderly patient presents in SE, he or she should receive the highest level of triage and acute management focusing on the ABCs and establishing IV access. Pharmacologic management of SE in the elderly follows the accepted guidelines of all patients with SE, including benzodiazepines as first line followed by a medication load with a specific AED (such as levetiracetam, phenytoin, or valproate).[91] If SE continues, the next line of treatment includes anesthetic agents (such as pentobarbital, midazolam, or propofol). Patients with refractory SE requiring this addition treatment will require intubation and urgent neurology consultation.[91–93]

---

**Box 8**
**Provoked etiologies for elderly patients suffering a seizure**

- Stroke
- Cerebrovascular arteriosclerosis
- Intracranial hemorrhage
- Traumatic brain injury
- Infection
- Brain mass
- Vascular malformation
- Neurodegenerative disorder (ie, dementia)
- Neuropsychiatric disorders (ie, depression, anxiety)
- Metabolic conditions
- Cardiac insufficiency
- Toxic ingestions
- Medication withdrawal
- Cerebral anoxia
- Normal aging

*Data from* Refs.[81,82,85,86]

---

**Box 9**
**Differential diagnosis for new-onset seizure in the elderly**

- Cardiac arrhythmia
- Transient global amnesia
- TIA
- Stroke
- Migraine
- Hypoglycemia
- Hyperglycemic nonketotic state
- Hyponatremia
- Hyperthyroidism
- Orthostatic hypotension
- Carotid sinus sensitivity
- Adverse drug effect
- Vasovagal episode
- Infection
- Drug withdrawal
- Vertigo

*Data from* Nentwich LM. Neurologic emergencies in the elderly. In: Kahn JH Jr, Magauran BG, Olshaker JS, editors. Geriatric emergency medicine. New York: Cambridge University Press; 2014. p. 170–84.

---

Nonconvulsive SE (NCSE) is a form of SE in which there may be minimal clinical seizure activity, but there is a pattern of seizure activity on EEG that disappears with treatment. NCSE is more common in elderly patients, and due to its subtle clinical presentations, many patients with NCSE suffer a delayed or missed diagnosis. NCSE may last for hours to days, and patients present with altered mental status from mild confusion to delirium to coma with varying associated clinical features (**Box 10**). A high degree of suspicion and early EEG is required for prompt recognition of NCSE in elderly patients.[93,94]

## CENTRAL NERVOUS SYSTEM INFECTIONS

Infections are more frequent and typically more severe in the elderly than in younger patients, and geriatric patients often present with more subtle signs and less symptoms. Fever, a cardinal sign of infection in younger patients, is absent or blunted in 20% to 30% of severe infections in the elderly. The most common signs of infection in the elderly are nonspecific, such as falls, delirium, anorexia, or generalized weakness.[95] This is especially true of CNS infections. Infectious diseases in the elderly are discussed in depth in the article by (see Liang SY: Sepsis and Other Infectious Disease Emergencies in the Elderly, in this issue), and this article includes a brief discussion of bacterial meningitis and spinal epidural abscesses in the elderly.

### Community-Acquired Bacterial Meningitis

The rates of bacterial meningitis have decreased dramatically since the advent of *Haemophilus influenzae* type b and pneumococcal vaccines. Patients 65 years and

---

**Box 10**
**Clinical features associated with nonconvulsive status epilepticus in the elderly**

- Reduction in level of arousal

- Aphasia or interrupted speech

- Mild rhythmic myoclonus

- Staring

- Automatisms

- Echolalia or perseveration

- Increased tone

- Nystagmus or eye deviation

- Emotional lability

- Disinhibition and anosognosia

- Psychosis or hallucinations

*Data from* Woodford HJ, George J, Jackson M. Non-convulsive status epilepticus: a practical approach to diagnosis in confused older people. Postgrad Med J 2015;91(1081):655–61.

---

older are second only to children younger than 2 years in the incidence of bacterial meningitis. Not only is bacterial meningitis more common in older patients, it is also more deadly, as the overall mortality rate increases linearly with age, from 8.9% in patients 18 to 34 years to 22.7% in patients 65 years or older.[96] Advanced age is associated with unfavorable outcome in patients with bacterial meningitis, and complications are more likely to occur in older patients than younger patients.[97–100]

Atypical infectious presentations are more common in the elderly. Elderly patients with bacterial meningitis may present with fever, altered mental status, neck stiffness, headache, seizure, shock, or focal neurologic abnormalities. Neck stiffness, headache, and fever, traditionally taught as the cardinal signs of meningitis, occur less frequently in the elderly.[101] Older patients with bacterial meningitis present more frequently with altered mental status or focal neurologic abnormalities than the general population.[97,101–103] If bacterial meningitis is suspected, LP is an important diagnostic step, but should never delay the administration of antibiotics. Due to the risk of brain herniation in the setting of diagnostic LP, neuroimaging before LP is recommended in select patients to detect signs of elevated ICP (eg, new-onset seizure, immunocompromised, papilledema, altered level of consciousness). Best practice dictates that if neuroimaging is performed before LP, antibiotic therapy and corticosteroids should be initiated before the patient is sent for neuroimaging.[104]

Empiric antibiotic therapy should target *Streptococcus pneumoniae, Staphylococcus* species, *Neisseria meningitidis*, and *Listeria monocytogenes,* which are among the bacterial organisms most commonly found in elderly patients with community-acquired bacterial meningitis.[100] Such coverage is best achieved through the combination of vancomycin plus a third-generation cephalosporin plus ampicillin. Additionally, due to a proven mortality benefit, adjunctive dexamethasone therapy should be initiated in all patients with suspected bacterial meningitis before or with the first dose of antibiotics.[100,104,105] Inappropriately selected empiric antibiotics have a greater effect on patients older than 65 and is an independent predictor of 28-day mortality.[106] Admission to the hospital with respiratory isolation for 24 hours is indicated for patients with suspected meningococcal infection.[104]

## Spinal Epidural Abscess

Spinal epidural abscesses (SEAs) are the accumulation of purulent material in the epidural space between the dura mater and the osseo-ligamentous confines of the vertebral canal.[107] SEA is a dangerous infection that is common in elderly patients and presents a diagnostic dilemma, as most patients do not present with the classic triad of back pain, fever, and neurologic deficit, and misdiagnosis and delayed diagnosis are common.[108] Further complicating the diagnosis of SEA in elderly patients is that elderly patients frequently present to the ED with back pain from degenerative disease.[109] Most patients with SEA have one or more predisposing condition, such as diabetes, alcoholism, infectious source, or spinal abnormality or intervention, and many of these conditions are commonly observed in elderly patients.[110]

Diagnosis of SEA is suspected of the basis of clinical findings and supported by laboratory data and imaging studies. The most common presenting symptoms include back pain, fever, and neurologic dysfunction. Other symptoms may include paravertebral muscle spasm, limited spinal motion, paresthesias, weakness, and difficulty ambulating.[107,110] Leukocytosis is detected in only approximately two-thirds of patients, but inflammatory markers (erythrocyte sedimentation rate and C-reactive protein) are almost uniformly elevated. Bacteremia as the cause of or arising from SEA is detected in approximately 60% of patients, and blood cultures can provide identification of the causative pathogen.[110] When SEA is suspected, gadolinium-enhanced MRI of the entire spine should be obtained emergently.[107]

Emergent surgical depression and drainage of the abscess together with systemic antibiotics is the treatment of choice for the vast majority of patients diagnosed with SEA. Pending results of the cultures, empiric antibiotic therapy should provide coverage of the most common causative organisms (ie, *Staphylococcus* and *Streptococcus* species) with additional coverage for gram-negative organisms, especially in patients who are immunocompromised, have a history of intravenous drug abuse, or have had recent infection or manipulation of the genitourinary tract.[107,109,110]

## SUMMARY

Given an aging population, the care of the elderly patient in the ED is becoming increasingly common. Neurologic emergencies are frequent in elderly patients and are associated with high morbidity and mortality. Complicated by the physiologic changes of aging as well as increased medical comorbidities in older patients, the care of the geriatric patients with neurologic emergencies is challenging and complicated. However, through aggressive and directed care in conjunction with proper specialist consultation, ED physicians can improve outcomes and quality of life in these patients.

## REFERENCES

1. Mozaffarian D, Benjamin EJ, Go AS, et al. Heart disease and stroke statistics–2015 update: a report from the American Heart Association. Circulation 2015; 131(4):e29–322.
2. Pare JR, Kahn JH. Basic neuroanatomy and stroke syndromes. Emerg Med Clin North Am 2012;30(3):601–15.
3. Russo T, Felzani G, Marini C. Stroke in the very old: a systematic review of studies on incidence, outcome, and resource use. J Aging Res 2011;2011: 108785.
4. Howard G, Goff DC. Population shifts and the future of stroke: forecasts of the future burden of stroke. Ann N Y Acad Sci 2012;1268:14–20.

5. Muangpaisan W, Hinkle JL, Westwood M, et al. Stroke in the very old: clinical presentations and outcomes. Age Ageing 2008;37(4):473–5.

6. Kothari R, Sauerbeck L, Jauch E, et al. Patients' awareness of stroke signs, symptoms, and risk factors. Stroke 1997;28(10):1871–5.

7. Jauch EC, Saver JL, Adams HP, et al. Guidelines for the early management of patients with acute ischemic stroke: a guideline for healthcare professionals from the American Heart Association/American Stroke Association. Stroke 2013;44(3):870–947.

8. NIH Stroke Scale - NIH_Stroke_Scale.pdf [Internet]. Available at: https://www.ninds.nih.gov/doctors/NIH_Stroke_Scale.pdf. Accessed February 12, 2016.

9. Nentwich LM, Veloz W. Neuroimaging in acute stroke. Emerg Med Clin North Am 2012;30(3):659–80.

10. Tissue plasminogen activator for acute ischemic stroke. N Engl J Med 1995; 333(24):1581–8.

11. Hemphill JC, Lyden P. Stroke thrombolysis in the elderly: risk or benefit? Neurology 2005;65(11):1690–1.

12. Longstreth WT, Katz R, Tirschwell DL, et al. Intravenous tissue plasminogen activator and stroke in the elderly. Am J Emerg Med 2010;28(3):359–63.

13. Hacke W, Kaste M, Bluhmki E, et al. Thrombolysis with alteplase 3 to 4.5 hours after acute ischemic stroke. N Engl J Med 2008;359(13):1317–29.

14. Sylaja PN, Cote R, Buchan AM, et al. Canadian Alteplase for Stroke Effectiveness Study (CASES) Investigators. Thrombolysis in patients older than 80 years with acute ischaemic stroke: Canadian Alteplase for Stroke Effectiveness Study. J Neurol Neurosurg Psychiatry 2006;77(7):826–9.

15. Mishra NK, Ahmed N, Andersen G, et al. Thrombolysis in very elderly people: controlled comparison of SITS International Stroke Thrombolysis Registry and Virtual International Stroke Trials Archive. BMJ 2010;341:c6046.

16. Pundik S, McWilliams-Dunnigan L, Blackham KL, et al. Older age does not increase risk of hemorrhagic complications after intravenous and/or intra-arterial thrombolysis for acute stroke. J Stroke Cerebrovasc Dis 2008;17(5):266–72.

17. Del Zoppo GJ, Saver JL, Jauch EC, et al, American Heart Association Stroke Council. Expansion of the time window for treatment of acute ischemic stroke with intravenous tissue plasminogen activator: a science advisory from the American Heart Association/American Stroke Association. Stroke 2009;40(8): 2945–8.

18. Berkhemer OA, Fransen PSS, Beumer D, et al. A randomized trial of intraarterial treatment for acute ischemic stroke. N Engl J Med 2015;372(1):11–20.

19. Goyal M, Demchuk AM, Menon BK, et al. Randomized assessment of rapid endovascular treatment of ischemic stroke. N Engl J Med 2015;372(11):1019–30.

20. Campbell BCV, Mitchell PJ, Kleinig TJ, et al. Endovascular therapy for ischemic stroke with perfusion-imaging selection. N Engl J Med 2015;372(11):1009–18.

21. Saver JL, Goyal M, Bonafe A, et al. Stent-retriever thrombectomy after intravenous t-PA vs. t-PA alone in stroke. N Engl J Med 2015;372(24):2285–95.

22. Jovin TG, Chamorro A, Cobo E, et al. Thrombectomy within 8 hours after symptom onset in ischemic stroke. N Engl J Med 2015;372(24):2296–306.

23. Campbell BCV, Hill MD, Rubiera M, et al. Safety and efficacy of solitaire stent thrombectomy individual patient data meta-analysis of randomized trials. Stroke 2016;47(3):798–806.

24. Vahedi K, Hofmeijer J, Juettler E, et al. Early decompressive surgery in malignant infarction of the middle cerebral artery: a pooled analysis of three randomised controlled trials. Lancet Neurol 2007;6(3):215–22.

25. Vahedi K, Vicaut E, Mateo J, et al. Sequential-design, multicenter, randomized, controlled trial of early decompressive craniectomy in malignant middle cerebral artery infarction (DECIMAL Trial). Stroke 2007;38(9):2506–17.

26. Jüttler E, Schwab S, Schmiedek P, et al. Decompressive Surgery for the Treatment of Malignant Infarction of the Middle Cerebral Artery (DESTINY): a randomized, controlled trial. Stroke 2007;38(9):2518–25.

27. Hofmeijer J, Kappelle LJ, Algra A, et al. Surgical decompression for space-occupying cerebral infarction (the Hemicraniectomy After Middle Cerebral Artery infarction with Life-threatening Edema Trial [HAMLET]): a multicentre, open, randomised trial. Lancet Neurol 2009;8(4):326–33.

28. Cruz-Flores S, Berge E, Whittle IR. Surgical decompression for cerebral oedema in acute ischaemic stroke. Cochrane Database Syst Rev 2012;(1):CD003435.

29. Zweckberger K, Juettler E, Bösel J, et al. Surgical aspects of decompression craniectomy in malignant stroke: review. Cerebrovasc Dis 2014;38(5):313–23.

30. Jüttler E, Unterberg A, Woitzik J, et al. Hemicraniectomy in older patients with extensive middle-cerebral-artery stroke. N Engl J Med 2014;370(12):1091–100.

31. Easton JD, Saver JL, Albers GW, et al. Definition and evaluation of transient ischemic attack: a scientific statement for healthcare professionals from the American Heart Association/American Stroke Association Stroke Council; Council on Cardiovascular Surgery and Anesthesia; Council on Cardiovascular Radiology and Intervention; Council on Cardiovascular Nursing; and the Interdisciplinary Council on Peripheral Vascular Disease. The American Academy of Neurology affirms the value of this statement as an educational tool for neurologists. Stroke 2009;40(6):2276–93.

32. Kleindorfer D, Panagos P, Pancioli A, et al. Incidence and short-term prognosis of transient ischemic attack in a population-based study. Stroke 2005;36(4):720–3.

33. Rothwell PM, Warlow CP. Timing of TIAs preceding stroke: time window for prevention is very short. Neurology 2005;64(5):817–20.

34. Giles MF, Rothwell PM. Risk of stroke early after transient ischaemic attack: a systematic review and meta-analysis. Lancet Neurol 2007;6(12):1063–72.

35. Wu CM, McLaughlin K, Lorenzetti DL, et al. Early risk of stroke after transient ischemic attack: a systematic review and meta-analysis. Arch Intern Med 2007;167(22):2417–22.

36. Siket MS, Edlow JA. Transient ischemic attack: reviewing the evolution of the definition, diagnosis, risk stratification, and management for the emergency physician. Emerg Med Clin North Am 2012;30(3):745–70.

37. Johnston SC, Nguyen-Huynh MN, Schwarz ME, et al. National Stroke Association guidelines for the management of transient ischemic attacks. Ann Neurol 2006;60(3):301–13.

38. Johnston SC, Albers GW, Gorelick PB, et al. National Stroke Association recommendations for systems of care for transient ischemic attack. Ann Neurol 2011;69(5):872–7.

39. Kernan WN, Ovbiagele B, Black HR, et al. Guidelines for the prevention of stroke in patients with stroke and transient ischemic attack a guideline for healthcare professionals from the American Heart Association/American Stroke Association. Stroke 2014;45(7):2160–236.

40. Rerkasem K, Rothwell PM. Carotid endarterectomy for symptomatic carotid stenosis. Cochrane Database Syst Rev 2011;(4):CD001081.

41. Qureshi AI, Tuhrim S, Broderick JP, et al. Spontaneous intracerebral hemorrhage. N Engl J Med 2001;344(19):1450–60.

42. Broderick J, Connolly S, Feldmann E, et al. Guidelines for the management of spontaneous intracerebral hemorrhage in adults: 2007 update: a guideline from the American Heart Association/American Stroke Association Stroke Council, High Blood Pressure Research Council, and the Quality of Care and Outcomes in Research Interdisciplinary Working Group. Circulation 2007;116(16):e391–413.

43. Weigele JB, Hurst RW. Neurovascular emergencies in the elderly. Radiol Clin North Am 2008;46(4):819–36, vii.

44. Nentwich L, Goldstein J. Intracerebral hemorrhage. In: Rogers R, Scalea T, Wallis L, et al, editors. Vascular emergencies. New York: Cambridge University Press; 2013. p. 18–29.

45. European Stroke Initiative Writing Committee, Writing Committee for the EUSI Executive Committee, Steiner T, et al. Recommendations for the management of intracranial haemorrhage—part I: spontaneous intracerebral haemorrhage. The European Stroke Initiative Writing Committee and the Writing Committee for the EUSI Executive Committee. Cerebrovasc Dis 2006;22(4):294–316.

46. Runchey S, McGee S. Does this patient have a hemorrhagic stroke? Clinical findings distinguishing hemorrhagic stroke from ischemic stroke. JAMA 2010; 303(22):2280–6.

47. Hemphill JC, Greenberg SM, Anderson CS, et al. guidelines for the management of spontaneous intracerebral hemorrhage: a guideline for healthcare professionals from the American Heart Association/American Stroke Association. Stroke 2015;46(7):2032–60.

48. Anderson CS, Huang Y, Wang JG, et al. Intensive blood pressure reduction in acute cerebral haemorrhage trial (INTERACT): a randomised pilot trial. Lancet Neurol 2008;7(5):391–9.

49. Qureshi AI, Palesch YY, Martin R, et al. Effect of systolic blood pressure reduction on hematoma expansion, perihematomal edema, and 3-month outcome among patients with intracerebral hemorrhage: results from the antihypertensive treatment of acute cerebral hemorrhage study. Arch Neurol 2010;67(5):570–6.

50. Anderson CS, Heeley E, Huang Y, et al. Rapid blood-pressure lowering in patients with acute intracerebral hemorrhage. N Engl J Med 2013;368(25): 2355–65.

51. Yates S, Sarode R. Reversal of anticoagulant effects in patients with intracerebral hemorrhage. Curr Neurol Neurosci Rep 2015;15(1):504.

52. Abo-Salem E, Becker RC. Reversal of novel oral anticoagulants. Curr Opin Pharmacol 2016;27:86–91.

53. Pollack CV, Reilly PA, Eikelboom J, et al. Idarucizumab for dabigatran reversal. N Engl J Med 2015;373(6):511–20.

54. Siegal DM, Curnutte JT, Connolly SJ, et al. Andexanet Alfa for the reversal of factor Xa inhibitor activity. N Engl J Med 2015;373(25):2413–24.

55. Becker KJ, Baxter AB, Cohen WA, et al. Withdrawal of support in intracerebral hemorrhage may lead to self-fulfilling prophecies. Neurology 2001;56(6):766–72.

56. Zahuranec DB, Brown DL, Lisabeth LD, et al. Early care limitations independently predict mortality after intracerebral hemorrhage. Neurology 2007; 68(20):1651–7.

57. Suarez JI, Tarr RW, Selman WR. Aneurysmal subarachnoid hemorrhage. N Engl J Med 2006;354(4):387–96.

58. Sedat J, Dib M, Rasendrarijao D, et al. Ruptured intracranial aneurysms in the elderly: epidemiology, diagnosis, and management. Neurocrit Care 2005;2(2): 119–23.

59. Edlow JA, Caplan LR. Avoiding pitfalls in the diagnosis of subarachnoid hemorrhage. N Engl J Med 2000;342(1):29–36.
60. Connolly ES, Rabinstein AA, Carhuapoma JR, et al. Guidelines for the management of aneurysmal subarachnoid hemorrhage: a guideline for healthcare professionals from the American Heart Association/American Stroke Association. Stroke 2012;43(6):1711–37.
61. Kolias AG, Chari A, Santarius T, et al. Chronic subdural haematoma: modern management and emerging therapies. Nat Rev Neurol 2014;10(10):570–8.
62. Adhiyaman V, Asghar M, Ganeshram KN, et al. Chronic subdural haematoma in the elderly. Postgrad Med J 2002;78(916):71–5.
63. Almenawer SA, Farrokhyar F, Hong C, et al. Chronic subdural hematoma management: a systematic review and meta-analysis of 34,829 patients. Ann Surg 2014;259(3):449–57.
64. Potter JF, Fruin AH. Chronic subdural hematoma–the "great imitator". Geriatrics 1977;32(6):61–6.
65. Santarius T, Kirkpatrick PJ, Ganesan D, et al. Use of drains versus no drains after burr-hole evacuation of chronic subdural haematoma: a randomised controlled trial. Lancet 2009;374(9695):1067–73.
66. Miranda LB, Braxton E, Hobbs J, et al. Chronic subdural hematoma in the elderly: not a benign disease. J Neurosurg 2011;114(1):72–6.
67. Thompson HJ, McCormick WC, Kagan SH. Traumatic brain injury in older adults: epidemiology, outcomes, and future implications. J Am Geriatr Soc 2006;54(10):1590–5.
68. TBI Data and Statistics | Concussion | Traumatic Brain Injury | CDC Injury Center [Internet]. Available at: http://www.cdc.gov/traumaticbraininjury/data/index.html. Accessed March 18, 2016.
69. Hukkelhoven CW, Steyerberg EW, Rampen AJJ, et al. Patient age and outcome following severe traumatic brain injury: an analysis of 5600 patients. J Neurosurg 2003;99(4):666–73.
70. Menon DK, Schwab K, Wright DW, et al, Demographics and Clinical Assessment Working Group of the International and Interagency Initiative toward Common Data Elements for Research on Traumatic Brain Injury and Psychological Health. Position statement: definition of traumatic brain injury. Arch Phys Med Rehabil 2010;91(11):1637–40.
71. Decuypere M, Klimo P. Spectrum of traumatic brain injury from mild to severe. Surg Clin North Am 2012;92(4):939–57, ix.
72. Holmes JF, Hendey GW, Oman JA, et al. Epidemiology of blunt head injury victims undergoing ED cranial computed tomographic scanning. Am J Emerg Med 2006;24(2):167–73.
73. Stiell IG, Wells GA, Vandemheen K, et al. The Canadian CT Head Rule for patients with minor head injury. Lancet 2001;357(9266):1391–6.
74. Haydel MJ, Preston CA, Mills TJ, et al. Indications for computed tomography in patients with minor head injury. N Engl J Med 2000;343(2):100–5.
75. Mower WR, Hoffman JR, Herbert M, et al. Developing a decision instrument to guide computed tomographic imaging of blunt head injury patients. J Trauma 2005;59(4):954–9.
76. Brain Trauma Foundation - coming soon | brain trauma splash page [Internet]. Available at: https://www.braintrauma.org/. Accessed March 18, 2016.
77. Brain Trauma Foundation, American Association of Neurological Surgeons, Congress of Neurological Surgeons. Guidelines for the management of severe traumatic brain injury. J Neurotrauma 2007;24(Suppl 1):S1–106.

78. Badjatia N, Carney N, Crocco TJ, et al. Guidelines for prehospital management of traumatic brain injury, 2nd edition. Prehosp Emerg Care 2008; 12(Suppl 1):S1–52.
79. Calland JF, Ingraham AM, Martin N, et al. Evaluation and management of geriatric trauma: an Eastern Association for the Surgery of Trauma practice management guideline. J Trauma Acute Care Surg 2012;73(5 Suppl 4):S345–50.
80. Faught E, Richman J, Martin R, et al. Incidence and prevalence of epilepsy among older U.S. Medicare beneficiaries. Neurology 2012;78(7):448–53.
81. Verellen RM, Cavazos JE. Pathophysiological considerations of seizures, epilepsy, and status epilepticus in the elderly. Aging Dis 2011;2(4):278–85.
82. Hauser WA. Seizure disorders: the changes with age. Epilepsia 1992;33(Suppl 4): S6–14.
83. Ferlazzo E, Sueri C, Gasparini S, et al. Challenges in the pharmacological management of epilepsy and its causes in the elderly. Pharmacol Res 2016; 106:21–6.
84. Hauser WA, Beghi E. First seizure definitions and worldwide incidence and mortality. Epilepsia 2008;49(Suppl 1):8–12.
85. Poza JJ. Management of epilepsy in the elderly. Neuropsychiatr Dis Treat 2007; 3(6):723–8.
86. Ramsay RE, Rowan AJ, Pryor FM. Special considerations in treating the elderly patient with epilepsy. Neurology 2004;62(5 Suppl 2):S24–9.
87. Stephen LJ, Brodie MJ. Epilepsy in elderly people. Lancet 2000;355(9213): 1441–6.
88. Brodie MJ, Kwan P. Epilepsy in elderly people. BMJ 2005;331(7528):1317–22.
89. Nentwich LM. Neurological emergencies in the elderly. In: Kahn JH Jr, Magauran BG, Olshaker JS, editors. Geriatric emergency medicine. New York: Cambridge University Press; 2014. p. 170–84.
90. Brodie MJ, Elder AT, Kwan P. Epilepsy in later life. Lancet Neurol 2009;8(11): 1019–30.
91. de Assis TMR, Costa G, Bacellar A, et al. Status epilepticus in the elderly: epidemiology, clinical aspects and treatment. Neurol Int 2012;4(3):e17.
92. Rossetti AO, Lowenstein DH. Management of refractory status epilepticus in adults: still more questions than answers. Lancet Neurol 2011;10(10):922–30.
93. Lowenstein DH. The management of refractory status epilepticus: an update. Epilepsia 2006;47(Suppl 1):35–40.
94. Woodford HJ, George J, Jackson M. Non-convulsive status epilepticus: a practical approach to diagnosis in confused older people. Postgrad Med J 2015; 91(1081):655–61.
95. Gavazzi G, Krause KH. Ageing and infection. Lancet Infect Dis 2002;2(11): 659–66.
96. Thigpen MC, Whitney CG, Messonnier NE, et al. Bacterial meningitis in the United States, 1998-2007. N Engl J Med 2011;364(21):2016–25.
97. Weisfelt M, van de Beek D, Spanjaard L, et al. Community-acquired bacterial meningitis in older people. J Am Geriatr Soc 2006;54(10):1500–7.
98. van de Beek D, de Gans J, Spanjaard L, et al. Clinical features and prognostic factors in adults with bacterial meningitis. N Engl J Med 2004;351(18):1849–59.
99. Wang AY, Machicado JD, Khoury NT, et al. Community-acquired meningitis in older adults: clinical features, etiology, and prognostic factors. J Am Geriatr Soc 2014;62(11):2064–70.
100. Hofinger D, Davis LE. Bacterial meningitis in older adults. Curr Treat Options Neurol 2013;15(4):477–91.

101. Domingo P, Pomar V, de Benito N, et al. The spectrum of acute bacterial meningitis in elderly patients. BMC Infect Dis 2013;13:108.
102. Lai W-A, Chen S-F, Tsai N-W, et al. Clinical characteristics and prognosis of acute bacterial meningitis in elderly patients over 65: a hospital-based study. BMC Geriatr 2011;11:91.
103. Cabellos C, Verdaguer R, Olmo M, et al. Community-acquired bacterial meningitis in elderly patients: experience over 30 years. Medicine (Baltimore) 2009; 88(2):115–9.
104. van de Beek D, de Gans J, Tunkel AR, et al. Community-acquired bacterial meningitis in adults. N Engl J Med 2006;354(1):44–53.
105. Brouwer MC, Tunkel AR, van de Beek D. Epidemiology, diagnosis, and antimicrobial treatment of acute bacterial meningitis. Clin Microbiol Rev 2010;23(3): 467–92.
106. Lee CC, Chang CM, Hong MY, et al. Different impact of the appropriateness of empirical antibiotics for bacteremia among younger adults and the elderly in the ED. Am J Emerg Med 2013;31(2):282–90.
107. Tompkins M, Panuncialman I, Lucas P, et al. Spinal epidural abscess. J Emerg Med 2010;39(3):384–90.
108. Pope JV, Edlow JA. Avoiding misdiagnosis in patients with neurological emergencies. Emerg Med Int 2012;2012:949275.
109. Kulchycki LK, Edlow JA. Geriatric neurologic emergencies. Emerg Med Clin North Am 2006;24(2):273–98, v–vi.
110. Darouiche RO. Spinal epidural abscess. N Engl J Med 2006;355(19):2012–20.

# Evaluation of Syncope in Older Adults

Teresita M. Hogan, MD[a],*, Stephen Tyler Constantine, MD[b], Aoko Doris Crain, MD[b]

## KEYWORDS

- Older adult • Emergency department • Syncope

## KEY POINTS

- Mixed cause syncope occurs frequently in older adults, so the emergency physician should continue the evaluation to uncover multiple contributing causes and ensure complete care.
- Medications commonly contribute to syncope. The emergency physician should routinely review prescription medications especially if no cause of syncope is clear from emergency department (ED) evaluation.
- All forms of syncope can have recurrence in elder patients. Even "benign" neurally mediated syncope/vasovagal syncope recur, and this is associated with injury and functional decline. The emergency physician should initiate standardized patient education from the ED in all discharged elder syncope patients, to help prevent recurrence.
- Structural heart disease and congestive heart failure are strongly associated with cardiac syncope. Patients with this history are at high risk.

## INTRODUCTION

Syncope is a sudden transient loss of consciousness (TLOC) and postural tone from rapid global cerebral hypoperfusion (RGCH) followed by full recovery to baseline function. Basing the definition of syncope on RGCH enables differentiation of syncope from other forms of TLOC, such as hypoxemia, hypoglycemia, seizure, vertebrobasilar ischemia, and psychogenic attacks. However, even elite medical publications apply variable definitions and inconsistent terminology for syncope, chiefly differing in the presence or absence of RGCH.[1] Using this confusing definition in clinical practice causes a huge variability in evaluation, diagnosis, treatment, and disposition. For example, without RGCH, syncope can be confused with seizure, hypoxia, or hypoglycemia. If the definition does not require full recovery, then it can overlap with cerebral vascular accidents. The above confusion begins by using the term syncope as a

Disclosure Statement: None of the authors has any conflicts of interest to disclose.
[a] Geriatric Emergency Medicine, University of Chicago Medicine, 5841 S Maryland Avenue, Chicago, IL 60637, USA; [b] University of Chicago Medicine, 5841 S Maryland Avenue, Chicago, IL 60637, USA
* Corresponding author.
*E-mail address:* thogan@medicine.bsd.uchicago.edu

Emerg Med Clin N Am 34 (2016) 601–627
http://dx.doi.org/10.1016/j.emc.2016.04.010
0733-8627/16/$ – see front matter © 2016 Elsevier Inc. All rights reserved.
emed.theclinics.com

diagnosis. However, syncope is not a diagnosis; it refers to the most dramatic presenting symptom of a variety of disease processes.

Emergency physicians evaluate the symptom of syncope in older adults on a daily basis. As with most emergent evaluations, the key tasks are to identify, stabilize, and admit life-threatening diagnosis, differentiate serious from benign causes in an efficient manner, risk stratify those who have an uncertain cause, and disposition patients to the appropriate subsequent level of care. This list of tasks is a tall order for the emergency provider because approximately 33% to 56% of syncope patients are discharged after a full hospital evaluation without definitive diagnosis.[2,3] Therefore, emergency physicians must become skilled in the detection of causes, prognostication of risk, and ensuring appropriate disposition of this varied population of syncope patients.

## EPIDEMIOLOGY

The true incidence of syncope is difficult to estimate because of the noted variation in its definition as well as differences in prevalence, and underreporting in the general population.[4] In the Framingham study, the age-adjusted incidence of syncope is 7.2 per 1000 person-years among both men and women. The lifetime cumulative incidence of syncope in women is almost twice that of men. The median peak of first syncope occurs around 15 years. The incidence rates increase with age, with a sharp increase at 70 years.[5] The increased risk of syncope in elder patients appears to be due to age and disease-related abnormalities that impair the normal response to certain physiologic stresses. The age-adjusted incidence in patients with cardiovascular disease is nearly twice that of patients without cardiovascular disease.[6] In the Framingham study, cardiac syncope increased the risk of nonfatal and fatal cardiovascular events and doubled the risk of death from any cause as compared with those without syncope. However, syncope itself does not increase risk of overall cardiac events or death except in the presence of heart disease, especially congestive heart failure (CHF). Patients with cardiac comorbidities are at increased risk of death after a syncopal event.

In the emergency department (ED), syncope is responsible for 1% to 3% of all patient visits and 6% of total hospital admissions. The elder population experiences disproportionately high hospitalization rates that increase by decade of life, with 58% of those over the age of 80 years admitted to the hospital when they present with the chief complaint of syncope.[7,8] The distributions of syncope causes in elder patients are divided as shown in **Fig. 1**.[9]

The epidemiology of syncope varies significantly with age. The primary causes of syncope in older adults are neurally mediated syncope (NMS) (which in the **Fig. 1** includes orthostatic hypotension [OH]), carotid sinus hypersensitivity (CSH), and dysrhythmias.[10] OH can be classed as a subtype of NMS or stand alone. In all of these classifications, syncope results from the lowering of peripheral resistance and/or cardiac output (CO).[11] NMS, inclusive of vagal, carotid, and situational events remains the most common cause of syncope even in the elder population. OH causes syncope in 20% to 30% of older adults.[12] Cardiac dysrhythmia incidence dramatically increases with age. Prevalence in patients over the age of 80 years is nearly 9% for atrial fibrillation/flutter alone.[13] Anyone with a history of rheumatic fever, CHF, or hypertension is at greater risk for a cardiac dysrhythmia as cause of syncope.[14]

Syncope can be remarkably debilitating and is associated with more than $2 billion in annual health care costs, and a mean cost of $5,400 per hospitalization.[4,15] Despite this high cost and resource utilization, the morbidity and mortality of syncope,

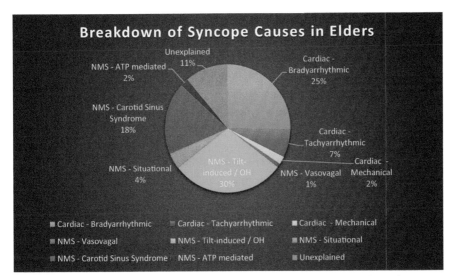

**Fig. 1.** Causes of syncope in the older adult population. (*Data from* McIntosh SJ, da Costa D, Kenny RA. Outcome of an integrated approach to the investigation of dizziness, falls and syncope in elderly patients referred to a syncope clinic. Age Ageing 1993;22:53–8.)

including those of cardiac cause, is minimally impacted by health care interventions.[16] Up to 60% of admitted syncope patients are discharged without receiving any therapeutic intervention for syncope.[17]

## PATHOPHYSIOLOGY

Once again, it can be seen why an important part of the syncope definition is that it results from RGCH. An approximate 20% drop in cerebral oxygen delivery is sufficient to cause loss of consciousness (LOC).[18] Cerebral perfusion pressure is dependent on mean arterial pressure, which is in turn dependent on CO and peripheral vascular resistance (PVR). The pathophysiology is not yet entirely known, and a topic of continued research, but it appears that alterations in CO and PVR contribute to most cases of syncope.[19]

NMS is due to abnormal autonomic regulation, resulting in hypotension, bradycardia, and ultimately, LOC. Humans have the exceptional ability to maintain stable blood pressures during physiologic stress and shifting fluid volumes through changes in vascular tone and CO. Decreased output sensed by arterial baroreceptors in the carotid sinus and aortic arch increase sympathetic output, resulting in increased heart rate and ventricular contractility. In addition, the vascular system responds by limiting blood flow to nonessential organs, thereby increasing PVR and causing a gradual increase in diastolic pressure.[20] In NMS, an abnormal autonomic nervous system overresponds to different stimuli, most commonly prolonged standing, heat, emotional stress, or carotid sinus stimulation. These stimuli increase heart rate and ventricular contraction. However, by unclear mechanism, neural signals reach the brainstem and result in a combination of sympathetic withdrawal and increased parasympathetic output, instead leading to bradycardia, hypotension, and syncope. Decreased venous filling due to hypovolemia from volume loss, inadequate intake, or medication effects causes OH. It can also be due to autonomic dysfunction. Cardiogenic syncope is due to structural heart diseases or dysrhythmias. Both impair CO and thus cerebral perfusion.

Aging patients are more prone to syncope because of the following:

1. Reductions in cerebral blood flow, CO, and thirst
2. Altered homeostasis of water and salt in the renal system
3. Altered baroreceptor function, diminished heart rate, and vasoconstriction response
4. Structural heart disease
5. The impaired diastolic filling and stroke volume with normal aging
5. Autonomic dysfunction
6. Polypharmacy

## CAUSE AND CLASSIFICATION OF SYNCOPE
### Main Causes of Syncope

Three main categories encompass most syncope causes: they are most commonly NMS, followed by OH, then cardiac cause. Mixed cause syncope is common in the older adult, but its exact incidence is not clear. It is therefore important to note that older patients may often have multifactorial causes of syncope. Emergency physicians, however, often stop once a single attributable cause has been identified; this fails to identify mixed cause syncope. Physicians should consider multiple causes in all patients with syncope. The most high-yield secondary causes are medication effect and comorbidities. Always consider these as causes of multifactorial syncope.

1. NMS includes functional disruption of CO by bradycardia or vasodilation; this is also termed reflex syncope. The mechanisms involved are divided into vasovagal syncope (VVS), situational, or carotid sinus sensitivity.
   a. VVS is the single largest cause of syncope. In this situation, syncope is triggered by an event such as pain, emotional upset, fear, or prolonged standing. Onset is associated with typical prodromal symptoms of diaphoresis, nausea, tunnel vision, and then LOC. VVS requires an intact autonomic nervous system, and therefore, should never be diagnosed in patients with autonomic dysfunction.
   b. Situational syncope follows specific events of micturition, defecation, coughing, laughing, or swallowing. However, lack of cerebral perfusion may wipe the memory of this precipitating event away and confound the history.
   c. CSH is an exaggerated response from stimulation of the carotid sinus causing asystole. It can be isolated or exist as part of a generalized autonomic disorder. It is most common in men and is often associated with falls, placing patients at higher risk for injury and fractures.
2. OH can be included under the category of NMS syncope. It can also be classed alone when it occurs from simple volume depletion such as poor intake, gastrointestinal (GI) loss, or hemorrhage. Drugs from several classes may also cause OH by lowering PVR. Finally, OH occurs when the normal autoregulatory processes of vasoconstriction and reflex heart rate increase fail to occur. OH can be a result of primary autonomic failure from neurodegenerative disease or secondary autonomic failure from other systemic diseases like diabetes, hepatic or renal failure, and chronic alcohol abuse. OH is an example of a geriatric syndrome and may be seen as part of the systemic dysregulation that occurs in frailty.[21] The clinical symptoms and signs of OH depend on its cause and severity. OH as a geriatric syndrome is a predictor of poor prognosis.[22]
3. Cardiac causes of syncope occur as decreased CO causes hypoperfusion. Events are either electrophysiological as in dysrhythmia, structural, or related to cerebrovascular steal syndromes.

a. Dysrhythmias include atrial fibrillation and flutter, high-grade atrioventricular (AV) block, ventricular tachycardia, sinus node dysfunction, sick sinus syndrome, and pacemaker dysfunction. The causes of the rhythm disturbance itself are most commonly ischemic, followed by hypertensive disease.

b. Structural heart disease, such as valvular stenosis, cardiomyopathies, cardiac masses, and pericardial effusions or other outflow obstructions.

c. Cerebrovascular steal syndromes occur when distal obstruction of an artery prevents normal forward flow, leading to retrograde flow, resulting in ischemia distal to the involved artery. These very rarely occur without associated focal neurologic deficits or seizurelike activity.

4. Multifactorial syncope is common in older adults and is an independent risk for adverse outcomes. When several causes may be in play simultaneously, consider this a high-risk patient and investigate multiple causes even when the first most likely cause has already been found.

## Unlikely Causes of Syncope

### Transient ischemic attacks

Transient ischemic attacks (TIAs) do not cause true LOC. The only possible exception is a TIA affecting the vertebrobasilar circulation. In this situation, other signs such as paralysis, eye movement disorders, and vertigo, should be noted by history or physical examination. Any syncopal events without these associated symptoms are not due to cerebrovascular ischemia, and typical syncope patients do not warrant a TIA evaluation.

### Psychogenic syncope

These episodes do not fit the full definition of syncope because LOC here is not caused by RGCH. However, up to 20% to 35% of more loosely defined syncope patients may have psychogenic syncope and require psychiatric evaluation to determine this cause. Emergency physicians should consider a psychiatric cause of these TLOC events that look like syncope. Understanding this distinction may result in better diagnosis and treatment.

## DIAGNOSTIC EVALUATION

### History

The main goal in syncope evaluation is differentiating benign versus life-threatening causes. The single most important tool in the syncope evaluation is a good history. A complete syncope history can reduce the need for additional testing, decrease costs, shorten ED stays, and improve patient satisfaction. A detailed syncope history may be the key to distinguishing benign from more concerning causes.

Step 1 is to establish syncope as a TLOC of rapid onset and short duration, with a complete and spontaneous recovery to presyncope level of function.[23] Beginning with an inconsistent definition leads to inappropriate diagnostic testing and inconsistent treatment.[24] The American College of Cardiology and the American Heart Association use the broader classification of syncope, whereas the European Society of Cardiology (ESC) definition is narrower.[25] Specific features may be difficult to establish by history, because cerebral hypoperfusion may cause amnesia of the event. In fact, 40% of elder patients have complete amnesia of a syncopal event.[26] Further complicating the history, witnesses to the event may not be present or may report inconsistent accounts. Moreover, syncope is often difficult to differentiate from seizure because of the convulsive activity seen in 4% to 40% of syncopal events.[27] LOC in syncope is due to RGCH, whereas in seizure, it is due to abnormal electrical activity. To facilitate this often difficult distinction, Sheldon[27] created a history-based scoring system that can differentiate between the 2 with a sensitivity and specificity for seizures of 94%. A history of tongue biting and confusion following the episode is more indicative of seizure, whereas light-headedness, sweating, and prolonged standing are more predictive of syncope (**Table 1**).

| Table 1 Questions to differentiate syncope and seizure | |
| --- | --- |
| **Question** | **Points** |
| Any tongue biting? | 2 |
| Any sense of déjà vu before the episode? | 1 |
| Association with emotional stress? | 1 |
| Anyone notice head turning during event? | 1 |
| Any unusual posturing, jerking limbs, or lack of memory afterwards? | 1 |
| Any confusion afterwards? | 1 |
| History of lightheaded episodes? | −2 |
| Sweating before episodes? | −2 |
| Any prolonged standing or sitting? | −2 |

Seizures are more likely if the point score is ≥1, and syncope if the point score is <1.

### History of present illness
Classically, VVS features a prodrome of warmth, nausea, sweating, and light-headedness.[28] Syncope without prodrome, or when associated with palpitations, supine position, or exercise, is concerning for cardiac cause.[29] It is also important to investigate for concurrent infection or illness, especially symptoms consistent with hypovolemia, such as vomiting, diarrhea, bleeding, and decreased appetite that may point to OH. The clinician should elicit any associated straining or coughing that could point to a situational cause and obtain any history of prior episodes. Evaluate medications for agents such as diuretics, antihypertensives, and others that may affect volume status, autonomic stability, or cardiac function. Inquire regarding any medication dose changes, new medications, and recent alcohol or drug use. Recent bed rest and deconditioning can also cause OH.

### Past medical history
After discussing the current episode, it is important to further risk stratify using the patient's past medical history. Obtain any history of heart failure, myocardial infarction, structural heart disease, and family history of heart disease or sudden death. Some common features that are predictive of low mortality following syncope are history not consistent with cardiac, abdominal, or focal neurologic symptoms; a normal physical examination; no evidence of CHF; no new neurologic deficits; normal glucose; and benign EKG.[30] In this study, there were no deaths or adverse outcomes in patients discharged from the ED who met these criteria.

Heart disease is an independent predictor of cardiac syncope (odds ratio 16, $P = .00001$), with a sensitivity of 95% and a specificity of 45%. In contrast, the absence of heart disease excludes a cardiac cause of syncope in 97% of the patients.[29] Also, solicit illnesses with dysautonomia such as Parkinson disease, multiple sclerosis, alcohol abuse, and diabetes.

### Medications
Medications are a major issue in the evaluation of syncope. OH alone may be caused by a long list of medications including diuretics causing volume depletion, α-blockers

for benign prostatic hypertrophy (BPH), sympatholytics and vasodilators impairing autonomic response, anti-Parkinson medications, tricyclics, atypical antipsychotics, and monoamine oxidase inhibitors. A careful review of medications is needed, and if suspected as a cause of syncope, consultation with a pharmacologist may be helpful.

### Structured syncope history

1. Define history of true syncope with global cerebral hypoperfusion
2. Distinguish from other transient LOC events (ie, seizure)
3. Treat near syncope the same as full syncope
4. Define precise details of the event/chief complaint
   a. Ask what the patient was doing at the time
   b. Ask about provocative triggers
   c. Ask if any prodromal symptoms occurred
   d. Establish series of events
   e. Determine duration of LOC
   f. Ask if associated symptoms occurred
   g. Ask if there is a current contributory illness/event (flu, fever, bleeding)
   h. Ask if there are symptoms of OH or autonomic dysfunction
5. Are there active traumatic complaints or risk of trauma
6. Specifically question any fall and falls in the prior year
7. Obtain a focused past medical history
   a. Prior syncope and its diagnosis
   b. Cardiovascular disease
   c. GI losses especially hemorrhage
   d. Diseases with autonomic failure
8. Medications: specifically review for drug effect syncope; class IA and IC antiarrhythmics are common causes of syncope; anticoagulants are critical if concurrent trauma exists

## Physical Examination

After a careful history, conduct a thorough physical examination. First, examine the vital signs, including orthostatic vital signs. Abnormal vital signs need to be addressed and warrant explanation. Those with persistent (>15 minutes) abnormal vitals are at higher risk for adverse outcome.[31] Furthermore, a careful cardiopulmonary examination should be done to evaluate for signs of heart failure or structural heart disease. Take note of any pericardial rubs, murmurs, extremity edema, jugular venous distension, or rales. Neurologic examination should evaluate for focal deficit or altered mentation. Focal neurologic examination may suggest an alternate diagnosis and should be further evaluated.[32] Because tongue biting is very specific (96%) for seizure, it is useful to examine the tongue.[33] A rectal examination for fecal occult blood should be performed if GI bleeding is a concern. It is also important to evaluate for signs of trauma, which accompany 39% of syncopal episodes in the older patient.[34]

## Testing

Initial testing will depend largely on information gathered on history and physical examination, with few exceptions. One exception is that all patients with syncope should have a 12-lead electrocardiogram (EKG) performed in the initial evaluation.[35]

### Electrocardiogram

The EKG is fast, inexpensive, and safe. With an EKG, the clinician can assess for signs of structural heart disease and arrhythmia. The Ottawa EKG Criteria identify patients at risk for 30-day serious cardiac outcome. Positive findings are second-degree Mobitz type 2 or third-degree AV block, bundle branch block with first-degree AV block, right bundle branch with left anterior or posterior fascicular block, new ischemic changes, non-sinus rhythm, left-axis deviation, or ED cardiac monitor abnormalities. The sensitivity and specificity of the Ottawa EKG Criteria were 96% and 76%, respectively.[36]

In addition, those with EKG showing any arrhythmia, premature atrial contraction, premature ventricular contraction, pacing, second- and third-degree AV blocks, and left bundle branch block may benefit from echocardiography. It is otherwise not useful in those with normal EKGs, who are unlikely to have structural heart disease.[37] Another important EKG diagnosis is Brugada syndrome (BS) (Fig. 2). BS is a channelopathy, caused by mutation in the cardiac sodium channel that can lead to tachyarrhythmia and sudden death in structurally normal hearts. It is characterized by signature ST elevation in the precordial leads. A coved-type ST-segment elevation (type I) in one of the right precordial leads (V1–2) is the basis for diagnosis. The saddleback type 2 and 3 Brugada patterns are suggestive, but not sufficient for diagnosis. The Brugada pattern type I occurs in between 0% and 0.3% of the population and is more common in Asians and in men.[38]

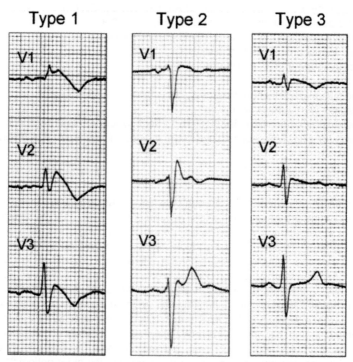

Fig. 2. BS EKG morphology. (*From* Napolitano C, Priori SG. Brugada syndrome. Orphanet J Rare Dis 2006;1:35.)

## Orthostatic vital sign evaluation

A simple addition to the syncope workup is orthostatic vital sign measurement in the well-appearing patient. OH is common in elders with a prevalence of 16.4% in community-dwelling patients and increasing to 50% in institutionalized patients.[39] It is critical to find OH because it is an independent predictor of mortality and falls.[40] OH is often overlooked, leading to falls, injury, recurrent syncope, loss of function, and even death.[41] OH is the physical finding of a greater than 20-mm Hg decrease in ystolic or greater than 10 mm Hg decrease in diastolic blood pressure within 3 minutes f standing.[42] Standing causes decreased venous blood return because 25% to 30% f the systemic circulation begins pooling in the lower extremities.[43] Subjective light-eadedness within 2 minutes of standing is also considered OH. There can be wide ariation in orthostatic vital sign changes for healthy and ill individuals alike, and there nay be poor correlation of vital signs with level of dehydration.[44] Nevertheless, positive rthostatic vital signs or those that reproduce symptoms can reinforce concerns about olume status or autonomic instability. OH is a common finding in elder patients. Older dults can have impaired ability to maintain blood pressure due to autonomic dysfunc-on, altered baroreceptor function, decreased cardiac contractility, and medication ffects in addition to peripheral vascular disease.[45] OH is present in up to 20% of atients older than 65 years, although as few as 2% of these patients were symptom-tic,[46] making it important to assess this finding when it is suspected.

### aboratory evaluation

nitial laboratory work should be catered to the individual patient. Routine blood work s low yield in the general evaluation of syncope. However, it is reasonable for all syn-ope patients to have a point-of-care glucose. This cheap, easy test can exclude an asily reversible cause of syncope.[47] Patients with clinical evaluations or histories con-erning for bleeding, acute coronary syndrome, or metabolic disturbance should be valuated for such diagnoses. However, in elder patients, the history can be unreveal-ng or unobtainable, and the physical examination is often nonspecific. Therefore, cli-icians should maintain high suspicion and order blood work on an individual basis. )ne test with high significance is the brain natriuretic peptide (BNP). Notably, elevation f the BNP has been associated with a significant increase in mortality.[48]

### naging

Jo imaging is routinely needed, again unless prompted by history or physical exam-nation. Routine computed tomographic (CT) scans, echocardiography, carotid ultra-ound, and electroencephalography all together affected diagnosis or management in ess than 5% of cases and helped determine the cause of syncope less than 2% of the me.[49] The American College of Emergency Physicians (ACEP) does not recommend outine CT head scan in asymptomatic adult patients with syncope, insignificant rauma, and a normal neurologic examination.[50] Nonetheless, 39% of elder patients vill present with trauma, which may necessitate individualized imaging.[34]

### Jon-emergency department testing

rrhythmia may be suspected in those syncopal patients with no prodrome, with pal-itations or arrhythmia on EKG, specifically those included in the Ottawa EKG criteria. 'atients with features concerning for arrhythmia should have telemetry monitoring. ollowing an ED telemetry observation period, some have proposed outpatient Holter nonitoring as a safe, effective means to diagnose arrhythmogenic syncope.[51] These levices are worn for 24 to 36 hours and should be considered in a carefully selected roup of patients who otherwise do not appear to have a life-threatening condition and lave frequent enough episodes that an event is likely to be detected during the Holter valuation timeframe. External or implantable loop recorders are potentially more use-ul devices in the detection of symptomatic arrhythmia during longer timeframes. 'hose at higher risk according to physician judgment or decision rules should be dmitted for telemetry monitoring.

A study by Kapoor and colleagues[52] found that prolonged monitoring could identify arious dysrhythmias, such as sinus bradycardia, supraventricular tachycardia, atrial ibrillation, ventricular tachycardia, or short sinus pauses. However, even in these patients with dysrhythmia, a definite cause of syncope was found in only 15% of subjects. Moreover, 1% to 4% of the normal populations exhibited asymptomatic periods of sinus pause, and up to 2% had short episodes of ventricular tachycardia.[52] Given this, one must be mindful that some arrhythmia findings during monitoring may be incidental and not the cause of syncope.

### Outpatient testing

Those discharged from the ED or from the hospital may require additional follow-up testing to clearly identify the cause of their syncope. Electrophysiology studies assess the integrity of the His Purkinje system. This study is rarely indicated for syncope, especially in those with a normal EKG and no structural heart disease. It is also not recommended for those with severe structural heart disease in which ICD instead is indicated. However, it may be reasonable in syncope patients with bifascicular block, when noninvasive tests fail to make the diagnosis.[53]

Tilt-table testing is a common outpatient procedure in the syncope workup. Many protocols exist, but it generally consists of passive head-upright tilt for 20 to 60 minutes, which can produce hypotension, bradycardia, presyncope, or syncope. Sometimes patients are also given isoproterenol, sublingual nitrates, or clomipramine to further provoke symptoms.[54] Tilt testing has been and remains a valuable tool for making correct and precise diagnoses of syncope and related conditions. It can be particularly helpful in distinguishing seizures versus syncope[27] and diagnosing VVS, OH, postural orthostatic tachycardia syndrome, and psychogenic pseudosyncope.[55]

### Treatment

Although the emergency physician's primary role in syncope is diagnosis, risk stratification, and determining safe disposition, it is important to be aware of some of the potential treatment modalities for syncope. Of course, specific interventions will be directed to the presumed or confirmed cause.

### Neurally mediated syncope

The emergency physician's most important role in the management of these patients is to diagnose the condition and educate the patient recognizing that patient misunderstanding and fear can severely impair quality of life and functioning. Education should include increased oral hydration and salt intake. This advice should be given with need to observe blood pressure elevation over time. Salt should be increased to 6 to 10 g of sodium chloride daily with 1.5 to 2 L of water. Physiologic counterpressure techniques, such as leg crossing and tensing calf muscles, are effective and can be done in any situation. The avoidance of trigger situations where identified should be advised. Finally, patients should be directed to lie flat at the onset of symptoms. Use of support stockings can alleviate symptoms and should be thigh or waist high to produce at least 15- to 20-mm Hg pressure.

It is critical to discontinue potentially offending medications; this may require pharmacology consultation, discussion with prescribing physicians, and ongoing patient evaluation. The emergency physician must take the time to ensure review of medications in every syncope patient. If the patient is to be discharged from the ED, it is critical for the emergency physician to ensure timely outpatient follow-up for ongoing evaluation and treatment. The primary goal is to reduce the incidence of recurrent syncope. In a structured follow-up setting, β-blockers, selective serotonin reuptake inhibitors, and midodrine have shown some potential benefit, especially in older patients with NMS. However, these medications are of questionable benefit and should not be initiated from the ED. Patients may also be referred for tilt-table testing, and consideration of pacemaker insertion if sinus arrest (carotid sinus syndrome) is the cause of NMS.[56] It is important to note that pacemaker insertion has shown proven benefit for NMS. In addition, there is consensus regarding benefit of pacer insertion for patients in whom carotid sinus massage triggers symptoms.[57] **Table 2** demonstrates vasovagal education.

**Table 2**
**Vasovagal management strategies**

| Prevention | Avoid Triggers | Aborting Strategies |
|---|---|---|
| Daily water and sodium intake | High temperatures | Squatting |
| Compression stockings | Prolonged standing | Leg crossing |
| Avoid diuretics and vasoactive drugs | Sudden posture changes | Quickly sit or lay supine |
| Avoid alcohol | Straining | — |
| Regular exercise | Blood draws | — |

*Adapted from* Coffin ST, Raj SR. Non-invasive management of vasovagal syncope. Auton Neurosci 2014;184:27–32.

*Arrhythmia monitoring*

There are 2 primary means of outpatient arrhythmia monitoring to consider when arrhythmia is the suspected cause of a syncopal event. Holter monitors are applied externally and monitored continuously for 24 to 48 hours. Unfortunately, these devices have shown low diagnostic yield and are likely inconclusive because of the low likelihood of recurrence within that period. Internal and external loop recorders offer the advantage of protracted monitoring. These devices record continuously, but only save abnormal rhythms. Patients can also manually activate the device when experiencing symptoms. Internal loop recorders in particular have been shown to be very effective, likely owing to their inherently excellent compliance: there are no electrodes to wear, and patients can have them in place operating for up to 3 years without battery change. This long timeframe and ease of use significantly increases the likelihood that abnormal rhythms will be detected. In some cases, these rhythms can be transmitted wirelessly to a receiving center, where the physician can make the diagnosis. ED utility of these devices is limited, but knowledge of their potential means of diagnosis is useful for specific outpatient follow-up strategies.

**RISK STRATIFICATION IN SYNCOPE**
*The High Risk Features of Syncope*

An emergency physician's disposition of patients after an ED syncope presentation substantially impacts health care cost, resource utilization, ED throughput, and patient satisfaction, among other metrics. Today, about a third of patients presenting to the ED with syncope are admitted. The criticism falling on emergency physicians is that roughly a third of these admitted patients are discharged without requiring any intervention. Numerous clinical decision rules (CDR) have been developed to help predict those patients that require hospitalization. These CDR instruments help predict the likelihood of morbidity and mortality following syncope as detailed in later discussion. Reviews of CDR performance indicate that following well-established guidelines results in a thorough and high-yield evaluation of these patients, but that strict adherence to these rules does not improve patient outcomes or other metrics.[58] Ultimately, it is the ED physician's responsibility to identify patients with intermediate- or high-risk features of syncope who may benefit from either observation or admission.

## Heart disease

Cardiac syncope carries the highest associated mortality; therefore, the emergency physician should attempt to identify potential cardiac causes of syncope. The forms of organic heart disease, which may cause syncope, include coronary artery disease, structural heart defects, valve disorders, conduction defects, diseases of the great vessels, and associated pulmonary disease.[59] Identification of these cardiac causes through history and physical examination and appropriate diagnostic measures would likely identify high-risk individuals with syncope who would benefit from hospital admission.

Other features indicative of cardiac syncope are an abnormal EKG, a history of heart disease, presence of palpitations, syncope occurring during effort or while supine, absence of an autonomic prodrome, and absence of associated predisposing factors such as micturition, defecation, or blood draw.[60] Inquiring about these components of the syncopal event during history is needed to appropriately risk-stratify patients with an underlying cardiac syncopal event.

## Arrhythmia

Arrhythmia is the most common cause of cardiac-related syncope and therefore must be considered high in the differential. The EKG can show findings indicative or diagnostic of a cardiac syncopal event.[61] These findings are summarized in **Table 3**. When present, EKG findings such as BS must be addressed. However, because noncardiac syncope is vastly more common than arrhythmogenic syncope, note that a noncardiac cause may be present and should still be excluded in patients with abnormal EKG findings such as BS.[62]

## Clinical Decision Rules

Clinical decision instruments rely on the principle that identifying one high-risk feature distinguishes patients with higher mortality, which is sufficient justification for hospital admission. The instruments are designed to predict short-term mortality (typically within 1 month) following syncope. The following is an overview of the commonly cited syncope rules and their approximate sensitivities and specificities. It is worth noting that these rules, although useful in identifying high-risk features of syncope, have varying sensitivities in validation studies and thus have questionable practical utility in risk stratification. What is perhaps most useful from each of these decision instruments is the targeting of high-risk features when taking a thorough history of patients with syncope. Identification of high-risk features will help formulate a thoughtful diagnostic and disposition strategy.

## San Francisco syncope rule

This risk-stratification tool uses the following parameters: abnormal EKG (defined as new changes or nonsinus rhythm), systolic blood pressure less than or equal to 90, hematocrit less than or equal to 30%, and signs or symptoms of CHF. If answers to any of these parameters are affirmative, the patient is not low risk. Although this instrument was initially considered to be 98% sensitive and 56% specific, subsequent validation studies demonstrated varying degrees of sensitivity and specificity in predicting short-term patient outcomes. One study applying the San Francisco syncope rule (SFSR) to patients older than the age of 65 deemed that sensitivity was only 76.5%, suggesting that this instrument is not useful in the elder syncope population.[63]

## Osservatorio epidemiologico sulla sincope nel lazio score

The Osservatorio Epidemiologico Sulla Sincope Nel Lazio score, derived from an Italian study, identified the following criteria as independent predictors of mortality within

**Table 3**
**Features indicative of cardiac syncope causes**

| Cardiac Causes of Syncope in the Older Adult Patient | Diagnostic/Risk Stratification Strategies |
|---|---|
| Arrhythmias (most common) | EKG changes, especially sick sinus syndrome, AV block, pacemaker or implantable cardioverter-defibrillator issues, supraventricular tachycardia, ventricular tachycardia<br>Palpitations preceding syncope<br>Exertional or occurring while supine<br>Persistent bradycardia<br>History of prolonged QT syndrome<br>History of implantable loop recorder displaying abnormal rhythm |
| Ischemic heart disease/ coronary artery disease | History consistent w/acute coronary syndrome<br>Abnormal EKG<br>Exertional |
| EKG findings suggestive of arrhythmia[11] | Bifascicular block or other intraventricular conduction delay (QRS widening)<br>Mobitz 1 2nd-degree AV block<br>Inappropriate sinus bradycardia (<50 bpm) or sinus pause >3 s in the absence of β-blockers or other rate controlling agents<br>Nonsustained ventricular tachycardia<br>Pre-excitation QRS complexes<br>Long or short QT interval<br>Early repolarization<br>BS<br>Negative T waves in right precordial leads, epsilon waves, and ventricular late potentials as in arrhythmogenic right ventricular cardiomyopathy<br>Q waves consistent with myocardial infarction |
| Structural heart disease | Known abnormal echocardiogram (especially ejection fraction <35%)<br>Family history of unexplained sudden death<br>Exertional, or occurring while supine<br>Signs or symptoms of CHF, pulmonary embolism, aortic dissection, or critical aortic stenosis<br>B-type natriuretic peptide >300 |

*Adapted from* Moya A, Sutton R, Ammirati F, et al. Guidelines for the diagnosis and management of syncope (version 2009). Eur Heart J 2009;30(21):2631–71; with permission.

1 year of initial syncope evaluation: age greater than 65, a history of cardiovascular disease, syncope without prodromal symptoms, and abnormal EKG.[64] The investigators here found the mortality with increasing score to be additive, that is, a higher score was associated with higher mortality, as in **Table 4**.

**Table 4**
**Mortalities associated with Osservatorio Epidemiologico Sulla Sincope Nel Lazio score**

| OESIL Score | Mortality (%) |
|---|---|
| 1 | 0.8 |
| 2 | 19.6 |
| 3 | 34.7 |
| 4 | 57.1 |

### Rose rule

The Rose rule uses BNP elevation 300 pg/mL or greater, rectal examination with positive fecal occult blood test, hemoglobin less than or equal to 90 g/L, oxygen saturation less than or equal to 94% on room air, Q waves on the EKG (except lead III), chest pain at the time of syncope, and bradycardia with heart rate less than 50 bpm to predict serious adverse events. Sensitivity from the initial study was 92.5%, specificity 73.8%. The same investigators also performed a validation study using a subsequent cohort, in which they found sensitivity to be 87.2%, specificity 65.5%. BNP elevation alone was independently predictive of serious adverse events. The mnemonic "BRACES" is useful to remember the components of this rule: BNP, Rectal examination, Anemia, Chest pain, EKG, Saturation.[48]

### Boston rule

Using the Boston rule, any of the following clinical factors increased short-term risk for adverse events within 30 days: signs and symptoms of acute coronary syndrome, signs of conductive heart disease, history of heart disease, valvular heart disease (by history or examination), family history of sudden death, persistent abnormal vital signs in the ED, volume depletion (including signs of dehydration or GI bleeding or low hematocrit), or primary neurologic symptoms. Researchers claimed a sensitivity of 97%, specificity of 62%, and postulated that adopting this rule would result in a 48% decline in hospital admissions.[31] The investigators performed a follow-up validation study and found an 11% reduction in admissions, with 100% sensitivity for adverse events, but there have been no larger validation studies.[65]

### Limitations of the Clinical Decision Rules

Multiple studies suggest that syncope CDRs fail to adequately risk stratify ED patients. Kessler[66] reports 2 main problems with these instruments. First, they lack sensitivity, so that some patients are discharged without identification of a clinically significant cause that may require intervention. This potentially negates the number of saved, unnecessary admissions. Second, these rules lack specificity, so they identify high-risk individuals at the expense of costly and potentially unnecessary admissions. The SFSR and others provide valuable insights into the risk stratification of ED syncope patients, but cannot be solely relied on to determine risk and disposition.

The systematic review and meta-analysis of Serrano and colleauges[67] revealed the sensitivities and specificities for each of the CDRs summarized in **Table 5.**

**Table 5**
**Syncope decision rule sensitivities and specificities**

| Rule | Sensitivity (%) | Specificity (%) |
|---|---|---|
| SFSR | 86 | 49 |
| OESIL risk score | 95 | 31 |
| ROSE | 90 | 70 |
| Boston | 97 | 62 |
| Syncope risk score | 88 | 32 |

Kessler[66] reported the commonality of the rules is a set of broad criteria that may identify high-risk patients and include the following:

- An abnormal EKG (variably defined)
- Signs or symptoms of heart failure or cardiac dysrhythmia

- Abnormal vital signs in the ED that do not correct with routine interventions
- Old age (this cutoff varies, but is generally greater than 60 years old)

## Outcomes in Syncope

### Mortality

The mortality from syncope-related causes can be thought of in various ways. Mortality after ED presentation, regardless of whether patients are admitted or discharged, is up to 2.3% within 6 months, and up to 4% to 7% within 1 year. Incidentally, about 78% of deceased patients at 1 year had been admitted from the ED.[7,68] About 37% of these deaths in one study were related to cardiac cause in stark contrast to a 7% to 9% all-cause mortality. Because cardiac causes carry the highest mortality, the emergency physician's effort is first directed at seeking and ruling out cardiac-related syncope.[2] Patients who are appropriately diagnosed with a benign cause of syncope fare well after ED discharge. Patients with underlying cardiac disease require additional monitoring and investigation. Mortality from unexplained syncope is 6%.[68] The mortality of unexplained syncope is significant and virtually mandates such patients be risk stratified and dispositioned thoughtfully.

Posthospitalization mortality for syncope patients is 4.4%, with 1.1% of these deaths attributed to cardiac cause.[2] One-year mortality in patients with cardiac syncope may be as high as 33%, compared with patients with noncardiac syncope in whom mortality ranges from 0% to 12%. This range suggests the cardiac issues are treated but not cured during the hospitalization. The emergency physician must be aware of this fact in the evaluation of patients who return to the ED after syncope-related hospitalization.

### Recurrence

Patients who present with VVS have low mortality, and the condition is generally considered benign. However, recurrent VVS syncopal episodes are common and often affect the quality of life, contribute to repeat ED visits, and lead to increased risk of fall-related injury, especially in frail elders. In the immediate period following an episode of VVS, up to 20% of patients experience recurring syncope.[69] Earlier onset of recurring VVS in these patients is associated with a higher likelihood of additional recurrence. One study that followed VVS patients to 30 months showed an approximate 30% recurrence rate.[70] The recurrence of syncopal events in patients with this common cause of syncope is likely to have an effect on quality of life, but does not appear to affect mortality.

The mechanism of syncope has no association with the timing or frequency of recurrent episodes.[71] Physicians must consider risk of recurrent episodes during patient education and while arranging follow-up evaluations.

### Falls

Cerebral hypoperfusion results in memory impairment, making it difficult, if not impossible, for patients to relate an accurate syncope history. With the substantial overlap between falls and syncope, the provider should consider syncope as a possible cause in unexplained older adult falls. In addition, near-syncope may be responsible for falls in this age group, which prompts an evaluation identical to that for true syncope.[72]

### Benign Syncope

It is important to identify the low-risk features that indicate benign syncope. The physician must note features of NMS and OH. Uncovering these features in the ED may facilitate a shorter ED stay, with limited testing, and identify those who do not require admission. Benign syncope is likely in patients with no history of heart disease, a long-standing history of syncope, or where the syncope occurs following exposure to a noxious stimulus. **Table 6** lists other features of low-risk syncope. When this cause can be readily identified, and a cardiac cause is not suspected, the patient will in general not benefit from hospital admission.[73]

**Table 6**
**Clinical features of benign syncope**

| Type of "Benign" Syncope | Clinical Features |
|---|---|
| VVS and NMS[11] | No significant cardiac history<br>Multiple episodes of recurring syncope<br>Occurring after sudden unexpected noxious stimulus<br>Prolonged standing/hot/crowded environment<br>Associated with nausea, vomiting<br>During eating/postprandial<br>After rotating head or pressure on the carotid<br>*After* (not during) exertion |
| OH[11] | After sitting → standing<br>Related to starting or changing dose of vasodepressive drugs<br>Prolonged standing<br>History of autonomic neuropathy/parkinsonism<br>Standing up after exertion |

### Near Syncope

Near syncope is an entity that is even less well characterized than true syncope. Near syncope has a varying definition and perception among patients and clinicians. It is therefore difficult to study and determine its prevalence and associated outcomes. A reasonable definition of near syncope proposed by Scharenbrock and colleauges[74] is "transient light-headedness so severe that the patient felt they might suffer loss of consciousness." Using this definition, Grossman and colleagues[72] showed that rates of adverse outcomes with near syncope are similar to those with true syncope (rate of 20% and 23%, respectively, in their study). As such, especially in the older adult population, the physician should consider near syncope to portend similar risk as a true syncope. When an elder patient with falls also identifies symptoms consistent with near syncope, this overlap is even more essential.

There is limited research to suggest a reliable clinical decision instrument to screen patients with near syncope. In the patient population of Grossman and colleagues,[75] the modified Boston Syncope Criteria were predictive of safe discharge home with no 30-day adverse events. The modified criteria do not take into account prior history, and in this study, patients who had a clear VVS or a hypovolemic clinical picture along with a normal ED workup were considered safe for discharge. It is important to note, however, that these results require validation.[75]

### EMERGENCY DEPARTMENT DISCHARGE OF ELDER SYNCOPE PATIENTS
#### Follow-up

The key to any successful ED elder discharge is linkage with follow-up care. A rate of 2.4% of serious adverse outcomes occurs in syncope patients discharged from the ED, many of whom were given no further follow-up.[76] Consider developing an stitution-specific process of care where intermediate-risk patients are either observed or followed within 24 to 48 hours according to a predetermined readily available pathway. Development of such policies and protocols ensures follow-up availability with the most ease and best assurance of patient safety. In general, elder syncope patients should have follow-up evaluation by a primary care or specialty physician. The urgency of this follow-up depends on risk stratification. Some hospitals are developing "Falls and Faint Clinics" as a model of health care delivery that has been found to improve outcomes and generate profit as well.[77] The current poor outcomes with older patients should trigger multidisciplinary evaluations. Emergency physicians should ensure a formal pharmacology review in any patient taking 6 or more medications, or more than 3 antihypertensive drugs. Consider joint cardiology and neurology evaluations in cases where cause is difficult to establish. Consider routine referrals for treatment and patient education by physical therapy (PT) and occupational therapy (OT) to maintain proper functioning and enhance quality of life in syncope patients when no other specific treatment is available. ED administrators can work with PT/OT for a predetermined order set, goals of care, and reporting to PCPs in this population.

## Driving After Syncope

Patients who experience syncope may inquire about the safety of returning to driving. A few individual states require physicians to report syncope to trigger a review of the patient's official driving privileges. Be aware that each state has relevant laws and regulations in this regard, and physician permission to drive may be relevant in civil or criminal cases. The key factors to identify when determining safe return to driving are the cause of the patient's syncope, the likelihood of syncope recurrence while driving, and the type of driving.[78]

In 1992, the *Canadian Journal of Cardiology* performed a mathematical computation determining that the risk of recurring syncope must be less than 22% in order for the patient to be permitted to drive.[79] It is unlikely that the average physician will be able to determine this calculation. It is important that driving safety is considered when dealing with the geriatric ED patient in whom the question of driving is likely already a topic of debate.[80] More useful is the existence of programs on safe driving evaluation now popping up through various hospitals. The typical evaluation requires evaluation of driving functions, speed of reflexes, coordination, and cognitive response by a physical/occupational therapist. If a patient passes this evaluation, then they are observed during a road test. Recommendations are made as to fitness for driving with or without the use of aids. This testing is quite useful because it provides an independent assessment of necessary functions. However, this evaluation tests the patient at baseline only and does not consider the risk of having a syncopal event.

NMS (including VVS) while driving does occur.[81] Interestingly, this can occur in the seated driver, most likely because of impaired venous return from the legs. When an ED evaluation determines that the patient is suffering from a mild form of VVS (based on symptom severity and cause), it is reasonable to advise safe return to normal driving without any waiting period. When the VVS is considered severe or recurrent, the physician should recommend a waiting period of 3 months before returning to driving. This waiting period can be especially helpful while the patient adopts recommended treatment strategies and learns to control symptoms.

When syncope is caused by arrhythmia, treatment should be complete before resumption of driving, and the time period differs significantly based on the rhythm treated. In the case of tachydysrhythmias, the common treatment modality is automatic implantable cardioverter-defibrillator (AICD) implantation. Professional societies recommend a 6-month period of driving restriction before resuming regular driving. One study suggests that patients with AICDs are at similar if not reduced risk of automobile accidents, with a 3.4% rate per patient-year, compared with 7.1% in the general driving population.[78] For patients with bradydysrhythmias, after implantable pacemaker insertion, a 1-week waiting period before resumption of regular driving is advised.

### Quality of Life

Although most elders return home after a syncopal event, they may experience significant morbidity. Even syncope from simple VVS may seriously impact subsequent well-being. Quality-of-life studies show that elders may do poorly after syncope and develop significant functional impairments.[82] Recurrent syncope has the most important effects on health-related quality of life (HRQL). The absolute number of events decreases HRQL perception. Decreases in HRQL are attributed to limited mobility: pain associated with trauma and associated symptoms, inability to carry out activities of daily living, as well as anxiety and depression. Interestingly, physical impairment from recurring syncope appears to have the greatest impact on HRQL. The fear of syncope recurrence causes decreased activity, especially walking, and lowers overall vitality as well as social functioning. These effects are most pronounced within the first 6 months after a syncopal episode and lead to further functional decline. The need for admission, consultation, and further testing was related to poorer functional outcomes; this stresses the significance that the emergency physician's decision to evaluate, hospitalize, or discharge has on quality of life. Physicians need to ensure patients understand the truly benign nature of a syncopal event if that is the determination.

### COST
### Overall Costs

The estimated annual health care cost in the United States associated with syncope is $1.7 to 2.4 billion.[28] Much of this cost represents the frequency of ED visits as well as hospital admissions, recalling that approximately one-third of patients presenting to the ED for syncope are admitted from the ED. Cost numbers are likely underestimated, because they are based on discharge diagnostic codes.

Approximately 460,000 syncope patients are admitted annually, and patients older than 60 years of age are admitted at a rate of about 60% when they present to the ED with this complaint. In fact, advanced age is one of the factors associated with increased cost of syncope workup, along with large hospital size, urban setting, and geographic location.[83] Of course, treatment of known causes of syncope with implantable defibrillators and pacemakers is also associated with increased cost.

Investigators have estimated the costs for individual, commonly used tests in the ED workup of elder syncope. Those results are included in **Table 7** and are specific to the tests ordered on patients over the age of 65 in whom the results provided meaningful diagnostic utility. Some of the easiest and quickest ED tests also have the highest utility per dollar spent. Furthermore, investigators found that ordering tests based on adherence to the SFSR was associated with decreased cost per diagnostic test. For example, to discover abnormal orthostatic vital signs, the cost is about $10. In contrast, to diagnose clinically significant intracranial abnormality costs about $24,000 per abnormal CT scan of the head. Although the physician

**Table 7**
**Approximate cost per clinically meaningful test in the workup of syncope**

| Test | Price |
| --- | --- |
| Postural blood pressure | $10 |
| Telemetry | $700 |
| EKG | $1000 |
| Echocardiogram | $6000 |
| Cardiac stress testing | $8000 |
| Head MRI | $8000 |
| Carotid ultrasound | $19,000 |
| Cardiac enzymes | $22,000 |
| Head CT | $24,000 |
| EEG | $33,000 |

*Data from* Mendu ML, McAvay G, Lampert R, et al. Yield of diagnostic tests in evaluating syncopal episodes in older patients. Arch Intern Med 2009;169(14):1299–1305.

should not necessarily restrict testing based on cost alone, the results here suggest that ordering tests only when they are clinically indicated (based on established guidelines, history, physical examination, or CDRs) may help drive down costs in the ED.[49]

### Observation Units and Cost Control

One potential for cost savings is the concept of the "Syncope Observation Unit." Recently, researchers used a simulation model to predict cost savings if observation units were used to monitor and evaluate syncope patients at intermediate risk. Patients were included if deemed by the emergency physician to require further evaluation. Briefly, most observation units are billed on an outpatient basis, and their patients are generally managed in a protocol-based manner. Using a simulation model, researchers found an estimated 235,000 fewer inpatient admissions would be required, at an estimated cost savings of $108 million annually. Much of this cost was likely related to fewer hours spent in the hospital.[84] The consideration of an observation unit, whether dedicated to syncope or inclusive of other evaluations, may be a prominent step in reducing the cost associated with this common complaint. It is unclear, however, whether this benefit would extend to the elder population, who are more likely to be admitted for evaluation and considered high risk by the emergency physician.

### SOLUTIONS, INNOVATIONS, AND GUIDELINES
### A Structured Approach

Rather than strictly rely on specific clinical decision instruments to determine safe disposition, the physician should use a structured approach to these challenging patients, which includes

- A well-rounded history and physical examination
- Guided diagnostic testing.

Some specific guidelines are reviewed in later discussion. Their goal is to limit the current widespread variation in how clinicians approach the syncope patient.

## EUROPEAN SOCIETY OF CARDIOLOGY GUIDELINES

The ESC guidelines article portrays an extremely organized, logical, and thorough approach to syncope.[11] In analysis of using this approach, investigators found that a definite diagnosis was made in 98% of patients, and 50% of cases could be diagnosed from the initial evaluation alone.[85] This resource is valuable in full detail and lists concerning clinical features, EKG findings, specific testing modalities, and so on. A summary of the ESC recommended approach is listed as follows:

- *Initial Evaluation:* The goal here is to differentiate true syncope from mimics, rule out heart disease, and identify relevant historical features leading to the diagnosis. This goal is accomplished via careful history taking, physical examination, and baseline EKG.
- *Certain or Suspected Diagnosis:* In many cases, no further testing is needed after the initial evaluation, and the workup identifies a "certain diagnosis." More commonly, when the clinician reaches a "suspected diagnosis," he or she can perform directed confirmatory testing.
- *Unexplained Syncope:* In cases where the cause remains undetermined, the clinician should focus on ruling out cardiac causes by provocative stress testing, echocardiography, or arrhythmia detection. If cardiac evaluation is negative, causes of NMS are examined with further testing such as use of the tilt table.
- *Reappraisal:* If still undetermined, the clinician should start from the beginning, retaking the history and physical examination and searching for clues as to additional directed testing.

In a simple 2-step guideline, Croci and colleagues[86] describe the task force on syncope approach to ED syncope evaluation. Step 1, or "the initial evaluation," consists of history, physical examination, orthostatic vital signs, and EKG in patients greater than 45 years old or with a history of heart disease. The clinician may determine from this step alone the cause of syncope, obviating any additional workup. Otherwise, he or she proceeds to Step 2, "laboratory investigations." Here, testing is guided by the initial evaluation in order to investigate potential causes of cardiac, NMS, or neurologic syncope. For example, if the history and physical examination suggested NMS, the patient might be sent for tilt-table testing.

Using this approach, the initial evaluation determined the diagnosis responsible for syncope in 23% of patients. In addition, 21% of patients required only one test to reach this diagnosis; another 21% required at least 2 tests, and 16% required at least 3 tests. Overall, the investigators concluded that following this approach allowed establishment of a diagnosis with a minimal amount of simple testing.

## A RECOMMENDED APPROACH TO EMERGENCY DEPARTMENT ELDER SYNCOPE EVALUATION

Based on a review of the literature, the authors suggest a stepwise approach to the evaluation of older adult patients presenting to the ED with syncope. **Fig. 3** demonstrates a suggested algorithm.

### Structured History

An orderly structured history should be repeated on every syncope patient that documents precise details of the syncopal event. What was the patient doing at the time, and what prodromal symptoms occurred? One should take extra caution in differentiating a reported fall from a syncopal episode in this patient population. Focus on aspects of the event, such as the circumstances leading up to it, eyewitness reports, and

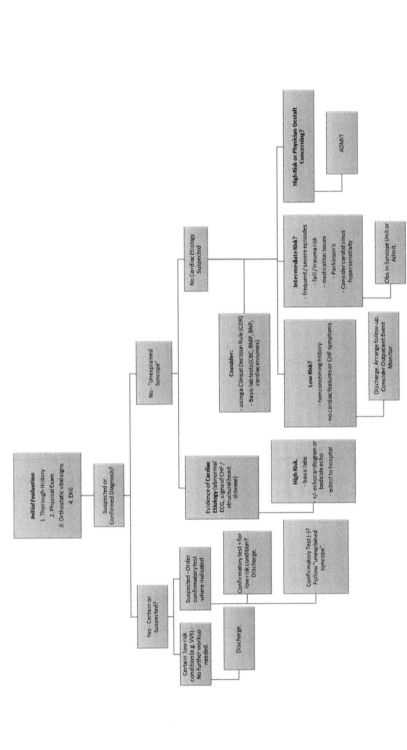

**Fig. 3.** Recommended approach to the older adult patient with syncope. BMP, basic metabolic panel; BNP, brain natriuretic peptide; CBC, complete blood count.

the speed and circumstances of recovery. A careful review of the patient's active medical problems, comorbidities, and medications is essential. The provider should search for clues that would suggest a cardiac cause in order to identify this high-risk population. In general, patients over the age of 65 years old are likely to be higher risk.

### Physical Examination

An important aspect of the examination is measurement of orthostatic vital signs. Orthostatic vital signs are omitted in the initial workup in almost two-thirds of patients, despite this being a rapid, low-cost test. Additional physical examination maneuvers may be guided by the history and the patient's age and be directed to uncover potential injuries sustained from falls.

### Electrocardiogram

Electrocardiogram is also a low-cost, rapidly performed test which, while often low yield, may quickly suggest a cardiac cause of syncope, imposing higher morbidity and mortality and the need for evaluation of structural heart disease.

### Specific Testing or Observation in the Hospital

If the above routine evaluation does not determine a cause of syncope, especially in the elder patient, further workup is needed. The current failures to diagnose syncope should be addressed and any hospital interventions on admitted patients should be performed. In addition, the high posthospitalization morbidities and mortalities must be decreased. ED leaders joined by key clinicians and administrators should develop institution-specific protocols for optimal observation, diagnosis, treatment, and disposition of this population. It is helpful to specify this approach via ED and hospital policies. For example, echocardiography may be indicated to rule out structural heart disease or valve disorder, but this may be unavailable in the ED. The same is true for tilt-table testing, carotid sinus massage, implantable loop recorders or Holter monitors, and other history-guided specific tests. If the institution delineates best practices to obtain such evaluation in a timely and safe fashion, more patients should be diagnosed more quickly with better safety and less cost.

At this point, the physician may decide to use a CDR to provide a framework of high-risk features that if present can guide further testing or the decision to discharge, observe, or admit. CDRs should not be used in isolation of these general guidelines or physician gestalt.

### Disposition

Once establishing either a diagnosis or a risk stratification, the emergency physician should make a careful disposition. Determination of low risk and discharge of patients incurs the further obligations of patient education, identification of suspect medications with plan to adjust or eliminate such drugs, plan to decrease recurrent syncope, and assurance of timely follow-up consistent with patient needs.

### SUMMARY

The older adult patient with syncope is one of the most challenging evaluations for the emergency physician. It requires clinical skill, patience, and knowledge of specific older adult issues. It demands care in the identification of necessary resources such as medication review, and potential linkage with several multidisciplinary follow-up services. Excellent syncope care likely requires reaching out to ensure that institutional resources align with ED patient needs; requiring us to stretch our administrative talents. Emergency physicians evaluate elders with syncope every day and should rise to the challenge to do it well.

## REFERENCES

1. Thijs RD, Wieling W, Kaufmann H, et al. Defining and classifying syncope. Clin Auton Res 2004;14(Suppl 1):4–8.
2. D'Ascenzo F, Biondi-Zoccai G, Reed MJ, et al. Incidence, etiology and predictors of adverse outcomes in 43,315 patients presenting to the emergency department with syncope: an international meta-analysis. Int J Cardiol 2013;167(1):57–62.
3. Getchell WS, Larsen GC, Morris CD, et al. Epidemiology of syncope in hospitalized patients. J Gen Intern Med 1999;14:677–87.
4. Getchell WS, Larsen GC, Morris CD, et al. A comparison of Medicare fee-for-service and a group-model HMO in the inpatient management and long-term survival of elderly individuals with syncope. Am J Manag Care 2000;6(10):1089–98.
5. Savage DD, Corwin L, McGee DL, et al. Epidemiologic features of isolated syncope: the Framingham Study. Stroke 1985;16(4):626–9.
6. Soteriades ES, Evans JC, Larson MG, et al. Incidence and prognosis of syncope. N Engl J Med 2002;347(12):878–85.
7. Quinn J, McDermott D, Kramer N, et al. Death after emergency department visits for syncope: how common and can it be predicted? Ann Emerg Med 2008;51(5):585–90.
8. Kapoor WN. Evaluation and management of the patient with syncope. JAMA 1992;268(18):2553–60.
9. Del Rosso A, Alboni P, Brignole M, et al. Relation of clinical presentation of syncope to the age of patients. Am J Cardiol 2005;96(10):1431–5.
10. McIntosh SJ, da Costa D, Kenny RA. Outcome of an integrated approach to the investigation of dizziness, falls and syncope in elderly patients referred to a syncope clinic. Age Ageing 1993;22:53–8.
11. Moya A, Task Force for the Diagnosis and Management of Syncope, European Society of Cardiology (ESC), et al. Guidelines for the diagnosis and management of syncope (version 2009). Eur Heart J 2009;30:2631–71.
12. Allcock LM, O'Shea D. Diagnostic yield and development of a neurocardiovascular investigation unit for older adults in a district hospital. J Gerontol 2000;55(8):458–62.
13. Wolf PA, Abbott RD, Kannel WB. Atrial fibrillation as an independent risk factor for stroke: the Framingham Study. Stroke 1991;22:983–8.
14. Adkisson WO, Benditt DG. Syncope due to autonomic dysfunction: diagnosis and management. Med Clin North Am 2015;99(4):691–710.
15. Sun BC, Emond JA, Camargo CA Jr. Direct medical costs of syncope-related hospitalizations in the United States. Am J Cardiol 2005;95:668–71.
16. Crane SD. Risk stratification of patients with syncope in an accident and emergency department. Emerg Med J 2002;19:23–7.
17. Blanc JJ, L'Her C, Touiza A, et al. Prospective evaluation and outcome of patients admitted for syncope over a 1 year period. Eur Heart J 2002;23:815–20.
18. Fu Q, Levine BD. Pathophysiology of neurally mediated syncope: role of cardiac output and total peripheral resistance. Auton Neurosci 2014;184:24–6.
19. Van Lieshout JJ, Wieling W, Karemaker JM, et al. Syncope, cerebral perfusion, and oxygenation. J Appl Physiol 2003;94(3):833–48.
20. Zaqqa M, Massumi A. Neurally mediated syncope. Tex Heart Inst J 2000;27(3):268–72.

21. Rockwood MR, Howlett SE, Rockwood K. Orthostatic hypotension (OH) and mortality in relation to age, blood pressure and frailty. Arch Gerontol Geriatr 2010; 54(3):255–60.

22. Fenech G, Safar M, Blacher J. Orthostatic hypotension: marker of severity and management of antihypertensive treatment. Presse Med 2012;41(11):1116–21 [in French].

23. Blanc J-J. Syncope. Card Electrophysiol Clin 2013;5(4):387–91.

24. Jhanjee R, van Dijk JG, Sakaguchi S, et al. Syncope in adults: terminology, classification, and diagnostic strategy. Pacing Clin Electrophysiol 2006;29(10): 1160–9.

25. Saal DP, Gert van Dijk J. Classifying syncope. Auton Neurosci 2014;184:3–9.

26. Kaufmann H. Syncope: a neurologist's viewpoint. Cardiol Clin 1997;15:177–94.

27. Sheldon R. How to differentiate syncope from seizure. Card Electrophysiol Clin 2013;5(4):423–31.

28. Angaran P, Klein GJ, Yee R, et al. Syncope. Neurol Clin 2011;29(4):903–25.

29. Alboni P, Brignole M, Menozzi C, et al. Diagnostic value of history in patients with syncope with or without heart disease. J Am Coll Cardiol 2001;37(7):1921–8.

30. Morag RM, Murdock LF, Khan Z, et al. Do patients with a negative Emergency Department evaluation for syncope require hospital admission? J Emerg Med 2004;27(4):339–43.

31. Grossman S, Fischer C, Lipsitz L, et al. Predicting adverse outcomes in syncope. J Emerg Med 2007;33(3):233–9.

32. Benditt DG, Adkisson WO. Approach to the patient with syncope: venues, presentations, diagnoses. Cardiol Clin 2013;31(1):9–25.

33. Brigo F, Nardone R, Bongiovanni LG. Value of tongue biting in the differential diagnosis between epileptic seizures and syncope. Seizure 2012;21(8):568–72.

34. Kapoor W, Snustad D, Peterson J, et al. Syncope in the elderly. Am J Med 1986; 80(3):419–28.

35. Strickberger SA, Benson W, Biaggioni I, et al. AHA/ACCF scientific statement on the evaluation of syncope: from the American Heart Association Councils on Clinical Cardiology, Cardiovascular Nursing, Cardiovascular Disease in the Young, and Stroke, and the Quality of Care and Outcomes Research Interdisciplinary Working Group; and the American College of Cardiology Foundation: in collaboration with the Heart Rhythm Society: endorsed by the American Autonomic Society. Circulation 2006;113(2):316–27.

36. Thiruganasambandamoorthy V, Hess EP, Turko E, et al. Defining abnormal electrocardiography in adult emergency department syncope patients: the Ottawa Electrocardiographic Criteria. CJEM 2012;14(4):248–58.

37. Anderson KL, Limkakeng A, Damuth E, et al. Cardiac evaluation for structural abnormalities may not be required in patients presenting with syncope and a normal ECG result in an observation unit setting. Ann Emerg Med 2012;60(4): 478–84.e1.

38. Adler A. Brugada syndrome: diagnosis, risk stratification, and management. Curr Opin Cardiol 2016;31(1):37–45.

39. Rutan G, Hermanson B, Bild D, et al. Orthostatic hypotension in older adults. The cardiovascular health study. CHS Collaborative Research Group. Hypertension 1992;19(6 Pt1):508–19.

40. Luukinen H, Koski K, Laippala P, et al. Prognosis of diastolic and systolic orthostatic hypotension in older persons. Arch Intern Med 1999;159:273–80.

41. Shibao C, Lipsitz L, Giaggioni I, On behalf of the American Society of Hypertension Writing Group. Evaluation and treatment of orthostatic hypotension. J Am Soc Hypertens 2013;7(4):317–24.

42. Freeman R, Wieling W, Axelrod FB, et al. Consensus statement on the definition of orthostatic hypotension, neurally mediated syncope and the postural tachycardia syndrome. Auton Neurosci 2011;161(1–2):46–8.

43. Monsuez J-J, Beddok R, Mahiou A, et al. Orthostatic hypotension: epidemiology and mechanisms. Presse Med 2012;41(11):1092–7 [in French].

44. Levitt MA, Lopez B, Lieberman ME, et al. Evaluation of the tilt test in an adult emergency medicine population. Ann Emerg Med 1992;21(6):713–8.

45. Grubb BP, Karabin B. Syncope: evaluation and management in the geriatric patient. Clin Geriatr Med 2012;28(4):717–28.

46. Lanier JB, Mote MB, Clay EC. Evaluation and management of orthostatic hypotension. Am Fam Physician 2011;84(5):527–36.

47. Brignole M, Alboni P, Benditt D, et al. Guidelines on management (diagnosis and treatment) of syncope. Eur Heart J 2001;22(15):1256–306.

48. Reed MJ, Newby DE, Coull AJ, et al. The ROSE (Risk Stratification of Syncope in the Emergency Department) Study. J Am Coll Cardiol 2010;55(8):713–21.

49. Mendu ML, McAvay G, Lampert R, et al. Yield of diagnostic tests in evaluating syncopal episodes in older patients. Arch Intern Med 2009;169(14):1299–305.

50. ACEP - Avoid head CT for asymptomatic adults with syncope | Choosing Wisely (Choosing Wisely). Available at: http://www.choosingwisely.org/clinician-lists/acep-avoid-head-ct-for-asymptomatic-adults-with-syncope/. Accessed January 4, 2016.

51. Probst M, Sun BC. How can we improve management of syncope in the Emergency Department? Cardiol J 2014;21(6):643–50.

52. Kapoor WN, Karpf M, Wieand S, et al. A prospective evaluation and follow-up of patients with syncope. N Engl J Med 1983;309(4):197–204.

53. Preminger M, Mittal S. Value of EP Study and other cardiac investigations. Cardiol Clin 2015;33(3):367–75.

54. Sheldon R. Tilt table testing and implantable loop recorders for syncope. Cardiol Clin 2013;31(1):67–74.

55. Sutton R. The value of tilt testing and autonomic nervous system assessment. Cardiol Clin 2015;33(3):357–60.

56. Moya A. Therapy for syncope. Card Electrophysiol Clin 2013;5(4):519–27.

57. Parry SW, Matthews IG. Update on the role of pacemaker therapy in vasovagal syncope and carotid sinus syndrome. Prog Cardiovasc Dis 2013;55(4):434–42.

58. Sheldon RS, Morillo C, Krahn AD, et al. Society position statement standardized approaches to the investigation of syncope: Canadian Cardiovascular Society position paper. Can J Cardiol 2011;27(2):246–53.

59. Olshansky B, Sullivan RM. Syncope in patients with organic heart disease. Card Electrophysiol Clin 2013;5(4):495–509.

60. Del Rosso A, Ungar A, Maggi R, et al. Clinical predictors of cardiac syncope at initial evaluation in patients referred urgently to a general hospital: the EGSYS score. Heart 2008;94(12):1620–6.

61. Marine JE. EKG Features that suggest a potentially life-threatening arrhythmia as the cause for syncope. J Electrocardiol 2013;46(6):561–8.

62. Olde Nordkamp LR, Vink AS, Wilde AA, et al. Syncope in Brugada syndrome: prevalence, clinical significance, and clues from history taking to distinguish arrhythmic from nonarrhythmic causes. Heart Rhythm 2015;12(2):367–75.

63. Schladenhaufen R, Feilinger S, Pollack M, et al. Application of San Francisco Syncope Rule in elderly ED patients. Am J Emerg Med 2008;26(7):773–8.
64. Colivicchi F, Ammirati F, Melina D, et al, OESIL (Osservatorio Epidemiologico sulla Sincope nel Lazio) Study Investigators. Development and prospective validation of a risk stratification system for patients with syncope in the emergency department: the OESIL risk score. Eur Heart J 2003;24(9):811–9.
65. Grossman SA, Bar J, Fischer C, et al. Reducing admissions utilizing the Boston Syncope Criteria. J Emerg Med 2012;42(3):345–52.
66. Kessler C, Tristano JM, De Lorenzo R. The emergency department approach to syncope: evidence-based guidelines and prediction rules. Emerg Med Clin North Am 2010;28(3):487–500.
67. Serrano LA, Hess EP, Bellolio MF. Accuracy and quality of clinical decision rules for syncope in the emergency department: a systematic review and meta-analysis. Ann Emerg Med 2010;56(4):362–73.e1.
68. Benditt DG. Syncope risk assessment in the emergency department and clinic. Prog Cardiovasc Dis 2013;55(4):376–81.
69. Barón-Esquivias G, Gómez S, Aguilera A, et al. Short-term evolution of vasovagal syncope: influence on the quality of life. Int J Cardiol 2005;102(2):315–9.
70. Barón-Esquivias G, Errázquin F, Pedrote A, et al. Long-term outcome of patients with vasovagal syncope. Am Heart J 2004;147(5):883–9.
71. Ungar A, Del Rosso A, Giada F, et al. Early and late outcome of treated patients referred for syncope to emergency department: the EGSYS 2 follow-up study. Eur Heart J 2010;31:2021–6.
72. Grossman SA, Babineau M, Burke L, et al. Do outcomes of near syncope parallel syncope? Am J Emerg Med 2012;30(1):203–6.
73. Dipaola F, Costantino G, Solbiati M, et al. Syncope risk stratification in the ED. Auton Neurosci 2014;184:17–23.
74. Scharenbrock C, Buggs A, Furgerson J, et al. A prospective evaluation of near syncope and syncope in the elderly. Acad Emerg Med 1999;6(5):532.
75. Grossman SA, Babineau M, Burke L, et al. Applying the Boston syncope criteria to near syncope. J Emerg Med 2012;43(6):958–63.
76. Thiruganasambandamoorthy V, Hess EP, Turko E, et al. Outcomes in Canadian Emergency Department syncope patients—are we doing a good job? J Emerg Med 2013;44(2):321–8.
77. Lund E, Sanders N, Brignole M, et al. Cost analysis of the faint and fall clinic: a new model in health-care delivery. J Innov Card Rhythm Mgmt 2013;1258–63.
78. Akiyama T, Powell JL, Mitchell LB, et al. Resumption of driving after life-threatening ventricular tachyarrhythmia. N Engl J Med 2001;345(6):391–7.
79. Assessment of the cardiac patient for fitness to drive. Can J Cardiol 1992;8(4):406–19 [in French].
80. Barbic F, Casazza G, Zamunér AR, et al. Driving and working with syncope. Auton Neurosci 2014;184:46–52.
81. Sakaguchi S, Li H. Syncope and driving, flying and vocational concerns. Prog Cardiovasc Dis 2013;55(4):454–63.
82. Van Dijk N, Sprangers MA, Colman N, et al. Clinical factors associated with quality of life in patients with transient loss of consciousness. J Cardiovasc Electrophysiol 2006;17:998–1003.
83. Sun BC. Quality-of-life, health service use, and costs associated with syncope. Prog Cardiovasc Dis 2013;55(4):370–5.
84. Baugh CW, Liang LJ, Probst M. National cost savings from observation unit management of syncope. Acad Emerg Med 2015;22(8):934–41.

85. Brignole M, Menozzi C, Bartoletti A, et al. A new management of syncope: pro-spective systematic guideline-based evaluation of patients referred urgently to general hospitals. Eur Heart J 2006;27(1):76–82.
86. Croci F, Brignole M, Alboni P, et al. The application of a standardized strategy of evaluation in patients with syncope referred to three syncope units. Europace 2002;4(4):351–5.

# The Geriatric Emergency Department

Mark Rosenberg, DO, MBA*, Lynne Rosenberg, PhD

## KEYWORDS

- Geriatric emergency department • GED • Emergency services • Geriatric • Senior

## KEY POINTS

- Population aging requires a shift in existing models of emergency care.
- Establishing the goals of a geriatric emergency department (GED) program provides guidance throughout the investigative and decision-making process but also provides the framework for improving emergency care for the elderly.
- A GED is more than just structural enhancements and should include operational enhancements focusing on the needs of the older patient.
- The GED guidelines provide a framework for providing emergency care to older patients.
- Older emergency patients benefit from comprehensive transition of care plans and case management.

## INTRODUCTION

"Change will happen. We can either cope with change or more desirably, we can lead change."[1] Change is the only constant in health care today, especially for emergency departments (EDs) and emergency services worldwide. Since its inception, the practice of emergency medicine has had to adjust to changing government regulations, insurance requirements, billing and reimbursements, technologies, politics, and an aging demographic. EDs continue to evolve and adapt while providing emergency care, urgent care, screenings, diagnostic testing, streamlining admissions, and providing a safety net for the most vulnerable.

All the while, professional and academic communities have been warning of the impact of global aging and longevity, as well as the need to start now to address the changing needs of the population.[2] The aging population has become the most important emerging group in health care for a multitude of reasons,[3] including political gains, financial means, medical resources, and social needs. With increasing longevity, it is in everyone's best interest to operationalize models of health care that address quality and cost-effectiveness, as well as population health measures.

Disclosure Statement: The authors have nothing to disclose.
a Department of Emergency Medicine, St. Joseph's Healthcare System, 703 Main Street, Paterson, NJ 07503, USA
* Corresponding author.
E-mail address: mark@markrosenberg.org

*Aging and Emergency Services*

As the world's population ages and life expectancy increases, hospitals are preparing for older adults to become a more significant part of the emergency care population. In the United States (US), the greatest number of ED visits are among patients 75 years and older compared with other age groups,[4,5] and approximately 17% of independent, older adults have 1 emergency services visit every year.[6] Fortunately, the US has an extensive health care delivery system and defined primary care networks; however, not all countries can provide the same level of health care access. Many patients in developing Asian countries do not have a regular family physician.[7] In some health care systems, emergency services may be the first encounter with the health care community.[7,8] Countries such as Canada, China, Singapore, South Korea, and the US are also developing and implementing geriatric ED (GED) initiatives[4] to support the growing older adult population.

There is a general consensus that health care costs need to be reduced while simultaneously improving outcomes for older adults. This is a challenging situation because older patients, in general, spend more time in the ED, require more time for assessment and diagnosis,[9–11] use more resources in terms of diagnostic studies,[9] are more than twice as likely to be admitted to the hospital,[12] and experience more adverse outcomes during or after their ED visit.[6,9,10,13–18]

The constraints inherent in providing emergency care for older patients may not be surprising considering that the modern ED design still adheres to principles by the Committee on Trauma of the American College of Surgeons set in 1962.[19] Each and every day, the typical ED provides care for patients of all ages. However, the patient flow and the actual physical design of the department have not kept pace with the special needs of an aging population.[9,13,19,20] When an elderly patient with "impaired memory, reduced mobility and impaired social support presents to the ED, the system experiences crisis, slows down, and becomes inefficient."[9]

## CONTEMPLATING A GERIATRIC EMERGENCY DEPARTMENT

Emergency medicine practitioners across the US recognize the need for a paradigm shift to focus on the needs of the older adult emergency patient. However, in an era of health care reform, regardless of shifting provider roles and services in emergency care, the ED needs seamless integration with the entire health care delivery system for maximum effectiveness and improved population health.

When considering a change in the delivery of emergency care, such as a GED, it is essential to gather as much information as possible. This includes speaking with as many stakeholders as possible, including hospital administrators, finance, clinical services, community outreach and, most importantly, older members of the community who will be using these services. Networking opportunities and field trips to hospitals with functioning GEDs provide valuable information and resources to further discussions. Key individuals need to be identified to guide the process and provide overall responsibility. **Box 1** provides potential questions to generate discussion. As the process continues, more questions will need to be investigated and answered to make an informed decision concerning the feasibility of a GED for the individual hospital and community.

### Reasons to Consider a Geriatric Emergency Department

Changes in how the older adult is cared for affect all levels of the health care system. The American College of Emergency Physicians (ACEP) and Society for Academic Emergency Physicians (SAEM) recommend reviewing the traditional ED model in light

> **Box 1**
> **Sample discussion questions when considering a geriatric emergency department**
>
> Does hospital administration recognize the need to improve geriatric emergency services?
>
> Does hospital administration support the design of a physical space within the ED for geriatric patients?
> Develop separate space?
> Redesign existing rooms?
>
> Who are potential champions to attain and sustain identified initiatives?
>
> Do space limitations and budgets require shifts in policy to accommodate the geriatric emergency population?
>
> What is the financial and logistic feasibility of structural modifications?
>
> What are the demographics of the older people living in the community?
>
> What is the current percentage of the community population 65 years of age and older? Are they living independently in the community, residing with family and/or friends, or residing in residential facilities?
>
> What medical resources are available for older people in the surrounding community?
>
> What are the overall goals of this project?
> Increase or decrease admissions?
> Maintain independence of older people in the community?
> Improve outcomes for seniors?
>
> What is the marketing strategy?

of the growing segment of elderly in the US.[19,21] Points to consider when discussing how to improve geriatric emergency services include the influence of contributing factors such as

- Medicare, as the primary insurance for 93% of noninstitutionalized people 65 years and older,[22] pays 25% to 31% less than private insurers[23]; and many physician practices are no longer accepting new Medicare patients. As the general population ages, medical providers are seeing a 50% reduction in family practice residents,[24] a decrease in internal medicine residents choosing primary care,[24] and a deficit of approximately 25,000 gerontologists by 2030,[24] directly impacting the medical management of older patients.
- Coordination of services to effectively manage an older patient's medical needs in a timely and cost-effective manner may not be available in a primary care physician (PCP) office. More PCPs are referring their patients to the ED because the work-up can be completed in 1 visit that includes laboratory tests, radiographs, and consultations, providing a diagnosis, and plan of care.[4] Data from the Agency for Healthcare Research and Quality show that the cost of ED visits, from the ambulance through disposition, account for 3% of health care costs.[25]
- Inpatient care consumes more than 30% of the health care budget. Therefore, to reduce health care costs, inpatient admissions must be reduced.[25] Nearly 50% of all admissions and 60% of admitted patients with Medicare come through the ED.[25] An ED visit is less expensive than a hospital admission[25] and, ultimately, the ED is positioned to play a pivotal role within the health care system by identifying those who require admission versus those who can be managed as an outpatient with appropriate resources.
- Middle-aged children of older patients may see value in a GED and drive to a hospital providing senior-friendly services. Public relations can focus marketing

efforts to attract this patient population that may also use higher reimbursing hospital-based programs such as cardiac, orthopedic, and neurologic services.[26]

## Defining Goals

Establishing the goals of a geriatric emergency program provides guidance throughout the investigative process and decision to build a GED but also provides the framework for improving emergency care for the elderly.[4] Defined goals help to maintain the focus when interacting with architects, consultants, and other vendors.

It is essential to maintain a broad perspective when considering a GED. All options for geriatric emergency care need to be investigated during the initial stages of discussion. Information gathered from site visits, colleagues, and the literature provides additional points of view for consideration.

Additionally, goals should address education, screening, and networking for a geriatric-friendly ED or a GED.[27] Education is the core component of all geriatric emergency care. Screening involves identification of older patients by residence (living independently in the community, in a residential facility, or in a skilled nursing facility), condition (trauma, frailty, dementia), or risk (polypharmacy, neglect), and intervening with a comprehensive evaluation and follow-up plan.[27] Networking identifies all resources, both in-house (case management, pharmacy, consultants) and in the community (visiting nurse services, meals on wheels).[27]

## Identifying Barriers

Barriers to implementing a GED include

- Most emergency physicians and nurses may think they can adequately care for any patient presenting for emergency treatment and question the growing push to change the model of care for older patients.[23] One of the largest hurdles is having staff recognize that geriatric patients present differently than other age groups.[4]
- Stereotypes of confused, dependent, elderly patients from nursing homes contribute to the reluctance of many health care providers to interact with these patients when they present for treatment.[4] Emergency patients are often referred to as a bed number or as a presenting complaint,[4] instead of addressing them by their name, adding to or creating confusion in an older patient.
- The ED environment itself is not conducive to eliciting a comprehensive history and work-up for these patients. Older patients spend more time in the ED, necessitating additional use of valuable personnel as well as preventing the use of an ED bed for an extended period of time.[23] Daily ED overcrowding, patient boarding, and ongoing nursing shortages contribute to the inability to perform screenings for geriatric syndromes[28] and implementation of effective interventions.[29]
- There is a reluctance to change an ED system of care that has existed for generations. As the care for geriatric patients continues to evolve and with the ongoing development of the Affordable Care Act, the GED possibly becomes more financially relevant. The potential benefits for patients and providers, as well as how the ED is being used by patients and providers, can be debated.

In spite of the barriers, ED use is increasing because it provides the following services:

- ○ Streamlining nonelective admissions through the ED[25]
- ○ Referral of complex patients for workup, diagnosis, and plan of care[25]

- o Coordination of resources for outpatient management of select patients[25]
- o Greater integration of the ED with PCPs and the surrounding community.[25]

## FINANCIAL ASPECTS

It is important to discuss the financial implications of providing geriatric emergency services, particularly in the current environment of health care reform. A few words regarding Medicare are needed because most elderly patients have Medicare as their primary insurance.

### Medicare

The current Medicare reimbursement structure does not recognize common problems, such as weakness, yet the admission rate for elderly patients presenting with weakness or other nonspecific complaints is 80% to 90%.[30] In the past, disposition was based on the clinical decision of the ED physician, regardless of the patient's billing status.[31] Now there are clinical decision support criteria for Medicare to determine the medical necessity of services, as well as appropriateness, for inpatient admissions.[31]

Medicare has fiscal intermediaries and area contractors that are hired to review each admission. This Center for Medicare or Medicaid Services (CMS) Recovery Audit may result in the loss of revenue for an entire hospital stay, along with substantial hospital penalties if the audit determines there was inappropriate level of care.[31] One of the areas of closest scrutiny is that of 1-day and 2-day hospital stays.[31]

As a result, hospitals need to prospectively screen eligible beneficiaries in the ED to determine appropriate level of care or service. The level of service, and where that service is delivered, involves a complex decision-making process. There are multiple options for transition of care from the ED, including inpatient, admit-to-home, placement in observation care, send home with home care, and so forth.

The Medicare rules and guidelines, McKesson's InterQual criteria[32] and Milliman[33] care guidelines are a complex system. Using a case manager in the GED as part of the transition of care process can decrease Medicare denials and improve resource utilization.

### Triple Aim

Although Medicare billing has become a complicated business, it is basically in synch with the goals of health care reform known as the Triple Aim. The goals of the Triple Aim are "improving the individual experience of care; improving the health of populations; and reducing the per capita costs of care for populations."[34] These goals are accomplished through incentives and penalties such as core measures, readmissions, or improving patient satisfaction. As hospital reimbursement moves into risk and bundled payment strategies, the GED will become more relevant financially because, by design, it meets the Triple Aim. **Box 2** provides examples of how a GED can meet the goals of the Triple Aim.

### Cost

The physical environment for a GED is only a small part of a geriatric program. The cost of building or renovating an ED varies according to each hospital's resources and needs. Improving the physical structure of an ED can range from a few hundred dollars to a capital improvement campaign. In most cases, major renovations are not needed.

---

**Box 2**
**The geriatric emergency department meets the triple aim of health care reform**

*Better health care*

- Patient experience of care
- Quality and core measures
- Patient safety
- Effectiveness
- Timeliness
- Efficiency

*Better population health*

- Geriatric screenings
  - Delirium
  - Dementia
  - Depression
  - Falls assessment
  - Functional decline risk
- Preventative care
  - Fall prevention
  - Vaccinations
- Nutritional assessments
- Increase physical activity

*Lower cost to beneficiaries*

- Decrease admissions
- Decrease iatrogenic complications

---

Staffing enhancements may be an additional cost, depending on existing hospital personnel. A GED will need a physician and nurse champion. Other potential staff include case managers, social workers, patient liaisons, and a pharmacist. Because many of these positions exist in the hospital, it may be beneficial to review existing personnel resources, their allocation, and how staff can be more responsive to the needs of a GED before allocating additional positions.

### Revenue

Reimbursement rates are the same for patients in a GED as a general ED. However, anecdotal evidence suggests reduced critical care admissions, reduced readmissions, and improved outcomes may provide additional sources of revenue.[26]

There is a growing trend towards increasing admissions through the ED and decreasing admissions from primary care and other settings.[35] This is mainly as a result of changing practice patterns evidenced by PCPs relying on EDs for complex work-ups, coverage after hours or weekends, and as a backup for overflow patients.[35] This change has resulted in the ED making decisions for nearly 50% of admissions.[35] The hospital and the patients benefit from a cost-effective streamlined process in the ED, leading to fewer hospital admissions, reduced length of stay, and less cost overall.[34] The unmeasured benefit to everyone is time saved in assessing and diagnosing the patient. The treatment plan that can take days or weeks as an outpatient can be done in a matter of hours through the ED.[4]

*Savings*

A GED creates opportunities for cost-savings through streamlined assessment, diagnosis, and care planning. Combining innovative admit-to-home or extended-home-observation programs with an observation program can save significant health care dollars. See later discussion of these programs.

## THE GERIATRIC GUIDELINES

The GED guidelines (http://www.acep.org/geriEDguidelines/) are the consensus-based collaborative work of the ACEP, American Geriatrics Society, Emergency Nurses Association (ENA), and SAEM, and have been approved by the board of directors from these organizations (http://www.saem.org/news-landing/2014/02/11/geriatric-emergency-department-guidelines-now-available-online). The recommendations, developed over 2 years, represent the first formal, joint organization and society approach to evidence-based guidelines for the care of older adults presenting for emergency care.[26,36,37]

The purpose of the guidelines is to provide a standardized set of guidelines that can effectively improve the care of the geriatric population and that is feasible to implement in the ED (http://www.acep.org/geriEDguidelines/; http://www.saem.org/news-landing/2014/02/11/geriatric-emergency-department-guidelines-now-available-online).

The guidelines, presented in 6 categories (**Table 1**), provide an opportunity to improve patient care, customer service, and staff education[26] (http://geriatricscareonline.org/ProductAbstract/geriatric-emergency-department-guidelines/CL013).

It needs to be remembered that currently the GED guidelines are not a mandate or a requirement for a GED. They are recommendations. Operationalizing the guidelines, in whole or in part, is the decision of each hospital community providing emergency services.

There are basically 2 approaches recommended to improve geriatric patient outcomes in the ED. One approach is to educate all staff from prehospital through disposition about geriatric patient care. This includes new policies, procedures, or protocols delineating care processes for emergency services.

The second approach incorporates all of the training for geriatric services but also includes infrastructure changes and ED redesign. It becomes each individual hospital's choice based on its specific demographics and budget. Ultimately, a GED is about the program design to support the elderly patient presenting for emergency treatment, not about new infrastructure.

Currently, there is not a database or registry to identify and forecast the growth of GEDs. Geriatric services may range from marketing strategies to senior-friendly EDs to full-service GEDs. In 2014, it was reported that there were 24 to 50 functioning GEDs with another 150 in development.[21,25]

## THE GERIATRIC EMERGENCY DEPARTMENT

It takes time and commitment to investigate geriatric emergency services and models of care. Each hospital and community needs to decide if its patient population can benefit from geriatric emergency services and in what capacity. Is a brand new GED feasible or is it more cost-effective to use existing infrastructure?

If the process leads to a decision to move forward with a GED, stakeholders will quickly discern that there is not a textbook approach to follow. This is because

**Table 1**
**Geriatric emergency department guidelines**

| General Category | Recommendation | Specific Examples |
|---|---|---|
| Staffing | ED availability of geriatric-trained physician and nursing leadership, including GED medical director who completes $\geq$8 h of geriatric CME every 2 years | GED medical director serves as liaison with hospital staff and outpatient-care partners, identifies needs and resources for staff geriatric education, and reviews and approves all hospital geriatric policies and procedures |
| Transitions of care | Transition-of-care protocols will facilitate timely communication of clinically relevant information appropriate for the level of geriatric syndrome (dementia, acute illness severity, frailty, sensory impairment) associated disability of the individual patient | Discharge instructions, available in large font, that provide HIPAA-compliant information to family or care provider, long-term care facilities, and surrogate decision makers |
| Transitions of care | Establish and maintain relationships with key community resources to access as needed in transition from ED to outpatient care | Medical home, case managers, home safety assessment by occupational therapy or home care nursing, medical transportation services, meal assistance programs, and prescription assistance |
| Education | Continuing medical education programs will increase physician and nursing staff awareness of unique geriatric emergency care needs, policies, and procedures | Multidisciplinary nature of effective geriatric heath recovery and maintenance, evidence-based geriatric syndrome screening instruments and interventions, atypical disease presentations balanced against overutilization of resources and goals of care, and palliative-medicine opportunities |
| Quality improvement | Geriatric quality improvement program will be developed and monitored by the GED medical director and nurse manager | Semiannual reviews targeting geriatric syndrome, prevalence of injurious falls, screening rates, and sequelae, as well as patient-centric outcomes, delirium screening and management, catheter-associated urinary tract infection prevention efforts, and inappropriate high-risk medication prescribing |
| Equipment and supplies | Physical infrastructure shall accommodate patients with mobility, continence, sensory, or cognitive impairment | Reclining chairs rather than gurneys to enhance comfort and minimize pressure ulcers, walking-assist devices and hearing aids at the bedside, patient-controlled lighting, and enhanced signage |
| Policies, procedures, and protocols | Department policies for prevalent geriatric syndromes should be developed by and readily available for staff | Delirium screening protocol, elder-abuse assessment strategy, urinary catheter placement criteria, transition-of-care priorities, and palliative-care triggers |

*From* Carpenter CR, Hwang U, Rosenberg M. New guidelines enhance care standards for elderly patients in the ED. ACEP NOW 2014;33(3):14–6, 28.

each GED reflects the hospital community's needs, including infrastructure resources, personnel, financial capabilities, patient volume, demographic mix, and the overall commitment of leaders to see the process through. Stakeholder expectations need to be managed. Quality programs need to mature to yield useful data to improve outcomes and all staff require ongoing education and feedback.

The goal of a GED is to improve emergency care for older patients in an efficient, safe, model of care[4] that is most conducive to positive outcomes.[26] Furthermore, a comprehensive GED program sets the plan of care for elderly patients by identifying those patients requiring admission and coordinating resources for those who can be safely managed as an outpatient (http://www.acep.org/geriEDguidelines/). The GED, similar to the ED for the general population, plays a central role in the continuum of care for older patients (**Fig. 1**).

## Infrastructure

It is not always feasible to use resources to provide bigger and better infrastructure for emergency services. Whether considering a new ED, renovating existing space, or replacing equipment and supplies, it is worth mentioning the concept of Universal Design. This concept as defined by Connell and colleagues[38] (including Ronald Mace) is "an approach to design that incorporates products as well as building features which, to the greatest extent possible, can be used by everyone."

Health care architects integrate Universal Design concepts as a rule in providing solutions that work for a larger number of people. Most Universal Design elements in a new ED are code requirements for hospitals, or just slightly more than what the code requires (Matthew Leonard, B Arch, personal communication, October 10, 2011). For example, the exterior entrance doors into the waiting area are automatically activated from both sides. This has been standard practice for EDs for quite some time, so it is not a new or uncommon concept.

There is growing recognition that the physical environment has a significant impact on elderly patients in terms of mobility, cognition, and independence.[39] Therefore, in considering specific modifications for geriatric emergency services, it is beneficial to invite patients who are representative of those who will be using these services to participate in the design process.

If given a choice, the GED should be located in a quieter area away from trauma alerts and high-volume traffic. Assessment areas should be located with attention to privacy concerns of the elderly during examinations and toileting.[3,5] Noise pollution can be reduced further with sound-absorbent flooring and/or ceiling tiles, decreased overhead announcements, and limited use of rolling equipment.

Geriatric emergency patient rooms should include the use of a variety of lighting solutions to accommodate not only bedside procedures performed but also the type of patients, whether for light-sensitivity or difficulty seeing in low-light conditions.[26] Physical discomfort is a general complaint among elderly patients, mainly due to lying on narrow stretchers, being unable to change positions, ambulate, toilet when needed, or feeling cold.[5,40] Purchasing thicker mattresses for new ED stretchers or gradually replacing stretcher mattresses benefits patients of all ages. Another option are wider stretchers or the use of hospital beds that allow patients to reposition themselves as needed.[40] Warm blankets and pillows provide additional comfort.

Orientation to physical surroundings, including the use of the call light, bathroom location or commode, and visual contact with ED staff, decreases anxiety and promotes positive patient satisfaction. Large-faced clocks, reading glasses, and hearing aids are assistive devices that help the patient orient in unfamiliar surroundings. Other

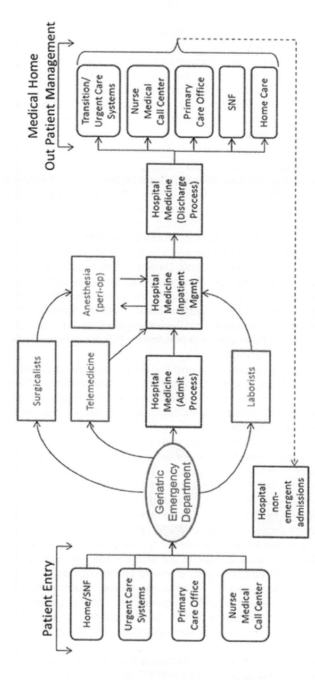

**Fig. 1.** GED continuum of care. Mgmt, management; Peri-op, perioperative; SNF, skilled nursing facility. (*Courtesy of* TeamHealth's Patient Care Continuum Model; with permission.)

areas worthy of consideration include patient waiting areas that allow eye contact with staff, large clear lettering on signs, strategic placement of handrails throughout, and clearly written discharge instructions.[3]

## Geriatric Care Issues

GEDs use specific interventions to improve patient satisfaction, comfort, and outcomes.[23] All care issues, including evaluating patient flow and supportive services, are magnified in a GED. Elderly patients cannot sit on hard chairs or lie on stretchers for hours.[40] Long wait times generate feelings of nervousness and confusion, intensified by feelings of abandonment and anxiousness when there is a lack of staff interaction during prolonged periods.[5] Many elderly are accompanied by and rely on their caregivers; therefore, the caregiver should have the ability to stay with the older patient if at all possible.[5]

Overall, communication is of great importance to the older emergency patient. Once they enter the system, elderly patients need to be updated during their emergency visit. If they speak a foreign language, it is preferred to use an interpreter rather than a family member or caregiver, to assure accurate translation of questions and responses, as well as the ability to freely discuss potentially sensitive issues.

Attention to small details may seem minor to busy ED staff, but to the elderly patient it can result in an overwhelmingly positive experience or a negative and frightening ED visit. Call light accessibility, frequency of offerings of meals or snacks, noise levels, lighting, and toilet availability are all sources of patient satisfaction or dissatisfaction.

## Staffing

In operationalizing a GED, it is essential to identify the available resources within the hospital itself. Staff resources within the ED and extending to the hospital system need to be evaluated and considered for their role in the GED. Most hospitals have social workers and case managers with access to physical therapy, occupational therapy, mental health staff, translation services, speech difficulties, spiritual care, and palliative care for consultations. Toxicologists may be available, if not within the hospital, then at the local poison control center. Some hospitals may have telemedicine capabilities available to access other resources or consultants. For a geriatric care process to be successful there must be a working relationship with these departments to provide services to the GED.

Currently, the professional organizations of ACEP, ENA, and SAEM do not require specific staffing models for a GED. There is, however, consensus that a multidisciplinary team should consist of a GED medical director, nurse manager, staff physicians, and nurses, complemented by medical staff specialists through consultation or transfer agreements (http://www.acep.org/geriEDguidelines/).

A geriatric case manager plays a vital role in navigating insurance requirements and documentation. As mentioned previously, Medicare reviews each admission retroactively. Case managers work in real time with the GED, helping to prevent costly insurance denials and decreased rates of admission.[41] Case managers, together with social services, work to improve discharge planning, decrease return visits, and increase referrals to community resources.[41]

A geriatric care coordinator, usually a registered nurse or social worker, oversees the care of the elderly ED patient. This position safeguards the transition of care for those patients being discharged into the community and maintains contact with the patient, "decreasing the potential for loss of follow-up care" (https://www.ena.org/practice-research/Practice/Documents/OlderAdultTopicBrief.pdf).

## Staff Education

Education and training of each and every staff member coming into contact with the geriatric patient is the cornerstone of any geriatric emergency or senior-friendly program. Education focuses on required changes in department culture, attitude, and everyday practices of staff in providing care for the elderly emergency patient.[5]

Resources include

- The Geriatric Emergency Department Guidelines education recommendations (http://www.acep.org/geriEDguidelines)
- ACEP's Academic Affairs Committee, in collaboration with SAEM's Academy of Geriatric Emergency Medicine, created 10 videos focusing on the unique circumstances of geriatric care in the ED (http://www.acep.org/Clinical—Practice-Management/Geriatric-Videos/)
- American Geriatrics Society Clinical Practice Guideline for Postoperative Delirium in Older Adults (http://geriatricscareonline.org/ProductAbstract/american-geriatrics-society-clinical-practice-guideline-for-postoperative-delirium-in-older-adults/CL018)
- The Geriatrics for Specialty Residents Toolkit: Emergency Medicine (http://geriatricscareonline.org/toc/the-geriatrics-for-specialty-residents-toolkit-emergency-medicine/TK008)
- ENA comprehensive geriatric online course consisting of 17 modules https://www.ena.org/education/education/GENE/Documents/Modules.pdf
- Geriatric education for emergency medical services (http://geriatricscareonline.org/ProductAbstract/geriatric_education_for_emergency_medical_services/B017)
- Beers criteria (http://www.americangeriatrics.org/health_care_professionals/clinical_practice/clinical_guidelines_recommendations/2012).

## Assessments

There are hundreds of assessment tools available for use from ED point of entry through discharge. This includes specific assessments for falls, delirium, mental status, depression, mobility, and so forth. There is not an endorsement for any specific instrument that allows each ED the ability to choose screening tools for their elderly population. The following 3 instruments are examples of assessment tools widely used with older patients.

The Emergency Severity Index (ESI) is the only 5-level triage instrument validated for people 65 years of age and older.[9,11] Frail elderly patients presenting without specific complaints are at risk of inappropriate or delayed evaluation due to undertriage. These patients have atypical presentations compared with younger patients.[42] Therefore, staff may underestimate the severity and acuity of their presenting complaint.[43] The ESI tool may improve care at the beginning of the ED visit by providing an accurate snapshot of the patient's acuity based on a decisional algorithm (www.ahrq.gov/research/esi).

The Identification of Seniors at Risk (ISAR) tool is a 6-item self-report screening tool to be completed by the patient, family, or caregiver.[26] It was developed for the ED population 65 years and older.[24] The 6 yes or no questions address self-care, hospitalizations, vision, memory, and medications. This screening tool demonstrates clinical relevance and validity,[24] and may be completed on the initial emergency visit regardless of presenting complaint.[24] In a systematic review of 10 studies, Yao and colleagues[44] (2015) reported poor validity in terms of ED revisits and hospital readmissions, as well as poor to fair predictive validity related to mortality and outcomes.

Many EDs use this tool as the first step in their transition of care (see later discussion) to identify those older patients who may be at risk of functional decline, need community services at home, or admission to long-term care or other facility.[45]

Comprehensive geriatric assessment (CGA), along with a multidisciplinary care plan, can lead to improved function and better health outcomes for elderly patients who are discharged from the ED.[46] CGAs prevent hospitalization by identifying appropriate resources when planning the transition of care[47,48] and addressing problems before they deteriorate to the stage at which admission is unavoidable.[48]

## TRANSITION OF CARE

The transition of care is perhaps the most critical phase in the care of elderly ED patients. There is an increased risk of adverse events each time an elderly patient transitions from a provider or setting to another.[14,48]

For those patients who are discharged from the ED, there is increased risk of functional decline, increased use of health services,[9] reduced health-related quality of life,[14] and death.[14] The greatest benefit to older patients is provided by early integration of home care services,[43,49] coordinating transition of care with family members and caregivers,[5] and considering consultative services such as palliative care.[5]

### Two-Step Assessment Program

A 2-step assessment program is a process to identify those older ED patients who have potential problems and may experience poor outcomes after discharge.[49] The program operates 24 hours per day, 7 days a week. There are many versions of a 2-step assessment program but the first step occurs during the ED visit and establishes the transition of care.[4] The initial evaluation may be done with the ISAR tool to identify those older patients who are at risk and require further evaluation and support at discharge.[49]

The second step occurs within 24 hours after discharge from the ED and is the most important step in the transition of care. During step 2, a member of the geriatric team calls the patient within 24 hours of discharge from the ED to determine whether the patient was able to comply with the discharge instructions. If the patient or their family is having difficulty with any of the instructions, other resources are made available. If the patient cannot follow-up with their primary physician, she or he is given a convenient time to return to the GED for re-evaluation. Continued contact is maintained with the patient until the patient has all of the resources needed to maintain functional status at home. Overall, the 2-step program results in greater utilization of home care services, increased communication and referrals to the PCP,[9,29,50] and significantly reduced functional decline.[9,29]

### Admitted or Transfer Patients

A transition plan of care is made for each GED patient who requires admission to the hospital. This plan is communicated to the patient's admitting physician and nursing staff on the clinical unit.

Patients who are boarded in the ED waiting for inpatient beds or those awaiting transfer to another institution are at increased risk because there are no clear delineations among staff concerning primary responsibility.[48] Patient tracking boards or dashboard systems may reduce the risk of transitional errors for these particular patients.[48] Additional factors, such as ED volume, time of day, and access to electronic records, may be normal in the course of a typical ED shift but pose additional risk for boarded and transfer patients.[48]

Of special note are those patients transferred to the ED from nursing homes. Lack of consistent communication from the nursing home to the ED and, conversely, from the ED to the nursing home are major obstacles in providing seamless care to the most vulnerable of the elderly population.[51,52] Factors contributing to communication difficulties include the cognitive status of the nursing home patient, lack of standard indicators for when to transfer to an ED, and minimum data requirements for transfer to and from an ED.[52] This allows individual nursing home facilities and EDs to operate without oversight for transfers to and from each institution.

Ultimately, the lack of standardization in communication regarding nursing home patients compromises patient care, contributes to medical errors, delays in emergency care, family distress, unnecessary treatments, and increases in morbidity and mortality.[53] The use of standardized transfer forms demonstrates improved documentation between facilities and the use of the electronic medical record holds promise as an effective communication tool but is not widely available.[53] In the interim, individual EDs can and should work with referring nursing homes to improve the transition of care for this vulnerable group of patients.

### Observation

Observation may be a status or unit located in the ED or on a clinical floor in the hospital. In the regulatory definition, observation is a billing status of a patient whether in the ED or on the floor of the hospital.[31] Observation allows time for testing, imaging, and other interventions while avoiding known risks associated with hospitalization.[9] This extended clinical period allows time to perform additional assessments, including a CGA, physical therapy assessment, and other assessments specific to the individual patient's medical, functional, and social situation.[31]

In 2008, ACEP supported ED-based observation units, which resulted in the availability of observation status in many EDs.[31] The use of observation units or beds has demonstrated decreased ED revisits and hospitalization rates.[31] However, ED physicians need to be familiar with the criteria for observation established by Medicare. According to 2016 CMS,[54] observation may be 48 hours or fewer than 2 midnights. Observation status is a level of care determination and billing status that is part of outpatient management. Patients admitted for observation must meet the established criteria and complex regulations for observation status. Although stated previously, case managers are an asset in navigating this challenging process.

### Home Services

Hospital-at-home services are an option to consider for older patients who would normally require acute care hospitalization.[55] Once older people are hospitalized, it is very difficult to arrange an early discharge.[46] Identifying those patients who can be safely managed outside of acute care becomes vital in supporting a healthy, elderly community population. The obvious advantages of caring for this population in their own homes include a significant reduction in mortality,[46,55] reduced functional decline,[46] reduced cost,[55] improved patient satisfaction,[55] seamless continuity of care,[4] and allowing the patient to be in the comfort of their own surroundings.[4]

Admit-to-home is for patients who would benefit from continued observation; however, patients with Medicare experience higher copays for outpatient services.[31] Therefore, programs such as admit-to-home offer a viable alternative. The patient receives written instructions to continue therapy at home and an appointment is made to return to the GED at a time convenient for the patient and their family. At return, a member of the geriatric team brings the patient directly to a bed, bypassing triage and registration. A re-examination is performed with repeat diagnostic studies, as the patient's condition warrants, and the transition of care is continued.

## QUALITY IMPROVEMENT

A quality improvement (QI) program for the GED may be a subcommittee of the existing ED quality committee or report as a separate entity to the hospital quality committee. Regardless of the reporting structure, the program should monitor clinical outcomes associated with the metrics identified for inclusion in the QI program.[4,26] As with any QI program, it is important that the program reflects the needs of the community's GED population in terms of metrics, committee composition or representation, and frequency of meetings (**Fig. 2**).

The patient experience of care deserves special attention within the GED setting. All patients expect quality care but quality metrics typically measure patient perception of care rather than outcomes and medical care. The Consumer Assessment of Healthcare Providers and Systems (CAHPS) surveys are designed specifically to measure the patient experience across diverse health care settings and are an integral part of CMS efforts to improve care (https://www.cms.gov/Research-Statistics-Data-and-Systems/Research/CAHPS/index.html).

The GED provides an opportunity to improve the patient experience because the CMS reimbursement strategies, known as value-based purchasing (VBP), use CAHPS surveys.[56] VBP withholds a portion of every hospital's Medicare payment for use as incentive payments. Under the VBP program, a hospital's performance determines Medicare reimbursement (http://www.cms.gov/Outreach-and-Education/Medicare-Learning-Network-MLN/MLNProducts/Downloads/Hospital_VBPurchasing_Fact_Sheet_ICN907664.pdf).

The patient experience of care domain currently includes

- Staff communication, including medical staff
- Staff responsiveness
- Pain management
- Patient hospital cleanliness and quietness
- Discharge information
- Overall hospital rating.

*Courtesy of* Jason Greenspan MD, FACEP, James De La Torre MD; Emergent Medical Associates; with permission.

## THE ELECTRONIC HEALTH RECORD

Broad application of information technology offers the possibility of a streamlined flow of information for the GED from the prehospital setting through discharge into the community. The key is to use the technology as an active delivery tool rather than as a database.[19]

The electronic health record (EHR) remains a relatively new system and, as the health care system matures, it is hoped that standards will be developed for the EHR. Specifically, for patient safety and quality care, it would be beneficial if every institution used the same EHR format. In that way, every ED or every PCP or every nursing home would know exactly where to look for essential information and every provider would have access to that information.[36] The numerous benefits of the EHR for the GED include[14]

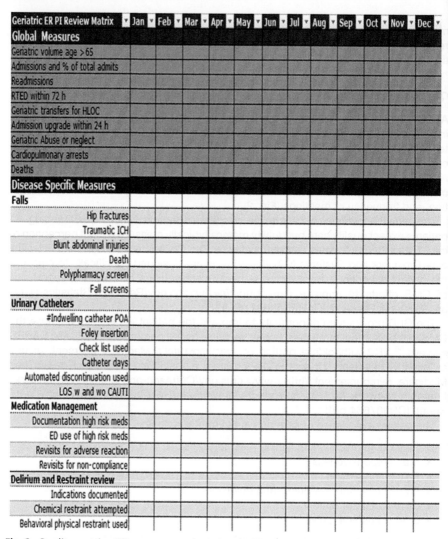

**Fig. 2.** Quality metrics. ED, emergency department; ER, emergency room; h, hour; ICH, intracranial hemorrhage; LOS, length of stay; PI, performance improvement; POA, present on admission; RTED, return; W, with; Wo, without. (*Courtesy of* Jason Greenspan MD, FACEP, James De La Torre MD; Emergent Medical Associates; with permission.)

- Reducing inappropriate medications and prescription errors
- Providing data for the QI program
- Capturing vital information from PCPs and transfer facilities
- Enhancing emergency care through preregistration and retrieval of relevant medical histories
- Improving the transition of care
- Improving communication networks.

## CONCLUDING REMARKS

For any geriatric emergency model to be successful, the support of the stakeholders is essential. This includes hospital administrators, medical staff, ED doctors and nurses, management, and other hospital community members with a vital interest in the success of the program. Education for all stakeholders and staff is essential.

To operationalize the new geriatric program there must be buy-in with the paradigm shift away from the old method of providing emergency care to a comprehensive model that is fluid. Every aspect of the ED process shifts to a geriatric-centric program. This makes the geriatric patient the ED's top priority: from intake and ED bed assignment to time seen by the provider, from inpatient bed admission to comprehensive discharge planning and transition of care, the older patient becomes the priority.

Many health care providers who visit a GED agree that they would prefer their parent, grandparent, or spouse be treated in a comprehensive ED that is designed to meet the needs of the geriatric population. Most enhancements are operational redesign and minor renovations that have minimal additional cost. These improvements, combined with continued education for every staff member, will ultimately produce a successful GED program.

## REFERENCES

1. Saba J, Bardwell P. Universal design concepts for the emergency department. J Ambul Care Manage 2004;27:224–36.
2. Lowenstein S, Crescenzi C, Kern K, et al. Care of the elderly in the emergency department. Ann Emerg Med 1986;15:528–34.
3. Banerjee J, Conroy S, Cooke M. Quality care for older people with urgent and emergency care needs in UK emergency departments. Emerg Med J 2013;30:699–700.
4. Rosenberg M, Rosenberg L. The geriatric emergency department. In: Kahn J, Magauran J Jr, Olshaker JS, editors. Geriatric emergency medicine principles and practice. Cambridge (United Kingdom): Cambridge University Press; 2014. p. 8–19.
5. Shankar KN, Bhatia BK, Schuur JD. Toward patient-centered care: a systematic review of older adults' views of quality emergency care. Ann Emerg Med 2014;63:529–50.
6. Hastings N, Whitson H, Sloane R, et al. Using the past to predict the future: latent class analysis of patterns of health service use of older adults in the emergency department. J Am Geriatr Soc 2014;62:711–5.
7. Foo CL, Siu VW, Tan TL, et al. Geriatric assessment and intervention in an emergency department observation unit reduced re-attendance and hospitalization rates. Australas J Ageing 2012;31:40–6.
8. Khan SA, Miskelly FG, Platt JS, et al. Missed diagnoses among elderly patients discharged from an accident and emergency department. Emerg Med 1996;13:256–7.
9. Salvi F, Morichi V, Grilli A, et al. The elderly in the emergency department: a critical review of problems and solutions. Intern Emerg Med 2007;2:292–301.
10. Aminzadeh F, Dalziel WB. Older adults in the emergency department: a systematic review of pattern of use, adverse outcomes, and effectiveness of interventions. Ann Emerg Med 2002;39:238–47.
11. Gilboy N, Tanabe P, Travers DA, et al. Emergency Severity Index, version 4: implementation handbook. Agency for Healthcare Research and Quality. Rockville (MD): AHRQ; 2005. Publication No. 05-0046-2.
12. Sinha S, Bessman E, Flomenbaum N, et al. A systematic review and qualitative analysis to inform the development of a new emergency department-based geriatric case management model. Ann Emerg Med 2011;57:672–82.

13. Salvi F, Morichi V, Grilli A, et al. A geriatric emergency service for acutely ill elderly patients: Pattern of use and comparison with a conventional emergency department in Italy. J Am Geriatr Soc 2008;56:2131–8.

14. Schoenenberger A, Exadaktylos A. Can geriatric approaches support the care of old patients in emergency departments? A review from a Swiss ED. Swiss Medical Weekly 2014.

15. Friedmann PD, Jin L, Karrison TG. Early revisit, hospitalization, or death among older persons discharged from the ED. Am J Emerg Med 2001;19:125–9.

16. McCusker J, Cardin S, Bellavance F. Return to the emergency department among elders: patterns and predictors. Acad Emerg Med 2000;7:249–59.

17. McCusker J, Bellavance F, Cardin S. Prediction of hospital utilization among elderly patients during the 6 months after an emergency department visit. Ann Emerg Med 2000;36:438–45.

18. Sanders AB. Older persons in the emergency medical care system. J Am Geriatr Soc 2001;49:1390–2.

19. Adams J, Gerson L. A new model for emergency care of geriatric patients. Acad Emerg Med 2003;10:271–4.

20. Hwang U, Morrison S. The geriatric emergency department. J Am Geriatr Soc 2007;55:1873–6.

21. Hogan T, Olade T, Carpenter C. A profile of acute care in an aging America: snowball sample identification and characterization of United States Geriatric Emergency Departments in 2013. Acad Emerg Med 2014;21:337–46.

22. Profile of Older Americans: 2013. Administration on Aging (AOA). U.S. Department of Health and Human Services. Available at: http://www.aoa.gov/Aging_Statistics/Profile/2013/docs/2013_Profile.pdf. Accessed November 16, 2015.

23. Fitzgerald R. The future of geriatric care in our nation's emergency departments: impacts and implications. Irving (TX): American College of Emergency Physicians; 2008. Available at: http://www.acep.org/workarea/DownloadAsset.aspx?id=43376. Accessed November 16, 2015.

24. Samaras N, Chevalley T, Samaras D, et al. Older patients in the emergency department: A review. Ann Emerg Med 2010;56:261–7.

25. ECRI. Available at: https://www.ecri.org/events/Pages/Annual-Conference-2014.aspx. Accessed December 1, 2015.

26. American College of Emergency Physicians, American Geriatrics Society, Emergency Nurses Association, Society for Academic Emergency Medicine and Geriatric Emergency Department Guidelines Task Force. Geriatric emergency department guidelines. Ann Emerg Med 2014;63:e7–25.

27. Walsh K, Stiles M. New age: why the world needs geriatric emergency medicine. Emerg Phys Inter 2013;11:23–5. Available at: http://www.epijournal.com/articles/100/new-age-why-the-world-needs-geriatric-emergency-medicine. Accessed May 10, 2016.

28. Carpenter C, Platts-Mills T. Evolving prehospital, emergency department, and "inpatient" management models for geriatric emergencies. Clin Geriatr Med 2013;29:31–47.

29. McCusker J, Verdon J, Tousignant P, et al. Rapid emergency department intervention for older people reduces risk of functional decline: results of a multicenter randomized trial. J Am Geriatr Soc 2001;49:1272–81.

30. Anderson R, Hallen S. Generalized weakness in the geriatric emergency department patient. Clin Geriatr Med 2013;29:91–100.

31. Moseley M, Hawley M, Caterino J. Emergency department observation units and the older patient. Clin Geriatr Med 2013;29:71–89.

32. Interqual Criteria. Available at: http://www.mckesson.com/payers/decision-management/decision-management-interqual/interqual-criteria/. Accessed November 3, 2015.
33. Health Cost Guidelines. Available at: http://us.milliman.com/Solutions/Products/Health-Cost-Guidelines-Suite/. Accessed December 1, 2015.
34. Berwick D, Nolan T, Whittington J. The triple aim: Care, health, and cost. Health Aff 2008;27:759–69.
35. Morganti K, Bauhoff S, Blanchard J, et al. The evolving role of emergency department's in the United States. Santa Monica (CA): The Rand Corporation; 2013. Available at: http://www.rand.org/content/dam/rand/pubs/research_reports/RR200/RR280/RAND_RR280.pdf.
36. Carpenter C, Bromley M, Caterino J, et al. Optimal older adult emergency care: Introducing multidisciplinary geriatric emergency department guidelines from the American college of emergency physicians, American Geriatrics Society, Emergency Nurses Association, and Society for Academic Emergency Medicine. Ann Emerg Med 2014;63:e1–3.
37. Carpenter C, Hwang U, Rosenberg M. New guidelines enhance care standards for elderly patients in the ED. ACEP Now 2014.
38. Connell BR, Jones M, Mace R, et al. The Center for Universal Design. The Principles of Universal Design. Available at: https://www.ncsu.edu/ncsu/design/cud/about_ud/udprinciplestext.htm. Accessed November 16, 2015.
39. Demirbilek O, Demirkan H. Universal design product design involving elderly users: a participatory design model. Appl Ergon 2004;35:361–70.
40. Rosenberg M, Rosenberg L. Improving outcomes of elderly patients presenting to the emergency department. Ann Emerg Med 2011;58:479–81.
41. Keyes D, Singal B, Dropf C, et al. Impact of a new senior emergency department on emergency department recidivism, rate of hospital admission, and hospital length of stay. Ann Emerg Med 2014;63:517–24.
42. Baumann MR, Strout TD. Triage of geriatric patients in the Emergency Department: validity and survival with the Emergency Severity Index. Ann Emerg Med 2007;49:234–40.
43. Rutschmann OT, Chevalley T, Zumwald C, et al. Pitfalls in the emergency department triage of frail elderly patients without specific complaints. Swiss Med Wkly 2005;135:145–50.
44. Yao JL, Fang J, Lou QQ, et al. A systematic review of the identification of seniors at risk (ISAR) tool for the prediction of adverse outcome in elderly patients seen in the emergency department. Int J Clin Exp Med 2015;8:4778–86.
45. David J. The life cycle of the banana: rethinking geriatric falls in the ED. Emerg Phys Monthly 2011. Available at: http://www.epijournal.com/articles/100/new-age-why-the-world-needs-geriatric-emergency-medicine. Accessed May 10, 2016.
46. Conroy SP, Ansari K, Williams M, et al. A controlled evaluation of comprehensive geriatric assessment in the emergency department: the 'Emergency Frailty Unit'. Age Ageing 2014;43:109–14.
47. Caplan GA, Williams AJ, Daly B, et al. A randomized, controlled trial of comprehensive geriatric assessment and multidisciplinary intervention after discharge of elderly from the emergency department—the DEED II Study. J Am Geriatr Soc 2004;52:1417–23.
48. Kessler C, Williams M, Moustoukas J, et al. Transitions of care for the geriatric patient in the emergency department. Clin Geriatr Med 2013;29:49–69.

49. McCusker J, Dendukuri N, Tousignant P, et al. Rapid two-stage emergency department intervention for seniors: impact on continuity of care. Acad Emerg Med 2003;10:233–43.
50. McCusker J, Verdon J. Do geriatric interventions reduce emergency department visits? A systematic review. J Gerontol A Biol Sci Med Sci 2006;61:53–62.
51. Terrell K, Hustey F, Hwang U, et al. Quality indicators for geriatric emergency care. Acad Emerg Med 2009;16:441–9.
52. Nelson D, Washton D, Jeanmonod R. Communication gaps in nursing home transfers to the ED: Impact on turnaround time, disposition, and diagnostic testing. Am J Emerg Med 2013;31:712–6.
53. Griffiths D, Morphet J, Innes K, et al. Communication between residential aged care facilities and the emergency department: a review of the literature. Int J Nurs Stud 2014;51:1517–23.
54. ACEP. Clinical & Practice Management. Observation Care Payments to Hospitals. Available at: http://www.acep.org/Clinical-Practice-Management/Observation-Care-Payments-to-Hospitals-FAQ/. Accessed December 26, 2015.
55. Ellis G, Marshall T, Ritchie C. Comprehensive geriatric assessment in the emergency department. Clin Interv Aging 2014;9:2033–43.
56. Centers for Medicare & Medicaid Services. Consumer assessment of healthcare providers & systems (CAHPS). Available at: http://www.cms.gov/Research-Statistics-Data-and-Systems/Research/CAHPS/index.html. Accessed December 26, 2015.

# Altered Mental Status and Delirium

Scott T. Wilber, MD, MPH*, Jason E. Ondrejka, DO

## KEYWORDS

- Delirium • Dementia • Elderly • Emergency medicine • Altered mental status
- Medical decision-making capacity

## KEY POINTS

- Altered mental status or change in behavior in an older patient presenting to the emergency department frequently represents delirium.
- Diagnosing delirium occurs at the bedside by the emergency physician and includes objective screening measures for level of consciousness and cognition followed by confirmatory testing.
- Delirium is often caused by a potentially life-threatening underlying condition and carries a poor prognosis if unrecognized.
- Determining the cause of delirium takes a thorough evaluation, including interviewing any available surrogates, reviewing medications, considering a broad differential, including infection, trauma, stroke, and performing comprehensive diagnostic testing.
- Treatment of delirium includes treating the underlying cause as well as careful administration of antipsychotic drugs when nonpharmacologic treatments are insufficient.

## INTRODUCTION

Older patients who present to the emergency department (ED) frequently have acute or chronic alterations of their mental status, including their level of consciousness and cognition. Recognizing both acute and chronic changes in cognition are important for emergency physicians. Chronic changes in cognition due to dementia may affect the reliability of patients' histories as well as their ability to follow discharge instructions.[1] Failure to recognize this chronic impairment may therefore affect patient outcomes.

Most importantly for emergency physicians is to recognize acute changes in mental status. When older patients present with change in mental status as a chief complaint, it is nearly always caused by delirium.[2] Delirium is characterized by an acute (hours to days) fluctuating change in attention, awareness, and cognition as defined by the

Disclosures: None.
Department of Emergency Medicine, Summa Health System-Akron City Hospital, Northeastern Ohio Medical University, 525 East Market Street, Akron, OH 44309, USA
* Corresponding author.
E-mail address: wilbers@summahealth.org

Emerg Med Clin N Am 34 (2016) 649–665
http://dx.doi.org/10.1016/j.emc.2016.04.012
0733-8627/16/$ – see front matter © 2016 Elsevier Inc. All rights reserved.
emed.theclinics.com

Diagnostic and Statistical Manual of Mental Disorders, Fifth Edition.[3] Older ED patients with delirium have an increased risk of mortality compared with nondelirious patients. The failure of ED physicians to diagnose delirium may also increase a patient's mortality, as mortalities are more than twice as high in patients in whom delirium was not diagnosed in the ED, compared with those in whom delirium was diagnosed and nondelirious patients.[4] Crucial to avoiding missed delirium is understanding the subtypes of delirium, which include hyperactive, mixed, and hypoactive states, with the most common being hypoactive.[5] Hypoactive delirium can be misinterpreted as "fatigue" or "not acting like themselves" by caregivers, making this subtype of delirium most challenging to recognize.

Consequently, it is the task of the emergency physician to recognize both acute and chronic mental status changes. A structured approach to the rapid assessment of cognitive status is required. Emergency physicians must have a high index of suspicion for delirium, and once suspected, conduct a thorough evaluation to find the underlying cause.

## Evaluation of Altered Mental Status and Delirium

### Delirium risk assessment

The emergency physician needs to gather predisposing risk factors for the development of delirium while taking the history of an elderly patient (**Table 1**).[6] Predisposing risk factors lower the threshold for a patient to become delirious when faced with a precipitating cause (**Fig. 1**). Furthermore, some predisposing risk factors can themselves cause delirium.

It is essential to include a review of the patient's active medication list for polypharmacy and for drugs that are known to cause confusion listed on the updated Beers criteria.[7,8] Notorious drug classes to screen for are anticholinergics, benzodiazepines, opiates, antidepressants, and muscle relaxants. A review of pharmacology in the geriatric patient can be found in the article by Welker KL, Mycyk MB: Pharmacology in the Geriatric Patient, in this issue.

### Assessing level of consciousness (arousal)

A bedside examination should assess the patient's level of consciousness using an objective bedside tool. These tools can assist in diagnosing delirium, and abnormal levels of consciousness are associated with mortality.

| Table 1 | | |
|---|---|---|
| **Predisposing risk factors for delirium** | | |
| **Demographics** | **Comorbid Disease** | **Drugs** |
| • Advanced age | • Number of comorbidities | • Polypharmacy |
| • Male gender | • Severity of comorbidities | • Baseline psychoactive medication use |
| | • Visual impairment | • Alcohol abuse |
| | • Hearing impairment | • Drug abuse |
| | • Dementia | |
| | • Depression | |
| | • History of delirium | |
| | • Cerebrovascular disease | |
| | • Falls | |
| | • Functional impairment | |
| | • Terminal illness | |
| | • Malnutrition | |

*Adapted from* Inouye SK. Delirium in older persons. N Engl J Med 2006;354(11):1160.

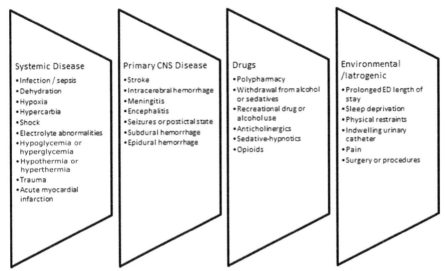

| Systemic Disease | Primary CNS Disease | Drugs | Environmental /Iatrogenic |
|---|---|---|---|
| •Infection / sepsis | •Stroke | •Polypharmacy | •Prolonged ED length of |
| •Dehydration | •Intracerebral hemorrhage | •Withdrawal from alcohol | stay |
| •Hypoxia | •Meningitis | or sedatives | •Sleep deprivation |
| •Hypercarbia | •Encephalitis | •Recreational drug or | •Physical restraints |
| •Shock | •Seizures or postictal state | alcohol use | •Indwelling urinary |
| •Electrolyte abnormalities | •Subdural hemorrhage | •Anticholinergics | catheter |
| •Hypoglycemia or | •Epidural hemorrhage | •Sedative-hypnotics | •Pain |
| hyperglycemia | | •Opioids | •Surgery or procedures |
| •Hypothermia or | | | |
| hyperthermia | | | |
| •Trauma | | | |
| •Acute myocardial | | | |
| infarction | | | |

**Fig. 1.** Precipitating causes of delirium. (*Adapted from* Inouye SK. Delirium in older persons. N Engl J Med 2006;354(11):1161.)

One of the simplest is the "AVPU" scale, which stands for alert, responsive to verbal stimuli, responsive to painful stimuli, or unresponsive.[9] However, this scale does not evaluate the level of response to the stimuli, limiting its usefulness. For example, patients who respond to verbal stimuli by waking and interacting with the examiner differ substantially from those whose response to verbal stimuli is groaning. In addition the AVPU scale has a lower ability to predict mortality in hospitalized patients compared with the Glasgow Coma Score (GCS) and the Richmond Agitation and Sedation Scale (RASS).[10]

The GCS was first described more than 40 years ago and is familiar to the emergency physician.[11] GCS is tabulated from 3 scores for best eye opening, best verbal response, and best motor response (**Table 2**). The advantage of GCS is familiarity due to the ubiquitous nature of the scale in the prehospital and hospital setting. There has been evidence that decreasing GCS in elderly trauma is associated with increased mortality, but this has not been widely studied in the nontraumatic elderly ED population.[12]

The RASS measures the patient level of arousal on a scale ranging from −5 (Unarousable) to +4 (Combative). A score of zero represents an alert and calm patient.[13] This simple tool takes less than 10 seconds to perform, and scores other than zero (alert and calm) have a high sensitivity for delirium.[13,14] In the ED setting, Han and colleagues[14] found that an RASS score of less than or equal to −1 or greater than or equal to 1 had a sensitivity of 84.0% and a specificity of 88%. An RASS of less than or equal to −2 or greater than or equal to 2 had a specificity of 99%, at the expense of a decreased sensitivity. The modified RASS provides an additional assessment of attention and provides additional anchors for scoring (**Table 3**).[13]

Patients who are awake and alert may also be inattentive, which represents a disturbance of consciousness. Inattention is a cardinal feature of delirium.[3] Inattention can be subjectively evaluated by simple observation of the patient, noting their ability to remain attentive to the process of taking a history. It is also evaluated in several delirium screening instruments (see later discussion). Objective tests of attention,

**Table 2**
**Glasgow Coma Scale**

| | | | | | |
|---|---|---|---|---|---|
| Eye opening response | 1 = No response | 2 = To pain | 3 = To speech | 4 = Spontaneous | |
| Best verbal response | 1 = No response | 2 = Incomprehensible | 3 = Inappropriate | 4 = Confused | 5 = Oriented |
| Best motor response | 1 = No response | 2 = Abnormal extension | 3 = Abnormal flexion | 4 = Withdraws from pain | 5 = Localizes to pain | 6 = Obeys commands |

**Table 3**
**Modified Richmond Agitation and Sedation Scale**

**Step 1: State the patient's name and ask patient to open eyes and look at speaker.**
**Ask: "Describe how you are feeling today"**
- If answers with short answer (<10 s), cue with second open-ended question.
- If no response to verbal cue, physically stimulate patient by shaking the shoulder.

**Step 2: Score Modified RASS**

| Score | Term | Description |
|-------|------|-------------|
| +4 | Combative | No attention; overtly combative, violent, immediate danger to staff |
| +3 | Very agitated | Very distractible; repeated calling or touch required to get or keep eye contact or attention; cannot focus; pulls or removes tube(s) or catheter(s); aggressive; fights environment not people |
| +2 | Slightly agitated | Easily distractible; rapidly loses attention; resists care or uncooperative; frequent nonpurposeful movement |
| +1 | Restless | Slightly distractible; pays attention most of the time; anxious, but cooperative; movements not aggressive or vigorous |
| 0 | Alert and calm | Pays attention; makes eye contact; aware of surroundings; responds immediately and appropriately to calling name and touch |
| −1 | Wakes easily | Slightly drowsy; eye contact >10 s; not fully alert, but has sustained awakening; eye-opening/eye contact to voice >10 s |
| −2 | Wakes slowly | Very drowsy; pays attention some of the time; briefly awakens with eye contact to voice <10 s |
| −3 | Difficult to wake | Repeated calling or touch required to get or keep eye contact or attention; needs repeated stimuli (touch or voice) for attention, movement, or eye opening to voice (but no eye contact) |
| −4 | Cannot stay awake | Rousable but no attention; no response to voice, but movement or eye opening to physical stimulation |
| −5 | Unarousable | No response to voice or physical stimulation |

*Reproduced from* Chester JG, Beth Harrington M, Rudolph JL, et al. Serial administration of a modified Richmond agitation and sedation scale for delirium screening. J Hosp Med 2012;7(5):451; with permission.

such as the Digit Span Forward or Digit Span Backwards tests, the Vigilance "A" test, or the Digit Cancellation test, may be useful in assessing delirium in hospitalized patients, but are too cumbersome for ED use.[15]

*Assessing cognition*
There are a variety of neuropsychiatric tests to score a patient's cognition. The most recognized test for 40 years is the Mini-Mental Status Examination (MMSE).[16] However, this test is difficult to perform in the ED, because it can take between 5 and 15 minutes to complete and requires a patient to have intact vision, hearing, and ability to write.

Other screening tests for cognition that have been studied in the ED include the Clock-Drawing Test, the Mini-Cog, the Brief Alzheimer's Screen, the Caregiver-completed AD8, the Short Blessed Test (also known as the Orientation Memory Concentration Test), the Six-Item Screener, and the Ottawa 3DY (**Table 4**).[17–20] Of these screening tests, the Six-Item Screener and the Ottawa 3DY have the advantage of being rapid, easily remembered, and simply scored, while having a reasonably high sensitivity and specificity. The Six-Item Screener consists of 3-item recall and

| Table 4 | | | | |
|---|---|---|---|---|
| **Screening tests for cognitive impairment in older emergency department patients** | | | | |
| Test | Sensitivity (%) | Specificity (%) | Time to Administer (min) | Scoring |
| Six-item screener[18-20] | 63–94 | 77–85 | 1 | Simple |
| Mini-Cog[19] | 77 | 85 | 2 | Moderately complex |
| Brief Alzheimer's Screen[17] | 95 | 52 | 5 | Complex, weighted |
| Short Blessed Test[17] | 95 | 65 | 2–5 | Complex, weighted |
| Ottawa 3DY[17] | 95 | 52 | 1 | Simple |
| Caregiver-completed AD8[17,18] | 63–83 | 63–79 | — | Simple |

orientation to year, month, and day of the week. The Ottawa 3DY consists of asking the patient the *D*ay of the week, spell "World" backward ("*D*LROW"), the *D*ate, and the *Y*ear.

### Assessing for delirium

There are many methods and approaches to diagnosing delirium in older ED patients. A simplistic test for the presence of delirium is the chief complaint of "altered mental status." In a study of 406 ED patients, Han and colleagues[2] found that this chief complaint had a 38% sensitivity and a 98.9% specificity for delirium. Consequently, the presence of this chief complaint is highly likely to rule delirium in, but its absence cannot reliably be used to rule delirium out. Similarly, single screening questions of informants ("'Do you think [name of patient] has been more confused lately?" or "How has your relative/friend's memory changed with his/her current illness?") have been studied in non-ED patients and have moderate sensitivities (77%–80%) and specificities (56%–71%).[21,22]

As noted above, an RASS of $\neq 0$ is 84.0% sensitive and 88% specific for delirium. A score of less than or equal to −2 or greater than or equal to 2 is 99% specific, but only 16% sensitive when performed by ED physicians.[14]

### The confusion assessment method and derivatives

The confusion assessment method (CAM) was first described by Inouye and colleagues[23] in 1990. The goal of the CAM was to "enable non-psychiatry trained clinicians to identify delirium quickly and accurately in both clinical and research settings."[23] A positive CAM requires the presence of acute onset *and* fluctuating course *and* inattention, and *either* disorganized thinking *or* altered level of consciousness. Studies have shown sensitivities ranging from 46% to 100% and specificities ranging from 63% to 100%. In an evaluation of high-quality studies in a recent systematic review, the investigators found an average sensitivity of 94% and an average specificity of 89%. However, to achieve these characteristics, it is recommended that formal cognitive testing such as the MMSE be performed, and that raters have formal training in the administration of the CAM.[24] For these reasons, the use of the CAM may be limited in ED settings.

The Confusion Assessment Method for the Intensive Care Unit (CAM-ICU) was developed for use in mechanically ventilated ICU patients.[24,25] The CAM-ICU uses brief and objective measurements for scoring and may be completed rapidly (in less than 2 minutes). For feature 1, the patient must have either an acute change OR a fluctuating course of their mental status. This requirement differs from the CAM, which requires an acute onset AND fluctuating course. For feature 2, inattention, the CAM-ICU presents a series of letters, and the patient is instructed to squeeze the rater's hand whenever an "A" is heard. More than 2 errors is considered abnormal. If the patient has negative evaluations for either feature 1 or feature 2, the test may be stopped, and the patient is considered CAM-ICU negative.

If the patient has an abnormal score for feature 1 AND feature 2, the patient is tested for altered level of consciousness using the RASS. If the RASS is not equal to zero, the patient is diagnosed with delirium. If the RASS is zero, 4 objective questions to evaluate disorganized thinking are asked. More than 1 error diagnoses delirium, 0 to 1 errors are consistent with no delirium.

The CAM-ICU was tested in ED patients, and emergency physicians applying this technique had a sensitivity of 72% and a specificity of 99%.[26] Consequently, this algorithm could be used to rule delirium in; however, the sensitivity is too low to use as a screening test in ED patients (**Fig. 2**).

Recently, Han and colleagues[27] described a 2-step approach for diagnosing delirium in the ED. The first step was to apply a brief, highly sensitive test for delirium. The investigators used the Delirium Triage Score (DTS), a combination of an RASS of less than or equal to −1 or greater than or equal to 1, or greater than or equal to 1 errors in spelling "Lunch" backwards. The DTS had 98% sensitivity and 55% specificity. If the patient was normal, they were not delirious.

If the patient was abnormal, the Brief Confusion Assessment Method (bCAM) was performed. Derived from the CAM-ICU, the bCAM is another objective method of assessing the 4 features of the CAM. Similar to the CAM-ICU, the bCAM uses altered mental status or fluctuating course for feature 1. For feature 2, inattention, the bCAM assesses the patient's ability to recite the months of the year backwards from December to July. Zero and 1 errors are consistent with no delirium. For feature 3, level of consciousness, the bCAM also uses the RASS. Finally, the bCAM uses the same questions for disorganized thinking as the CAM-ICU, but considers any error diagnostic of delirium. The bCAM was 84% sensitive and 96% specific. Combined, this 2-step approach had a sensitivity of 82% and a specificity of 96% (**Fig. 3**).[27]

## Evaluation for Precipitating Causes of Delirium

The discussion thus far has focused on what tools the emergency clinician can use to establish whether their patient is delirious. Simply recognizing delirium can seem daunting initially, but remember this evaluation is occurring in tandem with the comprehensive history and physical examination that is warranted. Once delirium is suspected, it is imperative that the emergency clinician acknowledges that they have recognized a potential life threat.

### Physical examination

The physical examination of the delirious patient should be a comprehensive effort to find clues as to the cause of delirium. Often this is in conjunction with the evaluation of their level of consciousness and cognition. Commitment to a systematic and thorough examination may provide a key piece of data to aid rapid diagnosis. Examination begins with vital signs, which can be critical for determining the underlying cause; for example:

- Hyperthermia—Infection, environmental exposure, thyroid storm, toxic ingestion (stimulants)
- Hypothermia—Infection, environmental exposure, myxedema coma, hypoglycemia

- Hypotension—Infection, cardiogenic shock (acute myocardial infarction/pericardial effusion/heart failure), hemorrhagic shock, dehydration, anaphylactic shock
- Hypertension—Hypertensive encephalopathy, intracranial hemorrhage
- Tachypnea—metabolic acidosis, pulmonary edema/effusion, pulmonary embolism, pneumonia

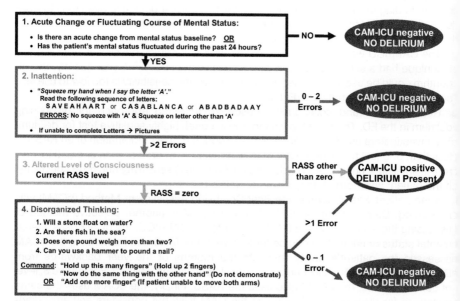

**Fig. 2.** Confusion assessment method for the ICU (CAM-ICU) flow sheet. (*Courtesy of* E. Wesley Ely, MD, MPH, Vanderbilt University.)

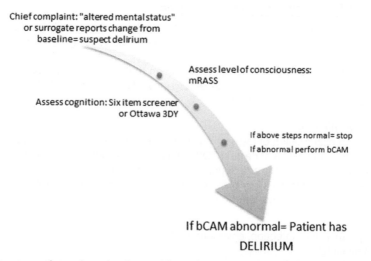

**Fig. 3.** Summary of steps based on best evidence for determining potential delirium in older ED patients.

Trauma is underrecognized in the elderly; therefore, if history is limited, it is reasonable to proceed with a primary survey as outlined by advanced trauma life support.[28,29] **Box 1** highlights key additional physical examination findings that are high yield or often missed and their association with causes of delirium. In addition, careful attention should be made to any indwelling devices such as pacemaker/implantable cardioverter defibrillator, central venous access, Foley catheters, and such.

A thorough neurologic examination is also necessary for both the diagnosis of delirium and identifying possible causes of delirium. The authors recommend a low threshold for performing a National Institutes of Health Stroke scale/score as part of the neurologic assessment because "confusion" could in fact be aphasia or hemineglect (**Table 5**). There is evidence to suggest that strokes in the elderly are less aggressively managed at onset with less use of MRI and referral to stroke units.[30] Faster recognition may improve the grim 1-year mortality of 27% in this population.

Comprehensive testing is usually indicated in the delirious elderly ED patient to evaluate for the precipitating causes of delirium, such as infection, acute stroke, cardiovascular disease, electrolyte disturbances, and medications, tailored to the patient's physical examination.[31–33] For example, most if not all delirious patients require electrolytes, complete blood count, urinalysis, electrocardiogram, and chest radiography, but certain patients will require further evaluation if clinically warranted, such as noncontrast computed tomography (CT) of the head, CT of abdomen and pelvis, and/or lumbar puncture. **Box 2** summarizes diagnostic tests ordered for delirium with clinical clues and causes of delirium. Comprehensive testing is needed at times when the patient presents with coma, multiple complaints, or nonspecific findings. Nonetheless, the authors recommend a targeted diagnostic approach when possible because unnecessary testing and increasing ED length of stay will contribute to further delirium, as discussed further in the next section.

## NONPHARMACOLOGIC TREATMENT

Nonpharmacologic approaches may be effective at reducing the incidence of delirium as well as reducing the symptoms of agitation in delirious patients.[34] In hospitalized patients, multicomponent interventions, which include cognitive stimulation and reorientation, early mobilization, hearing and vision aids, hydration and nutrition, and sleep strategies, significantly reduce the incidence of delirium. In addition, these interventions reduced the risk of falls and showed a trend toward reduction in hospital length of stay and rate of institutionalization.[34]

---

| Box 1 | |
|---|---|
| **Physical examination findings with associations to underlying causes of delirium** | |
| Head/facial trauma | Intracranial hemorrhage, cervical spine fracture |
| Pupillary/extraocular motor defects | Intracranial hemorrhage, seizure, medication toxicity |
| Cardiac murmur | Acute valvular heart failure, endocarditis |
| Asymmetric breath sounds | Pleural effusion, pneumonia |
| Abdominal tenderness/distention | Acute urinary retention or infection, bowel obstruction, cholecystitis, pancreatitis, appendicitis, abdominal aortic aneurysm, mesenteric ischemia |
| Skin hyperemia (including back) | Cellulitis, necrotizing fasciitis, anaphylaxis |
| Extremity tenderness/deformity | Fracture, dislocation, rhabdomyolysis, abuse |
| Peripheral extremity edema | Thromboembolic disease, heart failure, myxedema |
| Rectal bleeding | Gastrointestinal hemorrhage |

**Table 5**
**National Institutes of Stroke Scale**

| Item | Title | Responses and Scores |
|------|-------|----------------------|
| 1a | Level of consciousness | 0—Alert<br>1—Drowsy<br>2—Obtunded<br>3—Coma/unresponsive |
| 1b | Orientation questions | 0—Answers both correctly<br>1—Answers 1 correctly<br>2—Answers neither correctly |
| 1c | Response to commands | 0—Performs both tasks correctly<br>1—Performs 1 task correctly<br>2—Performs neither |
| 2 | Gaze | 0—Normal horizontal movements<br>1—Partial gaze palsy<br>2—Complete gaze palsy |
| 3 | Visual fields | 0—No visual field defect<br>1—Partial hemianopsia<br>2—Complete hemianopsia<br>3—Bilateral hemianopsia |
| 4 | Facial movements | 0—Normal<br>1—Minor facial weakness<br>2—Partial facial weakness<br>3—Complete unilateral palsy |
| 5 | Motor function (arm): a. Left; b. Right | 0—No drift<br>1—Drift before 5 s<br>2—Falls before 10 s<br>3—No effort against gravity<br>4—No movement |
| 6 | Motor function (leg): a. Left; b. Right | 0—No drift<br>1—Drift before 5 s<br>2—Falls before 5 s<br>3—No effort against gravity<br>4—No movement |
| 7 | Limb ataxia | 0—No ataxia<br>1—Ataxia in 1 limb<br>2—Ataxia in 2 limbs |
| 8 | Sensory | 0—No sensory loss<br>1—Mild sensory loss<br>2—Severe sensory loss |
| 9 | Language | 0—Normal<br>1—Mild aphasia<br>2—Severe aphasia<br>3—Mute or global aphasia |
| 10 | Articulation | 0—Normal<br>1—Mild dysarthria<br>2—Severe dysarthria |
| 11 | Extinction or inattention | 0—Absent<br>1—Mild (1 sensory modality lost)<br>2—Severe (2 modalities lost) |

*Adapted from* National Institute of Health, National Institute of Neurological Disorders and Stroke. Stroke Scale. Available at: http://www.ninds.nih.gov/doctors/NIH_Stroke_Scale.pdf.

---

**Box 2**
**Diagnostic test (clinical clue) matched with causes of delirium**

| | |
|---|---|
| Electrolyte panel | Hyponatremia, hypoglycemia/ hyperglycemia, acute kidney injury/failure, uremia |
| ECG | Myocardial infarction, dysrhythmia, medication toxicity |
| Complete blood count with differential | Leukocytosis/leukopenia (infection), thrombocytosis (acute phase reactant), elevated band count (infection), acute anemia/hemorrhage |
| Chest radiography | Pneumonia, pulmonary edema/heart failure |
| Cardiac enzymes (ischemic ECG, dyspnea, chest pain) | Myocardial infarction |
| Arterial blood gas (respiratory distress, chronic respiratory disease) | Hypercarbia, hypoxia, metabolic acidosis |
| Hepatic function panel ± ammonia level (vomiting, jaundice, abdominal tenderness) | Cholecystitis, cholangitis, hepatitis, pancreatitis, hepatic encephalopathy |
| CT abdomen/pelvis (abdominal pain/ tenderness) | Diverticulitis, appendicitis, complicated UTI/ obstructive uropathy |
| Abdominal ultrasound | Cholecystitis |
| Thyroid-stimulating hormone (thyroid mass, prior thyroid disease/surgery, peripheral edema, alopecia) | Myxedema, thyroid storm |
| Noncontrast CT head (trauma, focal neurologic deficits, coma) | Intracranial hemorrhage, ischemic stroke (subacute), mass |
| Lumbar puncture (fever, meningismus) | Meningitis, encephalitis |

*Abbreviations:* ECG, electrocardiogram; UTI, urinary tract infection.

---

In older patients at risk of developing delirium, ED-specific interventions may include the use of existing sensory aids, such as glasses and hearing aids. As EDs typically have little natural light, providing orientation cues such as large face clocks and calendars and reducing artificial light at night may be beneficial. Visitors should be encouraged to stay at the bedside with patients and to provide reorientation as necessary, reminding the patient where they are and why. Some investigators think that reorientation and short-term memory questions may agitate the patient and recommend that reorientation be attempted, but if that fails, to use distraction techniques or go along with the disorientation and other behaviors as long as they do not cause harm.[35] Adequate treatment of pain may reduce agitation in the patient with altered mental status. Long ED length of stays (LOS) is associated with an increased risk of developing delirium during hospitalization.[36] Avoiding long ED LOS, reducing ED boarding, and providing hydration and a meal may reduce the risk of developing delirium.

Unless absolutely necessary for patient care, medical devices that may tether the patient should be avoided. When feasible, vital signs should be obtained intermittently, and devices such as cardiac monitors, pulse oximeters, and blood pressure cuffs should be removed when not in use.[35] These items are commonly used in the ED and left in place even when continuous monitoring of vital signs is not required. In addition to tethering the patient, frequent false positive alarms can be disorienting and disturbing for delirious ED patients.

Other tethers can include intravenous lines, restraints, and indwelling urinary catheters. Intravenous (IV) fluids can be given by intermittent bolus rather than continuous infusion when necessary; the intravenous tubing can be removed, and the catheter can be locked. Locked intravenous catheters can be hidden beneath gauze, Ace wraps, or cast sleeves if the patient tries to remove them.

Physical restraints significantly increase the risk of developing delirium as well as its severity in hospitalized patients.[36] Consequently, nonpharmacologic or pharmacologic methods for addressing dangerous behaviors (such as trying to get out of bed or interfering with therapy) in patients with delirium should always be preferred. Physical restraints should be avoided unless absolutely necessary for patient or provider safety and used only for the briefest time possible. Frequent reorientation of patients and feedback that they should avoid dangerous behaviors may be provided by family, sitters, or staff. Answering call lights as quickly as possible may also reduce the risk of dangerous behaviors such as trying to get out of bed.

Indwelling urinary catheters are associated with an increased risk of developing delirium during hospitalization, increased length of hospitalization, and increased mortality.[36,37] In addition, catheters can increase agitation, are at risk for traumatic self-removal, and are associated with urinary tract infections. Urine for urinalysis should be obtained by voiding whenever possible, or by intermittent straight catheterization if the patient is incontinent, rather than by placing an indwelling catheter. Most older ED patients do not need strict measurement of intake and output by indwelling catheter. Bedside commodes are an alternative when patients need to urinate frequently, such as following the administration of diuretics. One appropriate indication for an indwelling urinary catheter is acute urinary retention, which itself can cause agitation in the patient with altered mental status.

## PHARMACOLOGIC TREATMENT

Hyperactive delirium commonly requires intervention to protect the patient and staff from harm. Pharmacologic treatment with atypical and typical antipsychotics can reduce delirium if nonpharmacologic measures have failed.[38] Although medications for delirium should be used cautiously, they play an important role in the safe care of the acutely delirious older patient. Most commonly, the initial treatment requires intramuscular (IM) administration because the patient will not cooperate with oral medications. The elderly patient often requires much smaller doses than adult counterparts and repeated low doses are preferred to a single large initial dose (**Table 6**). Serious side effects with antipsychotics are lower in the acute care setting (0.9%) as opposed to chronic use.[39] In the large study by Hatta and colleagues,[40] nonserious extrapyramidal symptoms were the most common side effects at 5.6%. The serious adverse events mentioned were led by aspiration pneumonia and followed by cardiovascular events, none of which were fatal, and none occurred with intravenous haloperidol.

| Table 6 | | |
|---|---|---|
| Medication, preferred dosing regimen, and special considerations | | |
| Haloperidol | 0.5–1 mg IM/IV every 30–60 min as needed; 0.5–1 mg orally twice daily and every 4 h as needed | Preferred agent |
| Olanzapine | 2.5–5 mg orally once per day | — |
| Risperidone | 0.5 mg orally twice daily | — |
| Quetiapine | 12.5–25 mg orally twice daily | Parkinson disease and hypoactive delirium |
| Ziprasidone | 2 mg–5 mg IM | — |

Haloperidol is one of the oldest treatments and continues to be a preferred agent for hyperactive delirium. Haloperidol is likely as safe and effective as newer atypical medications.[40,41] The oral and parenteral options of haloperidol make it a versatile treatment option. Quetiapine is recommended in patients with underlying Parkinson disease and has been found effective in hypoactive delirium.[42,43] Benzodiazepines may exacerbate delirium and agitation and should be avoided unless treating acute alcohol withdrawal or seizure.[44] Furthermore, in critically ill older patients requiring sedation, dexmedetomidine has less risk of delirium than benzodiazepines and is preferred.[45]

## Assessment of Decision-Making Capacity

Emergency physicians are often faced with determining whether an ED patient has the capacity to make medical decisions. In general, clinicians often fail to identify patients with incapacity.[46] Nearly all (97%) healthy older patients retain their medical decision-making capacity; however, the proportion retaining these abilities decreases as cognitive function declines. In patients with mild cognitive impairment, 80% retain decision-making capacity; in nursing home residents, about 55% retain this ability.[46]

To consent for medical treatment, a patient must be provided with the risks, benefits, and alternatives to the recommended treatment; they must be free of coercion, and they must have medical decision-making capacity. Decision-making capacity relies on (1) the ability to understand the risks, benefits, and alternatives; (2) the ability to understand the consequences of their decision; (3) the ability to use reason for decision making; and (4) the ability to express their choice.

Decision-making capacity exists on a continuum; a patient may have the capacity to consent or refuse minor procedures but may lack capacity for more serious or complicated medical procedures. Consequently, decision-making capacity must be assessed individually for each medical decision. When a patient lacks decision-making capacity, a surrogate should be used for decision making. Hospitals should have policies in place to guide surrogate decision-making decisions. Whenever possible, a patient should still participate in discussions regarding medical decisions. Surrogate decision makers should use "substituted judgment" rather than "best interest" when making medical decisions for a patient.[47] Substituted judgment relies on the decision maker's knowledge of the patient and the patient's preferences and beliefs to make decisions. Phrasing questions as, "what would the patient have wanted in this situation," is one way to promote the use of substituted judgment. Only when the patient's preferences and beliefs are unknown to the surrogate decision maker should the surrogate use "best interest" to make medical decisions.[47]

## OUTCOMES/DISPOSITION

Most causes of delirium require medical hospitalization. Even patients with equivocal testing but confirmed acute delirium are generally unsafe for discharge. Compared with nondelirious elderly patients presenting to the ED, those with delirium have longer average LOS (1 day vs 2 days).[1] The doubling of LOS persists in delirious patients admitted to the hospital (2 days vs 4 days).[48] There are higher utilization of resources in the delirious elderly population because they are more likely to require the ICU and be discharged to a new long-term care facility than those without delirium. Consistently poor outcomes are demonstrated in this population with higher 30-day mortality (6% vs 1%) and 30-day readmission (27% vs 13%) rates.[48] This 30-day mortality is higher than elderly patients with ST-elevation myocardial infarction.[49] Another study showed a 37% mortality at 6 months compared with 14% in nondelirious older patients, a 72% higher mortality even when controlling for age, comorbidity, severity of illness, functional dependence, and nursing home residence.[1] Interestingly the 6-month mortality of delirium is greater than that of stroke in the elderly (37% vs 27%).[30]

### Billing and Coding Considerations

This discussion has focused on the signs and symptoms of altered mental status and the subtype of delirium. This paradigm is appropriate for the ED physician because they are often presented a constellation of signs and symptoms and tasked with finding a cause to the best of their abilities. Current billing practices, namely International Classification of Disease–10th edition, call on providing the most specific diagnosis possible, which has significant financial ramifications for reimbursing providers and hospitals caring for these patients. Although altered mental status and delirium are the topics of conversation, they are commonly describing a form of encephalopathy that provides a more specific code for billing purposes (for example, metabolic encephalopathy secondary to acute hyponatremia). If a form of encephalopathy is not applicable, then it is important to link the delirium to the precipitating cause suspected, if possible (for example, acute delirium secondary to community-acquired pneumonia with sepsis).

### SUMMARY

- Suspect delirium if patient has chief complaint of "altered mental status" or report of change from baseline in mental status/behavior.
- Assess level of consciousness with modified RASS, assess cognition with Six-Item Screener, or Ottawa 3DY, and if abnormal, perform bCAM.
- Once delirium is diagnosed, acknowledge prompt evaluation for underlying life threats.
- Perform a comprehensive physical examination to identify potential causes, including trauma evaluation and stroke scale evaluation.
- Obtain diagnostic testing to confirm cause of delirium.
- Treat underlying cause of delirium as appropriate while addressing symptoms of delirium with nonpharmacologic means.
- If nonpharmacologic treatments fail, proceed with haloperidol for hyperactive delirium and quetiapine for hypoactive delirium or delirium with underlying Parkinson disease.
- Maintain low threshold for admitting patient with delirium for aggressive management given their high mortality and morbidity.

### REFERENCES

1. Han JH, Eden S, Shintani A, et al. Delirium in older emergency department patients is an independent predictor of hospital length of stay. Acad Emerg Med 2011;18(5):451–7.
2. Han JH, Schnelle JF, Ely EW. The relationship between a chief complaint of "altered mental status" and delirium in older emergency department patients. Acad Emerg Med 2014;21(8):937–40.
3. American Psychiatric Association. Diagnostic and statistical manual of mental disorders. 5th edition. Washington, DC: American Psychiatric Publishing; 2013.
4. Kakuma R, du Fort GG, Arsenault L, et al. Delirium in older emergency department patients discharged home: effect on survival. J Am Geriatr Soc 2003; 51(4):443–50.

5. Han JH, Zimmerman EE, Cutler N, et al. Delirium in older emergency department patients: recognition, risk factors, and psychomotor subtypes. Acad Emerg Med 2009;16(3):193–200.

6. Inouye SK. Delirium in older persons. N Engl J Med 2006;354(11):1157–65.

7. Hein C, Forgues A, Piau A, et al. Impact of polypharmacy on occurrence of delirium in elderly emergency patients. J Am Med Dir Assoc 2014;15(11): 850.e11–5.

8. By the American Geriatrics Society 2015 Beers Criteria Update Expert Panel. American Geriatrics Society 2015 updated Beers criteria for potentially inappropriate medication use in older adults. J Am Geriatr Soc 2015;63(11):2227–46.

9. Sanders AB. Emergency care of the elder person. St Louis (MO): Beverly Cracom Publications; 1996.

10. Zadravecz FJ, Tien L, Robertson-Dick BJ, et al. Comparison of mental-status scales for predicting mortality on the general wards. J Hosp Med 2015;10(10): 658–63.

11. Teasdale G, Jennett B. Assessment of coma and impaired consciousness. A practical scale. Lancet 1974;2(7872):81–4.

12. Caterino JM, Raubenolt A, Cudnik MT. Modification of Glasgow Coma Scale criteria for injured elders. Acad Emerg Med 2011;18(10):1014–21.

13. Chester JG, Beth Harrington M, Rudolph JL, et al. Serial administration of a modified Richmond Agitation and Sedation Scale for delirium screening. J Hosp Med 2012;7(5):450–3.

14. Han JH, Vasilevskis EE, Schnelle JF, et al. The diagnostic performance of the Richmond Agitation Sedation Scale for detecting delirium in older emergency department patients. Acad Emerg Med 2015;22(7):878–82.

15. O'Keeffe ST, Gosney MA. Assessing attentiveness in older hospital patients: global assessment versus tests of attention. J Am Geriatr Soc 1997;45(4):470–3.

16. Folstein MF, Folstein SE, McHugh PR. "Mini-mental state". A practical method for grading the cognitive state of patients for the clinician. J Psychiatr Res 1975; 12(3):189–98.

17. Carpenter CR, Bassett ER, Fischer GM, et al. Four sensitive screening tools to detect cognitive dysfunction in geriatric emergency department patients: brief Alzheimer's screen, short blessed test, Ottawa 3DY, and the caregiver-completed AD8. Acad Emerg Med 2011;18(4):374–84.

18. Carpenter CR, DesPain B, Keeling TN, et al. The six-item screener and AD8 for the detection of cognitive impairment in geriatric emergency department patients. Ann Emerg Med 2011;57(6):653–61.

19. Wilber ST, Lofgren SD, Mager TG, et al. An evaluation of two screening tools for cognitive impairment in older emergency department patients. Acad Emerg Med 2005;12(7):612–6.

20. Wilber ST, Carpenter CR, Hustey FM. The six-item screener to detect cognitive impairment in older emergency department patients. Acad Emerg Med 2008; 15(7):613–6.

21. Hendry K, Quinn TJ, Evans JJ, et al. Informant single screening questions for delirium and dementia in acute care–a cross-sectional test accuracy pilot study. BMC Geriatr 2015;15:17.

22. Sands MB, Dantoc BP, Hartshorn A, et al. Single Question in Delirium (SQiD): testing its efficacy against psychiatrist interview, the confusion assessment method and the memorial delirium assessment scale. Palliat Med 2010;24(6): 561–5.

23. Inouye SK, van Dyck CH, Alessi CA, et al. Clarifying confusion: the confusion assessment method. A new method for detection of delirium. Ann Intern Med 1990;113(12):941–8.
24. Wei LA, Fearing MA, Sternberg EJ, et al. The confusion assessment method: a systematic review of current usage. J Am Geriatr Soc 2008;56(5):823–30.
25. Ely EW, Inouye SK, Bernard GR, et al. Delirium in mechanically ventilated patients: validity and reliability of the confusion assessment method for the intensive care unit (CAM-ICU). JAMA 2001;286(21):2703–10.
26. Han JH, Wilson A, Graves AJ, et al. Validation of the confusion assessment method for the intensive care unit in older emergency department patients. Acad Emerg Med 2014;21(2):180–7.
27. Han JH, Wilson A, Vasilevskis EE, et al. Diagnosing delirium in older emergency department patients: validity and reliability of the delirium triage screen and the brief confusion assessment method. Ann Emerg Med 2013;62(5):457–65.
28. Werman HA, Erskine T, Caterino J, et al, Members of the Trauma Committee of the State of Ohio EMS Board. Development of statewide geriatric patients trauma triage criteria. Prehosp Disaster Med 2011;26(3):170–9.
29. Ryb GE, Cooper C, Waak SM. Delayed trauma team activation: patient characteristics and outcomes. J Trauma Acute Care Surg 2012;73(3):695–8.
30. Montout V, Madonna-Py B, Josse MO, et al. Stroke in elderly patients: management and prognosis in the ED. Am J Emerg Med 2008;26(7):742–9.
31. Rahkonen T, Mäkelä H, Paanila S, et al. Delirium in elderly people without severe predisposing disorders: etiology and 1-year prognosis after discharge. Int Psychogeriatr 2000;12(4):473–81.
32. Jitapunkul S, Pillay I, Ebrahim S. Delirium in newly admitted elderly patients: a prospective study. Q J Med 1992;83(300):307–14.
33. Han JH, Wilber ST. Altered mental status in older patients in the emergency department. Clin Geriatr Med 2013;29(1):101–36.
34. Hshieh TT, Yue J, Oh E, et al. Effectiveness of multicomponent nonpharmacological delirium interventions: a meta-analysis. JAMA Intern Med 2015;175(4): 512–20.
35. Flaherty JH, Little MO. Matching the environment to patients with delirium: lessons learned from the delirium room, a restraint-free environment for older hospitalized adults with delirium. J Am Geriatr Soc 2011;59(Suppl 2):S295–300.
36. Inouye SK, Charpentier PA. Precipitating factors for delirium in hospitalized elderly persons. Predictive model and interrelationship with baseline vulnerability. JAMA 1996;275(11):852–7.
37. Holroyd-Leduc JM, Sen S, Bertenthal D, et al. The relationship of indwelling urinary catheters to death, length of hospital stay, functional decline, and nursing home admission in hospitalized older medical patients. J Am Geriatr Soc 2007; 55(2):227–33.
38. Kishi T, Hirota T, Matsunaga S, et al. Antipsychotic medications for the treatment of delirium: a systematic review and meta-analysis of randomised controlled trials. J Neurol Neurosurg Psychiatry 2015. http://dx.doi.org/10.1136/jnnp-2015-311049.
39. Hatta K, Kishi Y, Wada K, et al. Antipsychotics for delirium in the general hospital setting in consecutive 2453 inpatients: a prospective observational study. Int J Geriatr Psychiatry 2014;29(3):253–62.
40. Maneeton B, Maneeton N, Srisurapanont M, et al. Quetiapine versus haloperidol in the treatment of delirium: a double-blind, randomized, controlled trial. Drug Des Devel Ther 2013;7:657–67.

41. Yoon HJ, Park KM, Choi WJ, et al. Efficacy and safety of haloperidol versus atypical antipsychotic medications in the treatment of delirium. BMC Psychiatry 2013; 13:240.

42. Goldman JG, Holden S. Treatment of psychosis and dementia in Parkinson's disease. Curr Treat Options Neurol 2014;16(3):281.

43. Michaud CJ, Bullard HM, Harris SA, et al. Impact of quetiapine treatment on duration of hypoactive delirium in critically ill adults: a retrospective analysis. Pharmacotherapy 2015;35(8):731–9.

44. Lonergan E, Luxenberg J, Areosa Sastre A, et al. Benzodiazepines for delirium. Cochrane Database Syst Rev 2009;(4):CD006379.

45. Riker RR, Shehabi Y, Bokesch PM, et al. Dexmedetomidine vs midazolam for sedation of critically ill patients: a randomized trial. JAMA 2009;301(5):489–99.

46. Sessums LL, Zembrzuska H, Jackson JL. Does this patient have medical decision-making capacity? JAMA 2011;306(4):420–7.

47. Drickamer M, Lai J. Hazzard's geriatric medicine and gerontology. 6th edition. New York: McGraw-Hill Professional; 2009.

48. Kennedy M, Enander RA, Tadiri SP, et al. Delirium risk prediction, healthcare use and mortality of elderly adults in the emergency department. J Am Geriatr Soc 2014;62(3):462–9.

49. Swaminathan RV, Rao SV, McCoy LA, et al. Hospital length of stay and clinical outcomes in older STEMI patients after primary PCI: a report from the National Cardiovascular Data Registry. J Am Coll Cardiol 2015;65(12):1161–71.

# Palliative Care in the Emergency Department

Alyssia McEwan, DO, Joshua Z. Silverberg, MD*

## KEYWORDS

- Palliative care • Geriatric • End of life • Emergency medicine • Surrogate
- Communication

## KEY POINTS

- Shared decision making between physicians and patients/surrogates should be the framework for all conversations and decisions involving palliative and end-of-life care.
- Patient autonomy is the gold standard for decisions pertaining to care. If patients are unable to communicate; focus on prospective autonomy through substitute decision makers and written directives.
- Alleviation of suffering owing to end-of-life symptoms, whether physical or existential, is the responsibility of the emergency physician.
- Familiarity with evidence-based recommendations about symptom management at end of life is essential.

## INTRODUCTION

Emergency medicine (EM) is generally thought of as a resuscitative specialty, one that revolves around the identification of life-threatening conditions and swift intervention with the goal of curative treatment. The American College of Emergency Physicians defines the specialty of EM as "a medical specialty dedicated to the diagnosis and treatment of unforeseen illness or injury."[1]

The inherent culture of EM makes discussion revolving around impending death and associated symptoms incongruous with some emergency physicians, because the mere acknowledgment of this discussion may be perceived as failure. "Emergency medicine physicians are trained to save lives, not to manage death" is a statement that resonates with some emergency physicians in training.[2] Statistically, EM residents place training in palliative care to be at a lower priority than do residents in other specialties such as pediatrics and internal medicine.[2]

Disclosure Statement: J.Z. Silverberg owns equity in Johnson and Johnson and Pfizer; A. McEwan has nothing to disclose.
Department of Emergency Medicine, Albert Einstein College of Medicine, 1400 Pelham Parkway South, Building 6, Suite 1B-25, Bronx, NY 10461, USA
* Corresponding author.
E-mail address: Joshua.Silverberg@nbhn.net

Emerg Med Clin N Am 34 (2016) 667–685
http://dx.doi.org/10.1016/j.emc.2016.04.013
0733-8627/16/$ – see front matter © 2016 Elsevier Inc. All rights reserved.
emed.theclinics.com

The reality is that, although the majority of people wish to die at home, a significant number of patients in the final stages of their life visit the emergency department and are under the care of an emergency physician.[3] This number is continually growing as the aging population increases. According to the World Health Organization (WHO), between 2015 and 2050, the proportion of the world's population over 60 years will double. By 2050, there will be more than 400 million people aged 80 and older worldwide.[4] Experts are acutely aware of this fact and structure is in place for addressing this. In 2006, hospice and palliative medicine was recognized as an EM subspecialty by the American Board of Medical Specialties.[2] In 2007, Education in Palliative and End-of-life Care for Emergency Medicine was implemented to teach clinical competencies in palliative care to EM professionals.[2]

The groundbreaking Study to Understand Prognoses and Preferences for Outcomes and Risks of Treatments (SUPPORT) Trial (*JAMA* 1995) raised awareness of many of the shortcomings of care for seriously ill and dying hospitalized patients. The principal investigators concluded through their research that the care of seriously ill or dying patients is far from ideal and that "One would certainly prefer to envision that, when confronted with life-threatening illness, the patient and family would be included in discussions, realistic estimates of outcome would be valued, pain would be treated, and dying would not be prolonged."[5]

## COMMUNICATION WITH PATIENTS AND SURROGATES

Being comfortable with conversations pertaining to end-of-life and palliative issues is imperative for all physicians working in the emergency department. It has even been proposed that that training in communication skills should be integrated with mandatory resuscitation training.[6]

To adhere to best practice communication skills, it is useful to understand the concept of shared decision making and decision frames, and to be aware of certain tools for embarking on a discussion with a patient and/or their surrogate.

### Shared Decision Making

End-of-life discussions should be centered around a shared decision making model. This approach is often the crux of patient-centered medicine.[7] Shared decision making was first coined in 1988 by the Picker Institute and introduced as one of the fundamental approaches to improving health care delivery in the United States.[8] The Institute of Medicine defines shared decision making as "care that is respectful of and responsive to individual patient preferences, needs and values, and ensuring that patient values guide all clinical decisions."[9]

### Decision Frames

The way information is presented by the physician can have a significant impact on the decisions patients and their surrogates make. This phenomenon of "decision frame" was described by Tversky and Kahneman in 1981 in their landmark publication on the psychology of choice. People often demonstrate preference reversal, depending on how the physician frames the information. When choices are presented in terms of gains, people are risk averse and when choices are presented in terms of losses, people are risk seeking.[10,11]

A 2013 Barnato study demonstrated this effect with a randomized simulation experiment exploring the effects of surrogate emotional state and physician communication strategies on surrogate code status decisions. One of the only factors that had an effect on the cardiopulmonary resuscitation choice was how the physician framed he decision. The physicians either used the language of do not resuscitate (DNR) or he alternative allow natural death. Using the alternative language caused people to choose that option more often.[12]

Physicians are not always aware of the way they frame their discussions. In 2015, Lu and associates conducted a high-fidelity simulation study with emergency physicians, hospitalists, and critical care involving an elder with end-stage cancer and life-threatening hypoxia. When debriefed, many of the physicians who used language strongly indicating the necessity of life-sustaining treatment (intubation), felt intubation was actually inappropriate for the patient. The result of this in the simulation was that many times the simulated patient was intubated contrary to their initial wishes and even contrary to what the physician felt was appropriate.[13]

## Tools and Models to Aid in Communication

Researchers in palliative care, geriatrics, and oncology have published several tools and models to aid in difficult discussions with seriously ill patients. The Education in Palliative and End-of-life Care 6-step model, also known as the SPIKES model (setup–perception–invitation–knowledge–empathize; **Box 1**) is one of the most widely

---

**Box 1**
**SPIKES model**

*Setup*

- Prepare yourself with the medical facts.
- Determine who will participate in the conversation.
- Determine the location of the discussion, preferably a quiet location.
- Obtain a translator if needed.
- Let other staff know what you are going to be doing to avoid interruptions.

*Perception*

- Determine the participant's current perception about the situation.

*Invitation*

- Determine how much information the participants want to find out.

*Knowledge*

- Give a *warning shot*, for example, "I have some serious news to tell you."
- Deliver information in small parts.
- Avoid medical jargon.
- Allow time for comprehension.

*Empathize*

- Address participants' emotions and allow time for participants to understand their emotions (NURSE mnemonic; see **Box 2**).
- Resist the temptation to make things better.

*Summary*

- Summarize everything discussed and allow time for questions.

*Data from* Back AL, Arnold RM, Baile WF, et al. Approaching difficult communication tasks in oncology. CA Cancer J Clin 2005;55(3):164–77; and Rodriguez V. Communication: the most valuable palliative care tool. 2015. Available at: https://www.quantiamd.com/player/yemeuzwgd?cid=1818. Accessed November 5, 2015.

used and accepted models for discussing unfavorable news in the health care setting. This is commonly used in the emergency department for sharing test results, but is also helpful when discussing how to proceed with either aggressive resuscitation or palliation for a patient with progression of an end-stage disease.

If you need to elicit information regarding advance directives or a care plan for something that is happening in real time, an appropriate time to do so would be after going through SPIKES.

Responding to the emotions of the patient is important for communication. The NURSE (naming–understanding–respecting–supporting) mnemonic can help a physician give appropriate responses to the patient's or surrogate's emotions (**Box 2**).

In the emergency department, "ask–tell–ask" (**Box 3**) is a useful technique for communication when time is limited. It has 3 main steps and is a collaborative way to discuss new developments and discuss a treatment plan. This is an efficient way to get the patient/surrogate information, short of just spouting facts about the current situation.

Similar to SPIKES, after going through ask–tell–ask, it is appropriate to then elicit information about advanced directives and to discuss a treatment plan.

### Communication Behaviors to Avoid

Just as there are communication behaviors to foster, there are also communication behaviors to avoid (**Table 1**).

---

**Box 2**
**NURSE mnemonic for responding to emotions**

*Naming*

- Name the emotion that the participant seems to be experiencing in a suggestive way, that is:
  - "Some people may feel frustrated in this situation."
  - "It seems that you might be feeling afraid of what is next."
- Avoid telling listener how they are feeling.

*Understanding*

- Try to summarize what you are hearing:
  - "I am hearing you say that you are afraid of telling your siblings about this change in condition."

*Respecting*

- Match the intensity of your acknowledgment to the intensity of the participant's display of emotion.
- Consider praising coping skills of the participant at this point:
  - "I'm impressed with the care you have been giving your father during his long battle with cancer."

*Supporting*

- Tell the participants how much longer you will be present in the emergency department for support and let them know that you are there for them.
- Consider involving social worker or another staff member for further support.

*Exploring*

- Ask focused questions or express interest in something that was mentioned to deepen the empathetic connection.

*Data from* Rodriguez V. Communication: the most valuable palliative care tool. Available at: https://www.quantiamd.com/player/yemeuzwgd?cid=1818. Accessed November 5, 2015; and Back AL. Approaching difficult communication tasks in oncology. CA Cancer J Clin 2005; 55(3):164–77.

Palliative Care in the Emergency Department

---

**Box 3**
**Ask–Tell–Ask**

*Ask*

• Ask the patient/surrogate to tell you their level of understanding about the current situation.

*Tell*

• Tell the patient/surrogate the information that they need to know.

• Avoid lecturing or giving large amount of information at 1 time.

*Ask*

• Ask the patient/surrogate if they understand what was just told to them; consider asking them to repeat back what they have heard.

*Data from* Rodriguez V. Communication: the most valuable palliative care tool. Available at: https://www.quantiamd.com/player/yemeuzwgd?cid=1818. Accessed November 5, 2015.

---

### Communicating News Over the Telephone

As emergency physicians, we are often faced with the task of conveying grave news. This is best done face to face. If a surrogate is not present in the emergency department, it is better to encourage them to come to the emergency department for a conversation in person than to deliver the news over the phone. If it is not possible

---

**Table 1**
**Communication behaviors to avoid**

| Behavior | Description | Example and/or Rationale Behind Behavior | Result |
|---|---|---|---|
| Blocking | Patient/surrogate raises concern; doctor fails to respond or redirects the conversation. | *Patient:* "How long do you think I have?" *Doctor:* "Do not worry about that, how's your breathing?" | Results in not addressing the patient's most important concerns. |
| Lecturing | Doctor delivers a large amount of information without giving patient chance to respond/ask questions. | Doctors often revert to discussing medical facts when in the face of emotion. | Patient does not absorb information and may result in perpetuation of negative emotions by patients owing to lack of understanding. |
| Collusion | Patients do not bring up difficult topics and physicians do not ask them specifically. "Don't ask, don't' tell". | Patient assumes that doctor will bring it up if it is important AND doctor assumes that if the patient wants to know, they will ask. | Important conversations do not occur. |
| Premature Reassurance | Doctor responds to patient's concern with reassurance before understanding the emotion. | Often occurs when doctors feel that they do not have enough time to explore patient concerns. | Patient does not feel that they were understood, often leads to repeated questioning. |

*Adapted from* Back A, Arnold RM, Baile WF, et al. Approaching difficult communication tasks in oncology. CA Cancer J Clin 2005;55:164–77.

to have a conversation in person, the SPIKES, ask–tell–ask, and NURSE tools can be used. Below are helpful considerations for delivering bad news over the phone.[14]

1. Confirm the clinical information and make sure that you are prepared for the discussion.
2. Prevent interruptions by letting others know what you are doing and if interruptions are unavoidable, inform the surrogate in advance.
3. Ask the person on the phone to identify themselves and their relationship to the patient.
4. Ask the surrogate whether it is an appropriate time and place to have a serious conversation. If possible, make sure that the surrogate is not driving or in another situation that could be dangerous for them.
5. Encourage them to express their emotions; ask, "How are you feeling?" Allow time for processing of information.
6. Ask them to explain their understanding of the situation.
7. If the patient has died, give them specific next steps to take. If the patient is living and you wish to ascertain information about advanced directives, do so while being cognizant of framing effects (see "Decision Frames").

## SUBSTITUTE DECISION MAKERS AND WRITTEN DIRECTIVES

The most widely accepted view of end-of-life decision making is that decisions should be made based on the beliefs, preferences, and values of the patient. This emphasis on patient autonomy in decision making is widely accepted. Despite the common perception that everyone wants to make their own decisions, there is a minority of the population that would like those decisions entrusted to a close family member. To ensure a truly patient-centered approach, it is important to first determine the preferences of the patient.[15]

Patient autonomy is considered the gold standard but cannot always be relied on. Many elderly patients arriving in the emergency department at the end of life are unable to answer direct questions about the care they would like provided, commonly owing to their immediate clinical condition and/or cognitive impairment. In situations where patients lose decisional capacity, we rely on the concept of prospective autonomy, which means that personal values and priorities of patients will continue to dictate decisions about their care. We rely on designated decision makers or written directives for guidance regarding the patient's wishes for care at the end of life.

To navigate decision making for patients who have lost capacity, it is important to understand the meaning of the terminology used to describe the decision makers, the documents, and implications of various advanced directives. Notably, staff members in the emergency department failing to recognize the significance of the legal decision maker has been cited as a criticism of some family members when questioned about their experiences.[16]

To defer to a surrogate decision maker, it is necessary for the physician to first determine that the patient has lost decisional capacity. Decisional capacity is the ability of a person to understand his or her medical situation and to weigh the benefits, burdens, and risks of various treatment options. It also requires that the decision(s) made are consistent over time and that the decisions can be communicated. If it is unclear whether the patient has decisional capacity, it may be beneficial to consult psychiatry to help with the determination.

### ubstitute Decision Makers

After determining that the patient lacks decisional capacity, physicians often turn to a substitute decision maker for guidance. The substitute decision maker steps in only if and when the patient loses capacity to make their own decisions and lasts for as long as that is the case. They evaluate the information and make decisions that they believe the patient would make if they were able. There are different types of substitute decision makers, including health care proxies (HCPs), surrogates, and next of kin.

### Health care proxy

The term "health care proxy" (HCP) refers to both the substitute decision maker and the legal document that is signed by the patient which appoints a person this distinction. The HCP must be at least 18 years of age and must be appointed by the patient.

### Surrogate

A *surrogate* is similar to an HCP, but without being legally appointed as the decision maker. They must be a competent adult at least 18, know the patient well, and be familiar with the patient's wishes regarding their care.

### Next of kin

The next of kin is the patient's closest living relative. The order of hierarchy in determining next of kin in the United States is as follows:

1. Spouse
2. Children
3. Parents
4. Siblings
5. Grandparents
6. Uncles and aunts
7. Cousins

Spouses in this list include same-sex couples following the recent United State Supreme Court decision (*Obergefell v Hodges*) granting same-sex couples the right to marry.

In the case of informal/unofficial substitute decision makers (surrogates, next of kin), there are ethical considerations about who to turn to for guidance. With the increased complexity of modern families, legal definitions and hierarchy do not necessarily adhere to the purpose of a substitute decision maker, which is to maintain patient autonomy. Moral criteria for surrogate selection include choosing an individual who is most likely to know the patient's wishes and who is closest to the patient.[17] This person may or may not be a blood relative of the patient, and the physician should consider this when determining which person will guide decision making.

### Written Directives

There are 3 main types of written directives that can guide treatment at the EOL. Regardless of the type, these directives become valid only if/when a person becomes unable to communicate the decisions that they make about their care.

- Advance directives
- Do-not-resuscitate/do-not-intubate orders (DNR/DNI)
- Physician orders for life-sustaining treatment (POLST)

### Advance directives

Advance directives are further subdivided into the living will and the durable power of attorney for health care (also known as health care power of attorney and HCP, see above).

The *living will* is a legal document that must be written and signed by the patient. For a living will to be honored, in addition to the patient being unable to communicate their own decisions, they must also have a terminal illness or be permanently unconscious. If there is a chance for recovery, a living will does not apply. These forms must be signed by witnesses and notarized. Refer to **Box 4** for a list of people who are usually excluded as witnesses for this document.[18] A living will generally has specifics about what the patient does and does not want to undergo at the end of their life. Examples of information included in living wills are provided in **Box 5**.

The *durable power of attorney for health care* is a legal document in which a person is named as an agent to make all health care decisions if the patient is unable to do so. The ultimate goal of surrogacy is to maintain patient autonomy in the situation of a patient being unable to communicate their wishes. If a patient has previously documented a DNR/DNI request, this durable power of attorney for health care may not override a decision that has been made and documented by the patient when they were able to do so.

### Do-not-resuscitate, do-not-intubate, and do-not-hospitalize orders

Simply, these orders are to withhold cardiopulmonary resuscitation or intubation and do not extend further than these 2 concepts. All other care would be continued as is standard of care unless further delineated by any advance directive the patient might have.[18]

There are DNR orders specifically for in-hospital and for out-of-hospital scenarios. Out-of-hospital DNR orders are primarily for emergency medical services personnel and are in the form of a written document and, in some states, a bracelet. Some hospitals require a new DNR each time a patient is admitted. There is state-by-state variation in laws pertaining to DNR orders, both in and out of hospitals. This information can generally be found on the Department of Health websites for each state.

DNR and DNI orders have different implications depending on whether cardiac or pulmonary arrest is present. In cardiac or pulmonary arrest, a DNR order inherently includes an order to not intubate the patient. In nonarrest situations, where intubation is indicated, a separate DNI order is required to forego intubation. See **Table 2** for further clarification.[19]

As evident in the third and most rare scenario of "DNI only," there is a severe limitation on the physician's ability to provide effective resuscitation.[19]

A do-not-hospitalize order is another type of advance directive that is relevant for some nursing home residents who are impaired in their ability to communicate. This order specifies that, in the case of an acute medical crisis, the resident should not be transferred to a hospital for care.

| Box 4 Witness exclusions |
| --- |
| Spouses |
| Potential heirs |
| Doctors caring for the patient |
| Employees of the patient's health care facility |

---

**Box 5**
**Examples of living will content**

Use of equipment (dialysis machines, ventilators)

Orders pertaining to resuscitation (do-not-resuscitate and do-not-intubate orders)

Artificial fluids and nutrition

Symptomatic relief of pain, nausea, other symptoms

Organ donation

---

**Table 2**
**Implications of variations in DNR/DNI orders based on scenario**

|  | Cardiac or Pulmonary Arrest | Nonarrest |
|---|---|---|
| 1. DNR and DNI | No CPR, No intubation | No intubation |
| 2. DNR only | No CPR, No intubation | Perform intubation |
| 3. DNI only | Perform CPR, No intubation | No intubation |

*Abbreviations:* CPR, cardiopulmonary resuscitation; DNI, do not intubate; DNR, do not resuscitate.

### *Physician orders for life-sustaining treatment*

The National POLST Paradigm is an approach to advanced care planning that provides patients and their families an opportunity to guide EM personnel actions. A POLST is a medium by which detailed plan about end-of-life care can be communicated. Essentially, it gives specific and actionable details of the care that the patient would or would not like to receive at the end of life. POLST complements advance directives and is not meant to replace it. The POLST form is filled out by a physician after a conversation with patient and their family and is meant to guide treatment that the patient wants to have carried out.[20]

There is substantial variation among different states in the United States regarding POLST. As of 2015, there are only 5 states that do not have some form of POLST: Alabama, Alaska, Arkansas, Nebraska, and South Dakota. Not only does the name of the program vary (ie, POLST, MOLST, MOST, TPOPP, LaPOST, POST, COLST), but the structure of each program has a lot of variation as well. The POLST website, www.polst.org is the primary resource to find out more about POLST in each individual state.

### CATEGORIES OF CARE

It is important to understand each category of care as they have different implications. The types of care to be discussed here are palliative care, end-of-life care, hospice care, and comfort measures only care.

### *Palliative Care*

The WHO defines Palliative Care as "an approach that improves the quality of life of patients and their families facing the problems associated with life-threatening illness, through the prevention and relief of suffering by means of early identification and impeccable assessment and treatment of pain and other problems, physical, psychosocial and spiritual."[21] A patient does not need to be at the end of their life to be a candidate for palliative care.

### End-of-Life Care

An obstacle when discussing issues surrounding the "end of life" is the lack of a coherent, widely accepted definition of this term. It can be defined by diagnosis, prognostic criteria, symptom expression, hospice eligibility, and other factors. Lorenz and colleagues[22] propose that "the broadest approach to 'end-of-life' refers to a chronologically indefinite part of life when patients and their caregivers are struggling with the implications (eg, symptoms, practical support needs) of an advanced chronic illness." Most commonly, the terms "end-of-life care" and "hospice care" are interchangeable.

### Hospice Care

Hospice care is care focused on symptom relief at the end of life and is most commonly provided for patients with a life expectancy of 6 months or less. According to the National Hospice and Palliative Care Organization, hospice care is defined as "a team-oriented approach to expert medical care, pain management, and emotional and spiritual support expressly tailored to the patient's needs and wishes. Support is provided to the patient's loved ones as well."[23]

The Medicare Hospice Benefits booklet (updated in January 2015) explains hospice further: "When you choose hospice care, you've decided that you no longer want care to cure your terminal illness and related conditions, and/or your doctor has determined that efforts to cure your illness aren't working." Once hospice care is chosen, Medicare ceases to pay for a multitude of health care related costs, including care in an emergency room (unless visit is unrelated to the terminal illness or related condition; **Table 3**).[24]

| Table 3 Comparison of palliative care and hospice | |
|---|---|
| **Palliative Care** | **Hospice** |
| Palliative and curative treatments can be provided at the same time. | Treatment is geared toward symptom relief at the end of life; cessation of curative treatments. |
| Some treatment and medications may be covered by Medicare/Medicaid. | Medicare pays all hospice charges. Medicaid pays in most states. |

### Comfort Measures Only

The Joint Commission National Quality Core Measures Manual defines comfort measures only as "medical treatment of a dying person where the natural dying process is permitted to occur while ensuring maximum comfort."[25] These actions are not designed to hasten the end of life; they are designed to make it less difficult. Although patients have the right to opt out of certain treatments, they may still choose to engage in other types of treatments and interventions. The emphasis should not be on "withholding care," but instead should be placed on providing care that is in line with the patient's wishes.[26]

## SYMPTOM RECOGNITION

It can be challenging for a physician to determine whether some geriatric patients are experiencing discomfort or unwanted symptoms, especially in patients with dementia. This is likely the reason that patients with dementia receive less pain medication than their cognitively intact counterparts.[27] Patients with dementia are less likely to be able to self-report symptoms owing to loss of language skills and other cognitive deficits.

Although self-report is the gold standard for identifying pain and other unwanted sources of suffering (such as hunger, emotional distress, constipation, and cold), it is crucial to modify your approach when dealing with patients with dementia. Relying heavily on self-reported symptoms may result in an increased risk of underdiagnosis and inadequate treatment.[26] This becomes increasingly important as the number of new cases of Alzheimer's disease and other dementias is projected to double by 2050 with increasing life expectancy in the United States.[28]

In this population, pain may manifest differently than in cognitively intact patients, often with decreased mobility and agitation, and increased confusion as the only signs indicating pain.[29] The PAINAD observational pain assessment tool was developed in 2003 by Warden as a way to identify pain in patients with advanced dementia who are noncommunicative.[30,31] Several studies have compared different pain scales and the PAINAD scale has fared well in comparison.[29,32] The PAINAD tool requires observation of the patient for 5 minutes, focusing on 5 different behaviors: breathing, negative vocalization, facial expression, body language, and consolability. The total score is a compilation of scores from individual categories: 10 being severe pain and 0 being no pain (**Table 4**) According to Zwakhalen,[33] a score of 2 on the PAINAD scale can be used as an indicator of probable pain and initiation of pain treatment.

Despite the potential usefulness of pain assessment tools, they must not be used to the exclusion of self-report. An attempt to elicit information regarding patient's level of comfort by speaking with the patient must be done first.

## SYMPTOM MANAGEMENT

At the end of life, managing unpleasant symptoms can often make more of a positive difference than aggressive interventions. When managing patients at the true end of life, there are some general considerations that can make the process easier for patients and their loved ones.

**Table 4**
**Pain assessment in advanced dementia (PAINAD) scale**

| Observation | 0 | 1 | 2 |
|---|---|---|---|
| Breathing independent of vocalization | Normal | Occasionally labored, short period of hyperventilation. | Noisy labored breathing, long period of hyperventilation, Cheyne–Stokes respiration. |
| Negative vocalization | None | Occasional moan or groan. Low level of speech with a negative or disapproving quality. | Repeated trouble calling out. Loud moaning or groaning. Crying. |
| Facial expression | Smiling or inexpressive | Sad, frightened, frown. | Facial grimacing. |
| Body language | Relaxed | Tense, distressed pacing, fidgeting. | Rigid, fists clenched, knees pulled up, pulling or pushing away, striking out. |
| Consolability | No need to console | Distracted or reassured by voice or touch. | Unable to console, distract, or reassure. |

*From* Warden V, Hurley AC, Volicer V. Development and psychometric evaluation of the pain assessment in advanced dementia (PAINAD) scale. J Am Med Dir Assoc 2003;4(1):9–15; with permission.

### General Considerations for the Dying Patient in the Emergency Department

When caring for dying patients in a busy and hectic emergency department, many challenges exist that may not exist if the patient were in their own home or even in an inpatient bed. The fact that the patient is dying in the emergency department does not mean that they do not deserve the maximum amount of dignity and respect possible.

In her 2013 EMCrit lecture on Critical Care Palliation, Dr Ashley Shreves offers some salient advice about selecting the appropriate environment for the dying patient in the emergency department: "When looking at a patient who is clearly at the end of their life, imagine that it is your family member and (ask yourself if you) would be comfortable with the environment that has been created for them."[34] The most appropriate place for these patients is a private quiet room. If this is not possible, try to arrange things such that the patient and their loved ones have some semblance of privacy. It is important that, after an ideal environment has been created for the patient and their loved ones, they are not then promptly forgotten. The families of dying patients should not be left feeling ignored after being placed in a quiet room.

"There is no place for monitors in the care of the actively dying patient who is endorsing comfort as their goal."[34] Alerts and other sounds from monitors have the potential to distract the patient's loved ones (during the dying process and take them out of their experience) during their last moments together. Dr Scott Weingart offers advice about monitors at the end of life in his EMCrit podcast discussing End-of-Life and Palliative care in the emergency department.[35] He suggests that leaving a pulse oximeter on the dying patient, with alarms turned off, can give you an unobtrusive way to assess the waveforms and oximetry, which can guide you about when the appropriate time is to reassess the patient's status.

### Selection of Therapy for the Symptomatic Geriatric Patient at the End of Life

Although many of the medications and treatments commonly used in younger, healthier adults are the same medications used in the geriatric population to manage symptoms at the end of life, there are additional pharmacokinetic considerations in this population.[36] Some physiologic changes that occur during aging may have a clinically significant effect on drug handling. Taking these changes into account is important when choosing the appropriate pharmacologic regimen to manage symptoms at the end of life in the geriatric population.[37]

Reduced blood flow to the gastrointestinal tract, liver, and kidneys cause medications to be absorbed and metabolized differently than they might in a younger person. Decreased blood flow to the gastrointestinal tract leads to an increased risk of gastrointestinal-related side effects, such as opioid-related decreased gut motility. Decreased hepatic blood flow causes a reduction in first pass metabolism that may lead to an increase in drug bioavailability. Decreased renal blood flow may reduce excretion of drugs and metabolites leading to accumulation and prolonged effects.[37]

Decreased body water, increased body fat, and a lower concentration of plasma proteins lead to changes in drug distribution. Thus, water-soluble drugs have reduced distribution, lipid soluble drugs have a longer half-life, and there is an increased potential for drug–drug interactions.[37]

Hepatic metabolism is affected not only because of reduced hepatic blood flow. There is also a reduction in liver mass and functioning liver cells, which may lead to a prolonged half-life owing to reduction in oxidation reactions.[37]

Pharmacodynamic changes of decreased receptor density and increased receptor affinity may lead to increased sensitivity to drug effect, both with therapeutic response and significance of side effects.[37]

## Most Common End-of-Life Symptoms

The WHO analyzed a tremendous amount of evidence to determine the symptoms occurring most commonly at the end of life (**Table 5**).[38] The WHO last updated their Model List of Essential Medications in palliative care based on most common end-of-life symptoms in July 2013. The list is created after extensive research about the most common causes of death, the most distressing symptoms in palliative care, and identification of medicines recommended for treatment of the symptoms based on evidence (**Table 6**).[39] Below are specific treatment options for dyspnea, a common symptom seen in the emergency department particularly at the end of life.[39]

## Treating Dyspnea

The most commonly used therapies for dyspnea at the end of life are oxygen, opioids, and noninvasive positive pressure ventilation. A "distress protocol" (DP) for acute respiratory emergencies in terminally ill patients has also been proposed.

### Oxygen

The use of oxygen for dyspnea in palliative care is controversial. There is clear evidence that oxygen for hypoxemia is an important and beneficial treatment; however, oxygen therapy for normoxemic patients is generally not beneficial for patients who are near death.[40,41] Although there is a significant body of evidence discussing the uncertainty of appropriateness of oxygen use in palliative care for normoxemic patients, there is an ongoing dilemma. Kelly[41] explored this phenomenon and discovered that there are multiple factors that lead to (possibly inappropriate) oxygen use in palliative care: to appease patients and families who expect oxygen, to help health care workers feel better about themselves in the caring role, and to appease health care workers' own frustration and guilt in futile situations.

The use of air provides similar relief of breathlessness to oxygen—the mechanism of which is based on facial cooling and airflow. A simple handheld fan with air directed toward the face can reduce dyspnea.[41] Using a nasal cannula can cause skin irritation and can be uncomfortable, especially if there is a significant amount of flow of oxygen through the nares.

### Opioids

Opioids are a mainstay treatment for dyspnea in palliative care because they diminish respiratory drive in response to hypoxia and hypercapnia. A Cochrane Review of opioids for dyspnea supports the use of oral and parenteral opioids for dyspnea in advanced disease.[42] Opioids have the added benefit of treating pain and anxiety, which are contributors to suffering during periods of breathlessness.[43] A peripheral mechanism acting on lung parenchyma also exists, inhibiting the bronchoconstrictive

| Table 5 | | |
|---|---|---|
| **Most common EOL symptoms** | | |
| Anorexia | Depression | Nausea |
| Anxiety | Diarrhea | Pain |
| Constipation | Dyspnea | Respiratory tract secretions |
| Delirium | Fatigue | Vomiting |

| Table 6 |
|---|
| **Medications to treat common symptoms at the end of life based on WHO EML** |

| Class of Medication (Specific Medication on EML) | Symptom(s) to Treat |
|---|---|
| Opioids (morphine) | Air hunger |
| | Acute pain |
| | Dyspnea |
| Benzodiazepines (diazepam, lorazepam) | Anxiety |
| | Immediate anterograde amnestic properties |
| | Sedative |
| Antipsychotics (haloperidol) | Agitation |
| Antiemetics (metoclopramide) | Nausea and vomiting |
| NSAIDs (ibuprofen) | Pain |
| Antimuscarinics (hyoscine butylbromide) | Respiratory secretions |

*Abbreviations:* EML, Model List of Essential Medications; NSAIDs, nonsteroidal antiinflammatory drugs; WHO, World Health Organization.

response provoked by vagal stimuli. Because of this, morphine for intractable cough in advanced cancer has been proposed as per 2 case studies with promising results.[44]

Many physicians are fearful that administering opioids for dyspnea in patients with terminal disease will hasten death by causing respiratory depression. Although there is a small risk of causing respiratory depression in opioid naive patients, respiratory depression is very unlikely and the effects can be easily reversed by administering naloxone. The most appropriate way to administer opioids is careful titration of long-acting opioids with the addition of intermittent short-acting opioids for breakthrough pain.

### Noninvasive positive pressure ventilation

A randomized control trial by Nava[45] studied the effectiveness and mortality rate after use of NPPV in elderly patients greater than 75 years old with a DNI order. This randomized, controlled trial concluded that NPPV should be considered and offered as an alternative in patients with DNI status and/or those considered poor candidates for intubation. Schettino[46] looked at this same topic and determined that in patients with a DNI order and chronic obstructive pulmonary disease and cardiogenic pulmonary edema, NPPV successfully reversed acute respiratory failure and in-hospital mortality, but this was not observed in patients with end-stage cancer, hypoxemic respiratory failure, or postextubation failure.

### Distress Protocol

Godbout[39] discussed the use of a "distress protocol" (DP) to induce transient sedation in respiratory emergencies in terminally ill patients with chronic obstructive pulmonary disease or lung cancer. This is different from palliative sedation; it is not aimed at prolonging sedation until death. This is emergency sedation to treat unbearable symptoms that are common in terminal illness and at the end of life. The protocol involves subcutaneous injection of a combination of 3 medications: an anxiolytic, an opioid, and a muscarinic antagonist. The specific protocol discussed by Godbout can be found in **Box 6**. This cocktail may be repeated after 15 minutes if not effective in minimizing distress. Use of this cocktail did not hasten death, because there was no difference between time to death from admission in patients who did and did not receive DP.[39] The

| Box 6 |
| --- |
| **Distress protocol (in combination, subcutaneous route)** |
| 5 mg midazolam |
| 10 mg morphine |
| 0.4 mg scopolamine |

ndividual effects of the medications in the DP are aimed at relieving the most likely symptoms the patient is experiencing. If the DP does not induce sedation, it will likely at least alleviate some of the distressing symptoms that the patient is experiencing. Before widespread acceptance in the United States of this protocol, further evaluation s necessary, but it has the potential for decreasing distress in patients experiencing respiratory emergencies caused by terminal illness (see **Box 6**).

## Palliative Sedation

End-of-life symptoms can be extremely distressing and at times unbearable. Respiratory distress, intractable pain, and severe hemorrhage are some of the most traumatizing symptoms for patients and their families, and unfortunately, are very common at the end of life. Palliative sedation is defined as using medications to lessen patient consciousness for the purpose of limiting intractable and intolerable suffering.[47] It is on the spectrum of palliative and hospice care and is an appropriate therapy to consider in very specific circumstances.

Palliative sedation is most commonly used for situations of refractory pain, dyspnea, agitated delirium, and convulsions. The definition of a refractory symptom is one that cannot be controlled adequately despite aggressive efforts to identify a tolerable therapy that does not compromise consciousness.[48] Cherny and Portenoy[48] further define a refractory symptom to be one in which further invasive and/or noninvasive interventions meet any of the following criteria:

- Incapable of providing adequate relief
- Associated with excessive and intolerable acute or chronic adverse effects
- Unlikely to provide relief within a tolerable time frame

There are many ethical considerations that arise regarding palliative sedation. One of the primary discussion points is whether it hastens death. A 2015 Cochrane review assessing evidence for the benefit of palliative pharmacologic sedation discussed this issue. Although there were some methodologic limitations to the studies, 13 studies (of 14 reviewed) measured survival time to death from time of admission or referral and found no differences between the groups of sedated versus nonsedated patients.[49–51]

The other most common ethical consideration for palliative sedation is that family members and staff may have concerns that it is a form of euthanasia. Euthanasia is the "deliberate termination of life of a patient by active intervention at the request of the patient in a setting of uncontrolled suffering."[52,53] The goal of palliative sedation is not to hasten death or to terminate life; it is to provide relief from intolerable and intractable suffering. Thus, the distinction between palliative sedation and euthanasia is intent. The use of palliative sedation is supported by legal precedent if appropriate informed consent is obtained for this therapy. Supreme Court rulings (*Vacco v Quill*, 1997 and *Washington v Glucksberg*, 1997) supported the concept of sedation to relieve intractable suffering.[54] Informed consent must include the discussion about sedation preventing them from being able to eat and drink; implementation of artificial feeding and hydration should be discussed and considered.[54]

---

**Box 7**
**Proposed guidelines for considerations before sedation for existential suffering**

- The patient must have a terminal illness.
- All palliative treatments must be exhausted, including treatment for depression, delirium, anxiety, and so on.
- Psychological assessment by skilled clinician.
- Spiritual assessment by skilled clinician or clergy.
- A do-not-resuscitate order is in effect and informed consent has been obtained and documented.
- Informed consent obtained from patient/surrogate.
- Nutrition/hydration issues must be addressed before sedation.
- Consideration given to a trial of respite sedation.

*Adapted from* Rousseau P. Existential suffering and palliative sedation: a brief commentary with a proposal for clinical guidelines. Am J Hosp Palliat Care 2001;18(3):151–3.

---

The impetus for intolerable and intractable suffering is not confined to physical suffering. There is a large body of literature discussing the issue of existential suffering at the end of life and whether palliative sedation would be appropriate in this situation. Rousseau[55] proposed a set of guidelines by which sedation for existential suffering would be appropriate (**Box 7**).

Once it has been determined that palliative sedation is appropriate and agreed on by all deciding parties, the medications can be selected. There are no controlled trials comparing the efficacy of medications with sedating side effects. See **Table 7** for proposed agents and dosages.[56] The infusion should be initiated and titrated until the patient seems to be comfortable.

Many patients undergoing palliative sedation are already prescribed opioids, and they should not be withheld during sedation. Although opioids themselves are not used generally as a primary agent for sedation, some physicians believe that they are most appropriate in the care of the patient with a terminal disease who is primarily seeking comfort care because most symptoms are due to pain.[29]

The most appropriate course of action is to assess the patient fully and do your best to elucidate the cause of their emergent intractable and intolerable suffering—overwhelming pain crisis, asphyxiation, terminal dyspnea, and massive hemorrhage—and then tailor therapy to address the particular problem which they are facing.

---

**Table 7**
**Medications for palliative sedation**

| Medication | Bolus Dose | Infusion Dose |
|---|---|---|
| Midazolam (SC, IV) | 5 mg | 1 mg/h |
| Lorazepam (SC, IV) | 2–5 mg | 0.5–1.0 mg/h |
| Thiopental (IV) | 5–7 mg/kg/h | 20–80 mg/h |
| Pentobarbital (IV) | 1–2 mg/kg | 1 mg/kg/h |
| Phenobarbital (IV, SC) | 200 mg (can repeat q10–15 min) | 25 mg/h |
| Propofol (IV) | 20–50 mg (may repeat) | 5–10 mg/h |

*Abbreviations:* IV, intravenous; SC, subcutaneous.

## SUMMARY

As an emergency physician, it is just as important to be prepared to care for the geriatric patient suffering at the end of their life as it is to care for the young trauma patient. There is always something that we can do, and we should never tell a patient or their loved one that there is "nothing that we can do." Even if it is something as simple as actively listening to a patient, to acknowledge their suffering and to offer them compassion. By understanding how our communication can have an effect on outcomes, how to navigate advance directives, and how to recognize and treat common symptoms in the geriatric population, we can provide better care to this ever-increasing population.

## REFERENCES

1. American College of Emergency Physicians (ACEP). Definition of emergency medicine. Available at: https://www.acep.org/Clinical—Practice-Management/Definition-of-an-Emergency-Service/. Accessed August 19, 2015.
2. Meo N, Hwang U, Morrison RS. Resident perceptions of palliative care training in the emergency department. J Palliat Med 2011;14(5):548–55.
3. Shreves A. End of life/palliative care/ethics. Emerg Med Clin North Am 2014;32: 955–74.
4. World Health Organization (WHO). 10 facts on ageing and health. Available at: www.who.int/features/factfiles/ageing/en/. Accessed August 19, 2015.
5. A controlled trial to improve care for seriously ill hospitalized patients. The study to understand prognoses and preferences for outcomes and risks of treatments (SUPPORT). The SUPPORT principal investigators. JAMA 1995;274(20):1591–8.
6. Stupple A. Training in communication skills should be integrated with mandatory resuscitation training. BMJ 2015;350:h1405.
7. Stacey D. Decision aids for people facing health treatment or screening decisions. Cochrane Database Syst Rev 2014;(1):CD001431.
8. Barry MJ, Edgman-Levitan S. Shared decision making — the pinnacle of patient-centered care. N Engl J Med 2012;366(9):780–1.
9. Committee on Quality of Health Care in America. Crossing the quality chasm a new health system for the 21st century. Washington, DC: National Academy Press; 2001.
10. Tversky A, Kahneman D. The framing of decisions and the psychology of choice. Science 1981;211(4481):453–8.
11. Gamliel E. To end life or not to prolong life: the effect of message framing on attitudes toward euthanasia. J Health Psychol 2012;18(5):693–703.
12. Barnato AE, Arnold RM. The effect of emotion and physician communication behaviors on surrogates' life-sustaining treatment decisions: a randomized simulation experiment. Crit Care Med 2013;41(7):1686–91.
13. Lu A, Mohan D, Alexander SC, et al. The language of end-of-life decision making: a simulation study. J Palliat Med 2015;18(9):740–6.
14. Ngo-Metzger Q. Breaking bad news over the phone. Am Fam Physician 2009; 80(5):520.
15. Braun UK, Beyth RJ, Ford ME, et al. Decision-making styles of seriously ill male veterans for end-of-life care: autonomists, altruists, authorizers, absolute trusters, and avoiders. Patient Educ Couns 2014;94(3):334–41.
16. Morphet JJ, Decker K, Crawford K, et al. Aged care residents in the emergency department: the experiences of relatives. J Clin Nurs 2015;24:3647–53.

17. Watson AA. Biologically-related or emotionally-connected: who would be the better surrogate decision-maker? Med Health Care Philos 2015;18:147–8.
18. American Cancer Society 2015. Advanced directives. Available at: www.cancer.org/acs/groups/cid/documents/webcontent/002016-pdf.pdf. Accessed December 13, 2015.
19. Post LF, Blustein J. Handbook for health care ethics committee. 2nd edition. Baltimore: Johns Hopkins University Press; 2006.
20. What is POLST? National POLST. Available at: www.polst.org. Accessed December 12, 2015.
21. World Health Organization (WHO). Definition of palliative care. Geneva: WHO. Available at: www.who.int/cancer/palliative/definition/en/. Accessed December 12, 2015.
22. Lorenz KA, Lynn J, Morton SC, et al. Methodological approaches for a systematic review of end-of-life care. J Palliat Med 2005;8(Suppl 1):S4–11.
23. National Hospice and Palliative Care Organization (NHPCO). National hospice and palliative care organization. Available at: www.nhpco.org/about/hospice-care. Accessed August 15, 2015.
24. Centers for Medicare and Medicaid Services. Medicare Hospice Benefits Booklet. Revised 2015. Available at: http://www.medicare.gov/Pubs/pdf/02154.pdf. Accessed December 15, 2015.
25. Comfort Measures Only. Comfort measures only. Available at: https://manual.jointcommission.org/releases/tjc2015a/dataelem0031.html. Accessed August 15, 2015.
26. van der Steen JT, Sampson EL, Block LVD, et al. Tools to assess pain or lack of comfort in dementia: a content analysis. J Pain Symptom Manage 2015;50(5): 659–75.
27. Oosterman JM, Hendriks H, Scott S, et al. When pain memories are lost: a pilot study of semantic knowledge of pain in dementia. Pain Med 2014;15(5):751–7.
28. Alzheimer's Association. 2015 Alzheimer's disease facts and figures. 2015. Available at: https://www.alz.org/facts/downloads/facts_figures_2015.pdf. Accessed August 19, 2015.
29. Pautex S, Michon A, Guedira M, et al. Pain in severe dementia: self-assessment or observational scales? J Am Geriatr Soc 2006;54(7):1040–5.
30. Klapwijk MS, Caljouw MA, Soest-Poortvliet MCV, et al. Symptoms and treatment when death is expected in dementia patients in long-term care facilities. BMC Geriatr 2014;14:99.
31. Warden VV. Development and psychometric evaluation of the pain assessment in advanced dementia (PAINAD) scale. J Am Med Dir Assoc 2003;4:9–15.
32. Ngu SS. Pain assessment using self-reported, nurse-reported, and observational pain assessment tools among older individuals with cognitive impairment. Pain Manag Nurs 2015;16:595–601.
33. Zwakhalen SS. Which score most likely represents pain on the observational PAINAD pain scale for patients with dementia? J Am Med Dir Assoc 2012;13:384–9.
34. Shreves, A. Critical Care Palliation. 'Emcrit Conference 2013' N.P. 2013. Available at: http://emcrit.org/podcasts/critical-care-palliation/. Accessed October 25, 2015.
35. Weingart, Scott. 'EMCrit Podcast 25'. End of Life and Palliative Care in the ED. N.P. 2010. Available at: http://emcrit.org/podcasts/end-of-life-care/. Accessed August 15, 2015.
36. Wagner BB. Pharmacokinetics and pharmacodynamics of sedatives and analgesics in the treatment of agitated critically ill patients. Clin Pharmacokinet 1997;33: 426–53.

37. Abdulla AA. Guidance on the management of pain in older people. Age Ageing 2013;42(Suppl 1):i1–57.

38. World Health Organization (WHO). Essential medicines in palliative care. 2013. Available at: www.who.int/selection_medicines/committees/expert/19/applications/PalliativeCare_8_A_R.pdf. Accessed August 22, 2015.

39. Godbout KK. A distress protocol for respiratory emergencies in terminally ill patients with lung cancer or chronic obstructive pulmonary disease. Am J Hosp Palliat Care 2015. [Epub ahead of print].

40. Campbell ML, Yarandi H, Dove-Medows E. Oxygen is nonbeneficial for most patients who are near death. J Pain Symptom Manage 2013;45(3):517–23.

41. Kelly CC. Difficult decisions: an interpretative phenomenological analysis study of healthcare professionals' perceptions of oxygen therapy in palliative care. Palliat Med 2015;29(10):950–8.

42. Kamal AH, Maguire JM, Wheeler JL, et al. Dyspnea review for the palliative care professional: treatment goals and therapeutic options. J Palliat Med 2012;15(1):106–14.

43. Jennings A, Davies A, Higgins J, et al. A systematic review of the use of opioids in the management of dyspnoea. Thorax 2002;57(11):939–44.

44. An HH. Nebulized morphine for intractable cough in advanced cancer: two case reports. J Palliat Med 2015;18:278–81.

45. Nava SS. Non-invasive ventilation in elderly patients with acute hypercapnic respiratory failure: a randomised controlled trial. Age Ageing 2011;40:444–50.

46. Schettino GG. Noninvasive positive pressure ventilation reverses acute respiratory failure in select "do-not-intubate" patients. Crit Care Med 2005;33:1976–82.

47. National Quality Forum. A national framework and preferred practices for palliative and hospice care quality. Washington, DC: National Quality Forum; 2006.

48. Cherny NI, Portenoy RK. Sedation in the management of refractory symptoms: guidelines for evaluation and treatment. J Palliat Care 1994;10:31.

49. Beller EM, van Driel ML, McGregor L, et al. Palliative pharmacological sedation for terminally ill adults. Cochrane Database Syst Rev 2015;(1):CD010206.

50. Maltoni M, Pittureri C, Scarpi E, et al. Palliative sedation therapy does not hasten death: results from a prospective multicenter study. Ann Oncol 2009;20(7):1163–9.

51. Levy MH, Cohen SD. Sedation for the relief of refractory symptoms in the imminently dying: a fine intentional line. Semin Oncol 2005;32:237.

52. Cherny NI. The use of sedation in the management of refractory pain. Prin Pract Support Oncol Updates 2000;3:1–11.

53. Salacz M, Weissman D. Controlled sedation for refractory suffering – part I. CAPC Fast Facts and Concepts #106. 2009. Available at: www.capc.org/fast-facts/106-controlled-sedation-refractory-suffering-part-i/. Accessed November 1, 2015.

54. Gevers S. Terminal sedation: a legal approach. Eur J Health Law 2003;10:359.

55. Rousseau P. Existential suffering and palliative sedation: a brief commentary with a proposal for clinical guidelines. Am J Hosp Palliat Care 2001;18(3):151–3.

56. Salacz M, Weissman D. Controlled sedation for refractory suffering – part II. CAPC Fast Facts and Concepts #107. 2009. Available at: https://www.capc.org/fast-facts/107-controlled-sedation-refractory-suffering-part-ii/. Accessed November 1, 2015.

# Index

Note: Page numbers of article titles are in **boldface** type.

Emerg Med Clin N Am 34 (2016) 687–694
http://dx.doi.org/10.1016/S0733-8627(16)30043-8
0733-8627/16/$ – see front matter

emed.theclinics.com

# *Moving?*

## *Make sure your subscription moves with you!*

To notify us of your new address, find your **Clinics Account Number** (located on your mailing label above your name), and contact customer service at:

Email: **journalscustomerservice-usa@elsevier.com**

**800-654-2452** (subscribers in the U.S. & Canada)
**314-447-8871** (subscribers outside of the U.S. & Canada)

Fax number: **314-447-8029**

**Elsevier Health Sciences Division**
**Subscription Customer Service**
**3251 Riverport Lane**
**Maryland Heights, MO 63043**

*To ensure uninterrupted delivery of your subscription, please notify us at least 4 weeks in advance of move.

Printed and bound by CPI Group (UK) Ltd, Croydon, CR0 4YY

08/05/2025

01864686-0003